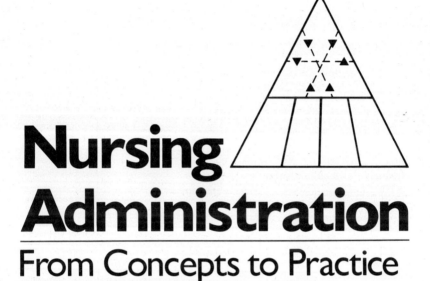

Nursing Administration
From Concepts to Practice

Laura C. Young, RN, MSN
Assistant Administrator
Bay Medical Center
Panama City, Florida

Arlene N. Hayne, RN, MSN
Doctoral Candidate
University of Alabama
Birmingham, Alabama

1988
W.B. SAUNDERS COMPANY
Harcourt Brace Jovanovich, Inc.

Philadelphia / London / Toronto
Montreal / Sydney / Tokyo

W. B. SAUNDERS COMPANY
Harcourt Brace Jovanovich, Inc.

West Washington Square
Philadelphia, PA 19105

Library of Congress Cataloging-in-Publication Data

Young, Laura C.

Nursing administration.

1. Nursing services—Administration. I. Hayne,
   Arlene Nash. II. Title. [DNLM,: 1. Leadership—
   nurses' instruction. 2. Nursing Services—
   organization & administration.
   3. Nursing, Supervisory. WY 105 Y73n]

RT89.Y68 1988   610.73'068   87–23547

ISBN 0–7216–1810–3

Editor: Dudley Kay
Designer: Terri Siegel
Production Manager: Bob Butler
Manuscript Editor: Tom Stringer
Illustrators: Glenn Edelmayer and Risa Clow
Illustration Coordinator: Walt Verbitski
Indexer: Dennis Dolan

NURSING ADMINISTRATION: From Concepts to Practice   ISBN 0–7216–1810–3

Last digit is the print number: 9   8   7   6   5   4   3   2   1

*To All the Nursing Administrators
Who Persevere Today
and Anticipate the Future*

PREFACE

Any endeavor of this magnitude is accomplished despite the many obstacles that occur in the everyday world of living and being. Despite these obstacles, these authors have been assisted in many ways. Our compatibility as two individuals, who lived over three hundred miles apart for the majority of the project, is noteworthy. We began as professional associates, and became friends before beginning this project. We are even better friends now. Our husbands, David Young and Van Hayne, are our greatest supporters and encouragers. They suffered the most in this process, but perhaps better than anyone else, truly understand what this project represents to us as professionals and as women. Someday, our young children, John Young (9) and Marian (6) and Matthew (3) Hayne, may be proud of us. Laura will always feel and remember the encouragement and support of her parents, Lawrence and Evelyn Childree.

We appreciate the contribution of Mrs. Bonita A. Pilon, R.N., M.N., in reworking the chapter on nursing theory. It was exceedingly helpful to have another doctoral student's perspective on this difficult chapter. All of our typists—Bonnie Lawley in Birmingham, and Cathy Taylor, Brenda Miller, Dorothy Walsingham, and Karen Salares in Panama City—are gratefully acknowledged for their tremendous work.

The Lord has truly blessed us with many abilities, loved ones, and special friends!

LAURA YOUNG
ARLENE HAYNE

CONTENTS

FOUNDATION FOR NURSING ADMINISTRATION

I

CONCEPTUAL FRAMEWORK

It is our intent that this book, by identifying and building on trends in today's changing health care climate and by utilizing basic theories and principles, would provide an in-depth guide for nursing administrators facing the current and future challenges in health care administration. Because of the complexities present in today's and tomorrow's health care environment, and recognizing the wide range of organizational size and degree of sophistication that exists within nursing organizations, there is no "one best way" to practice nursing administration. Therefore, various theories are presented as illustrations of available knowledge bases in the hope that nursing leaders, regardless of their needs and backgrounds, will (1) be able to increase their knowledge and understanding of the concepts, and (2) identify relevant concepts that are useful for application in their particular practice.

Now, more than at any time in its past, nursing faces issues that threaten not only its own management and direction but its very existence. It is our assumption that the future of the profession as a whole, as well as the future of the health of our society, will be significantly affected by the quality and type of nursing leadership that is practiced in health care organizations. Both nursing and society hold in their minds' eyes a preferred future state, what they would rather have, as well as what future state is not desired. The underlying theme of this book concerns moving nursing, and thereby ultimately society, deliberately forward to a desired future state. In this state, society experiences an above standard level of health as compared with the rest of the world, and nursing is a valued, powerful, prestigious profession because of its well-defined contribution to that standard of health.

The nursing administrator historically has been the nurse who endured, who followed the administrator's and physician's directions well, and who characteristically was seen as having less power and competence than other administrators. With today's pressures, that nursing administrator cannot long exist. Trends in the nursing community have now produced nursing administrators who can think independently and can solve problems as well as direct others in goal setting and achievement. Unfortunately, the issues

1

facing nursing today and in the coming years are extremely complex and involve more than just nursing.

Nursing administrators have been ill prepared to face these issues. There are nursing programs currently offering graduate education in nursing service administration, but the programs are somewhat limited by available books on the subject. Resources are frequently borrowed from other disciplines without adequate translation or adaptation to the administration of nursing practice. Likewise, these resources are used in isolation, like a tree within a large, thick forest, but there is no perspective of the whole forest. The changes in health care today have occurred so rapidly that much of what is available does not reflect these changes. Only literature from a wide variety of periodical sources is contemporary, let alone futuristic. There are a few resources that provide essential references for the nursing leader of today, and this text is intended to enhance and complement these resources. *Nursing Administration: From Concepts to Practice* provides a theoretical perspective on the nursing administrator's functional behaviors as well as a variety of theories and concepts that do not limit nursing leadership to one particular approach.

In the futuristic approach planned for our book, we will examine not only what has and is happening, but will also carefully identify future expectations based on cultural, health care, and nursing trends. We will then propose proactive responses to those trends by nursing administrators. We will suggest adaptive strategies for addressing the environment and the critical issues that are changing health care and the practice of nursing. We will identify principles and theories relevant to the practice of nursing administration, as well as the application of these principles.

This text is directed primarily at nursing administrators and at faculty and students in graduate or doctoral programs of nursing service administration. The nursing service administrator practicing in the majority of the small- to medium-sized health care institutions does not always have the time to research a topic of relevance to her practice, in order to facilitate her practice, or to augment a mentoring relationship with a nursing service administration student. Each chapter, in addition to the bibliography and reference list at the end of each chapter, provides the big picture as well as the specific content of all relevant concepts. Thus, it also provides one common reference point for nursing service administrators regardless of their organizational level or location. Faculty and students will find this text helpful as a common focus that pulls all relevant concepts together in an organized method provided through the conceptual framework. Doctoral students may also find this text a useful reference book in their library because it is based on a conceptual framework that has guided its development. Thus, it is an illustration of the need and placement of nursing theory in the practice of nursing leadership and management. As Stevens (1985) points out, all models, even the more sophisticated three-dimensional models, are incomplete. However, models and conceptual frameworks can serve as a device to assist learners and readers to get a grasp on a difficult subject.

The complexity of the practice of nursing administration arises from the purpose for which nursing administration exists, from the domains of knowledge and skills that compose its practice, and from the environment that exerts tremendous external forces.

The conceptual framework developed for this text is drawn from theoretical bases from several disciplines and from actual practice and experience at all levels of nursing service administration. The framework identifies the variables that are the foundation of nursing leadership and management. The framework also illustrates the contribution and effect of other variables such as the health care environment on nursing leadership and management. At the same time, the interactive effect that nursing has on and with these variables is illustrated. The large center triangle within the conceptual framework conceptualizes how the various components interact for nursing service administration to occur within the health care environment. Nursing leadership and management occur within the context of today's issues and trends. The active, not passive, role of the nursing administrator is illustrated in the conceptual framework. Finally, the proactive as well as the reactive relationship of nursing leadership and management in developing tomorrow's strategies is illustrated in the conceptual framework.

The conceptual framework for nursing administration is presented in Figure 1–1. The conceptual framework for nursing administration defines the limits and boundaries wherein nursing leadership and management occur; the forces or variables driving them; and the interaction among the key elements. Not infrequently, discussions occur concerning what kind of knowledge is required and essential for a nursing administrator to perform successfully. There is disagreement about how and the type of programs in which nursing administrators should be prepared. This conceptual framework illustrates the relevant fields of knowledge and their contribution to nursing leadership and management. The conceptual framework also demonstrates the uniqueness of the nursing administrator role in the delivery of patient care services.

The conceptual framework identifies four sets of major concepts that serve as foundations within nursing administration. These major concepts—ethics, nursing leadership, management, and the environment—provide basic knowledge and essential tools in the administration of patient care services.

Ethical concepts define the essential values and motives for nursing as a profession as well as for the individual nursing administrator. Nursing's responsibilities to society are the result of the values identified by our society (Uustal, 1977). The impact of ethical concepts on decision making is assuming a larger proportion in our technologically complex world (Tucker, 1979). Nursing administrators need to understand the role and purpose of ethical concepts in decision making for routine matters as well as in dealing with ethical dilemmas. Nurses are moral agents by nature of their humanity, to which is added the societal responsibilities of their profession. Ethics and values touch every aspect of human life from birth through death, reaching

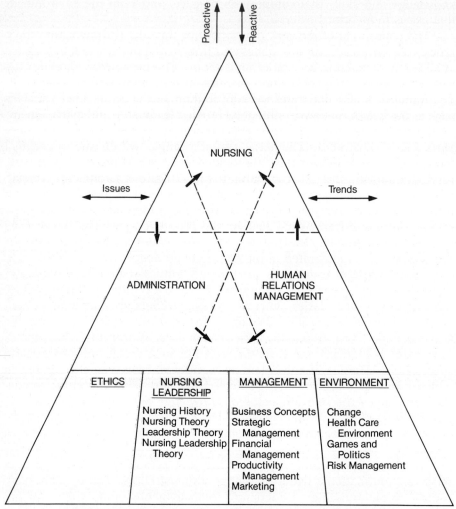

FIGURE 1-1. Conceptual framework for nursing administration.

into every action an individual experiences. Despite this, individuals continue to have difficulty articulating these complex concepts. As the complexity of societal ethical issues increases, and ethics have a continually greater impact on the choices or decisions affecting the nurse and the nurse executive, the greater is the need for the nurse executive to understand the ethical basis of decision making. Since the importance and significance of ethics to every nursing leader's practice cannot be minimized, a discussion of ethical theory and dilemmas as well as a proposed process for reaching ethical decisions are included in the first section of this book.

The concept of nursing leadership is a foundational concept for nursing administration. The concept of nursing leadership is composed of four major subconcepts. Nursing history serves to define what nursing has been over the centuries and reflects the results of the decisions and choices made by nursing leaders. Nursing as a profession and nursing administration cannot divorce itself from its past successes and failures. Nursing history did not occur in a vacuum, but felt the influence of past issues and trends affecting societies, health, and women (Sheahan, 1978).

The concept of nursing theory serves as a relevant foundation for nursing administration for several reasons. The essential purpose of nursing theory, to define and progress the unique body of knowledge that is nursing, is of primary importance. The development of nursing theory also provides the vehicle for the application and integration of knowledge from other disciplines into nursing. Nursing theory also allows for the orderly transition of these new ideas into the practice setting, which, in many circumstances, is the realm of the nursing administrator (Ellis, 1982). Therefore, the nurse administrator uses the concept of nursing theory not only to define practice but also to enhance it. The nurse administrator contributes to the development of nursing theory by conducting and encouraging nursing research in the practice setting.

A significant portion of the concepts and theories that compose the concept of nursing leadership have been defined by other disciplines. Leadership theories from the behavorial and social sciences as well as others serve as the basis for what has been done by managers, including nurse managers (McFarland, 1986). Therefore, the contribution of leadership theory is identified in the conceptual framework as a subconcept within nursing leadership. Within the context of this conceptual framework, leadership theories consist of such concepts as leadership, power, communication (including networking and mentoring), decision making, group dynamics, motivation, and organization.

The uniqueness of nursing leadership theory is also defined as a basic element of nursing administration. The uniqueness is a function of the role of nurse and the social context of the complementary roles that surround the role of nurse leader, which include other nurses, non-nurses, and patients. Nursing leadership theory is defined largely through the behaviors of deciding, relating, influencing, and facilitating (Yura, 1984). This theory of nursing leadership successfully addresses all groups encountered by the nursing administrator role, regardless of the level or type of health care organization.

The third major concept that serves as a foundation to nursing administration is the concept of management. Included in this concept are the subconcepts of business, strategic management, financial management, productivity, and marketing. The advantage of this conceptual framework over earlier models of nursing administration is its ability to show the relationship and fit of the concept of nursing to the concept of business (Holyfield, 1983). The conceptual framework illustrates them in a complementary relationship that becomes synergistic when actualized in the role of the nursing administrator.

The principles related to business and the importance of these principles to businesses in general and health care institutions specifically are basic to the discussion of nursing administration because of the current emphasis on health care institutions as businesses. The need for the nurse executive to successfully manage departments that operate effectively and at high levels of productivity is obvious when one considers that the measure of success in the business world depends highly upon these criteria.

Strategic management as a theoretical approach to thinking and planning is an important part of the foundation for management. Basic principles of strategic management are applied to organizations and businesses, and the specific application to health care and nursing administration is emphasized. The process of strategic management is illustrated with a model that outlines and explains the steps by which the process is carried out and how it applies to nursing administration.

Financial management has gained in importance as a basic foundation in health care management because of the increasing costs of health care in recent years. The factors that have influenced these health care costs and, thus, have influenced the role of financial management in nursing administration are discussed. Productivity has not always been a consideration within the field of nursing, but its importance in management is emphasized. Productivity measurement and management are major responsibilities for managers and have become a significant portion of the process of management.

Marketing has until recently not been considered of significance in planning for the future of health care. Principles of marketing and the ethical-legal implications of marketing are important for the nursing administrator as plans for the future are developed. Marketing, previously considered by many as only "selling," was often viewed with distaste by the service-oriented health care providers. However, marketing has a much broader scope in the identification of markets, the placement within the market, changing of positions to influence the market, as well as in program development, elimination or addition of services, or generally in accurate forecasting and ultimately success in the business of health care.

These principles or concepts related to management are essential to build the foundation for nursing administration. Combined with other building blocks described and the influence of the environment, the foundation may be made solid to produce outcomes in nursing administration that are desired.

The role of the environment as a driving force upon nursing administration is illustrated in the conceptual framework. Distinct from the ethical and historical perspective, the environment in this conceptual framework is defined differently than the forces being exerted by today's issues and trends. The environment includes the contribution and role of change theory for the nursing administrator (Lancaster, 1982). Change is a major variable affecting the practice of nursing administration. Strategies for accomplishing and controlling change place emphasis on the role of the nursing administrator in the process.

Defining the health care environment contributes to a better understanding of the issues and trends that rise and peak. Multiple factors in the health care environment are creating a synergistic effect on health care and nursing. In addition to the larger, more global variables within the health care environment, the contribution of the human environment, especially the games and politics that occur, significantly impact on the successful performance of every nursing administrator. Health care "games" play a major role in goal achievement within these health care institutions and as such must be recognized and dealt with by the nursing administrator.

With the somewhat hostile, external environment that institutions and nursing administrators are facing, there is an increasked risk. Risk management, defined as a planning approach to risk problems or loss exposures, has become a necessary component of nursing administration.

These driving forces and basic elements contribute to the concept of nursing administration. The foundations upon which nursing administration is built are not only important for the nurse executive of today, but will also influence the direction and scope of that practice tomorrow. The areas of practice that compose nursing administration—nursing, human relations, and administration—are interacting and overlapping concepts, and they are affected not only by the foundation on which they are built but also by the trends and issues within society.

These three roles—nurse, administrator, and human relations manager—are the major roles performed by the nursing administrator. As a leader, the nursing administrator interacts with today's issues and trends in each of the three described roles. The nursing administrator as leader and manager then determines reactive and proactive strategies that shape and direct the nursing, administration, and human relations management for tomorrow.

Administrative strategies for practice are presented within each individual chapter. Specific nursing strategies are presented in the chapter on patient care management. Similarly, strategies for human relations management are addressed in a separate chapter.

The conceptual framework has served as the basis for the development and presentation of this book. Admittedly, this conceptual framework has not been tested. This conceptual framework of nursing administration has evolved over time, based on actual practice as well as existing theory. Now that this conceptual framework for nursing administration has been articulated, it can be tested. The authors encourage research and practice utilizing this model and would welcome feedback concerning its application and use.

References

Ellis, R. (1982). Conceptual issues in nursing. *Nursing Outlook, 30*(7), 406–410.

Holyfield, D. (1983). The cost of doing business. *Horizons* (Fall) 2–8.

Lancaster, J. (1982). Change theory: An essential aspect of nursing practice. *In* Lancaster, J., and Lancaster, W. (eds). *Concepts of advanced nursing practice: the nurse as change agent*. St. Louis: C. V. Mosby.

McFarland, D. E. (1986). *The managerial imperative: The age of macromanagement.* Cambridge, MA: Ballinger.
Rowland, H., and Rowland, B. (1985). *Nursing administration handbook,* 2nd ed. Rockville, MD: Aspen.
Sheahan, Sister Dorothy (1978). Scanning the seventies. *Nursing Outlook, 26,* 33–7.
Stevens, B. J. (1985). *The nurse as executive* (3rd ed.). Rockville, MD: Aspen.
Tucker, R. W. (1979). The value decisions we know as science. *Advances in Nursing Service, 1*(2), 1–12.
Uustal, D. B. (1977). Searching for values. *Images, 9*(1), 15–17.
Yura, H. (1984). Nursing leadership evaluation. *The Health Care Supervisor, 12*(3), 16–28.

ETHICAL PERSPECTIVES

INTRODUCTION

Because every individual's life is a conscious or unconscious expression of his or her underlying values and ethics, this section, in some respects, could be near the beginning of any book. Despite the magnitude of their presence in individual and societal existence, values and ethics are difficult and complex concepts to articulate. Yet, as society becomes more complex there are more alternatives, more choices to be made, and consequently ethical decisions seem to be necessary more frequently. This section will provide the nursing leader with a theoretical understanding of values, rights, and ethics. A brief overview of several schools of ethical thought is presented. Ethics in health care will then be presented, including what constitutes an ethical dilemma. Finally, a model for ethical decision making will be presented.

VALUES

Values are a set of beliefs and attitudes about the truth, beauty, or worth of any thought, object, or behavior. Every decision made or course of action taken is based consciously or unconsciously on such beliefs and values. In other words, what is really important, what are the priorities in life, what is one willing to sacrifice or suffer in order to achieve, obtain, protect, or maintain oneself are basic issues for everyone. The majority of people in today's society have not had to answer these kinds of tough

2

questions consciously. As a result, there is a lot of unnecessary confusion, inconsistency, and ambivalence exhibited in people's behavior. Confusion and ambivalence concerning a person's own values are frequently confronted during difficult health care decisions.

Values provide individuals with the ideological justification for roles and norms within society (Uustal, 1977). Without values, there are no standards and hence no moral code, no right or wrong, and ultimately chaos. When one has at least a tentative idea of what is considered to be truth, beauty, and right or wrong, one is able to act in a manner consistent with those values. This behavior is more organized and predictable, not only for the individual but for the society as well. Jourard (1964) wrote

That until an individual knows his values he cannot know himself. Until one knows what he values or what lines in life he is not going to cross, an individual doesn't know himself very well.

Louis Raths (Raths et al, 1966) identified three processes that individuals go through as they attempt to clarify their values. The first process is the choosing process. Values are considered completely unique to each individual. Although two people may share the same value, they each arrived at that value individually. Theoretically, the choice of these values is made freely without indoctrination or coercion. Since values involve choosing, it is explicitly assumed that alternative values exist simultaneously. Because alternatives exist and because all decisions have consequences, the individual considers the consequences of all choices in making the ultimate decision.

The second process Raths identified in the value clarification process is labeled prizing. This occurs when the individual acknowledges first to himself and then publicly what his choice has been and how he feels about it. Generally, the individual is proud of his choice. In addition to publicizing his values, the individual will also actively support his values.

The third process in value clarification is called acting (Raths et al, 1966). It is at this point that the individual has truly internalized the value. In this respect, the individual's behaviors are a direct reflection of that value. Likewise, as an integral part of the individual's behavior, the value is then expressed not just episodically, but repeatedly.

Once individuals have developed values, generally their decisions are made in terms of those values. Value decisions or value judgments occur in three dimensions, referred to as rational, logical, or factual (Tucker, 1979). The judgment dimension goes from an extreme subjective, personal value judgment to the most objective factual consideration. A value judgment in this dimension may include a personal subjective value of chartreuse socks to a value of gold over silver because of their physical and societal properties.

Another dimension of value judgments deals with subscribership. This refers to an individual versus a collective or group value. The difficulty with this dimension is that it is related to the trouble with the discrete point at which one stops valuing something as an individual and begins valuing something because of his membership in a group. The value that individuals place on religion might be used as an example in this dimension. Some individuals value God on a very personal intimate level, having nothing to do with their membership in an organized church. Others, however, may value God because of their membership in an organized church.

The third and final dimension of value judgments concerns the explicitness of the value judgment. An example of a formal or highly explicit value judgment would be the signing of a petition. The other extreme or less explicit example of a formal value judgment would be the daily living of values.

When the three dimensions of value judgments are considered simultaneously, it is easy to understand the magnitude and extent of the effect that values have on lives. Values have significance for people as individuals and collectively as societies. Values are useful because they provide order and predictability. Values can be considered as a means to a good end. Inherently, values can make an individual feel good inside. Finally, values contribute to social order and societal maturation (Beckstrand, 1978).

As an individual grows, develops, and matures, values are defined and clarified, tested and revised, and gradually become all pervasive to the individual's existence. As such, the individual becomes an agent of value or, more commonly, a moral agent. The terms value and moral are frequently used interchangeably because they both deal with human behavior and values. In order for nurses to function optimally in complex settings and to act responsibly as moral agents, it is necessary for nurses to progress through the various stages of moral development as defined by Kohlberg.

In Kohlberg's (1971) model of moral growth and development, he described three levels with two stages within each level (Table 2–1). The first level is called the preconventional level. Within this level, the first stage is characterized by fear of punishment and recognition of authority. These are the principles that guide moral thoughts and actions. The second stage is the "do unto others" stage. This level has also been associated with the preadolescent age group.

The second level is called the conventional level and contains stages three and four. Moral behavior in stage three is characterized by conformance to peer group approval. This stage is associated with the adolescent age group. Stage four moves to a larger societal influence by acceptance of the need for law and order. The age group associated with this stage has been the early twenties.

The third level is called postconventional and has been associated with the late twenties and older population. Stage five is characterized by what is called a "social contract or constitutional-legal orientation." Stage six describes the most complex principled and autonomous behavior because it consists of "universal-ethical principled" influences.

Kohlberg's theory is considered biased because his research dealt primarily with boys. When Kohlberg's theory was applied to girls and women, discrepancies were attributed to the females, not the theory. Carol Gilligan (1982) has developed an integrative theory of women's moral development

TABLE 2–1
The Six Moral Stages

Level and Stage	What is Right	Context of Stage Reasons for Doing Right	Social Perspective of Stage
Level I: Preconventional Stage 1—Heteronomous morality	To avoid breaking rules backed by punishment, obedience for its own sake, and avoiding physical damage to persons and property.	Avoidance of punishment, and the superior power of authorities.	Egocentric point of view. Doesn't consider the interests of others or recognize that they differ from the actor's; doesn't relate two points of view. Actions are considered physically rather than in terms of psychological interests of others. Confusion of authority's perspective with one's own.
Stage 2—Individualism, instrumental purpose, and exchange	Following rules only when it is to someone's immediate interest; acting to meet one's own interests and needs and letting others do the same. Right is also what's fair, what's an equal exchange, a deal, and agreement.	To serve one's own needs or interests in a world where you have to recognize that other people have their interests, too.	Concrete individualistic perspective. Aware that everybody has his own interest to pursue and these conflict, so that right is relative (in the concrete individualistic sense).
Level II: Conventional Stage 3—Mutual interpersonal expectations, relationships, and interpersonal conformity	Living up to what is expected by people close to you or what people generally expect of people in your role as son, brother, friend, etc. "Being good" is important and means having good motives, showing concern about others. It also means keeping mutual relationships, such as trust, loyalty, respect, and gratitude.	The need to be a good person in your own eyes and those of others. Your caring for others. Belief in the Golden Rule. Desire to maintain rules and authority which support stereotypical good behavior.	Perspective of the individual in relationship with other individuals. Aware of shared feelings, agreements, and expectations which take primacy over individual interests. Relates points of view through the concrete Golden Rule, putting yourself in the other person's shoes. Does not yet consider generalized system perspective.

Stage 4—Social system and conscience	Fulfilling the actual duties to which you have agreed. Laws are to be upheld except in extreme cases where they conflict with other fixed social duties. Right is also contributing to society, the group, or institution.	To keep the institution going as a whole, to avoid the breakdown in the system "if everyone did it," or the imperative of conscience to meet one's defined obligations. (Easily confused with Stage 3 belief in rules and authority; see text.)	Differentiates societal point of view from interpersonal agreement or motives. Take the point of view of the system that defines roles and rules. Considers individual relations in terms of place in the system.
Level III: Postconventional, or principled Stage 5—Social contract or utility and individual rights	Being aware that people hold a variety of values and opinions, that most values and rules are relative to your group. These relative rules should usually be upheld, however, in the interest of impartiality and because they are the social contract. Some nonrelative values and rights like life and liberty, however, must be upheld in any society and regardless of majority opinion.	A sense of obligation to law because of one's social contract to make and abide by laws for the welfare of all and for the protection of all people's rights. A feeling of contractual commitment, freely entered upon, to family, friendship, trust, and work obligations. Concern that laws and duties be based on rational calculation of overall utility, "the greatest good for the greatest number."	Prior-to-society perspective. Perspective of a rational individual aware of values and rights prior to social attachments and contracts. Integrates pespectives by formal mechanisms of agreement, contract, objective impartiality and due process. Considers moral and legal points of view; recognizes that they sometimes conflict and finds it difficult to integrate them.
Stage 6—Universal ethical principles	Following self-chosen ethical principles. Particular laws or social agreements are usually valid because they rest on such principles. When laws violate these principles, one acts in accordance with the principle. Principles are universal principles of justice; the equality of human rights and respect for the dignity of human beings as individual persons.	The belief as a rational person in the validity of universal moral principles, and a sense of personal commitment to them.	Perspective of a moral point of view from which social arrangements derive. Perspective is that of any rational individual recognizing the nature of morality or the fact that persons are ends in themselves and must be treated as such.

Reprinted with permission from Kohlberg, L.: The Psychology of Moral Development, Vol. II. Harper and Row Publishers, 1984.

that challenges the completeness of Kohlberg's work. According to Gilligan, author of *In a Different Voice: Psychological Theory and Women's Development*, men and women have different ways of moral development. Women put an emphasis on relationships. Moral development for women concerns the woman's recognition that although being responsible and doing for others is important, her individual needs are important also. In contrast, men fear intimacy and view responsibility as not doing what they want because of others. Moral development for males involves the male regarding the other individual as equal to the self. Equality then provides the mechanism for making the intimacy safe. Masculinity is defined as separateness because of the difference between the male and the primary care giver, the female mother. Femininity is defined by attachment or similarity. Therefore, men value themselves as individuals and females value themselves as part of a relationship. New psychological studies of both females and males on the understanding of moral development are providing new insight into theories of moral development.

Moral development theories help us to understand why various age groups make the moral or value decisions that they do. Moral development occurs in relationship to the development of total personality. It is directly linked to the development of logical reasoning or intelligence. Logical reasoning occurs in three major stages: the intuitive, the concrete operational, and the formal operational. Since moral reasoning is reasoning, advancement in moral reasoning is dependent on development in logical reasoning. Likewise, moral reasoning is directly related to stages of social perception or role taking. How individuals perceive themselves and their relationship to others and their roles in society also affects their level of moral development.

Kohlberg's levels and stages of moral development are a useful model for nurses for several reasons. This model can be helpful for nurses in their relationships with patients as well as with co-workers. Secondly, this model suggests the importance of nurses maturing in their moral development in order to effectively deal with the complex situations they are faced with daily. If nurses are functioning at a pre-conventional level of moral development, they will not have adequate problem solving and critical thinking abilities to deal with complex ethical dilemmas. It is only by developing to the post-conventional level of moral development that nurses will be equipped to deal with the situations they are involved in.

Moral development occurs as the result of several factors. Cognitive stimulation is a necessary part of moral development. More importantly, however, is the presence of factors of general social experience and stimulation that Kohlberg labels as "role-taking" opportunities. Additionally, the presence of an environment that embodies a high stage of moral development can stimulate moral development. Thirdly, the presence of cognitive-moral conflict encourages moral development. Kohlberg states (1984, pp. 202–203):

Structural theory stresses that movement to the next stage occurs through reflective reorganization arising from sensed contradictions in one's current stage structure. Experiences of cognitive conflict can occur either through exposure to decision situations that arouse internal contradictions in one's moral reasoning structure or through exposure to the moral reasoning of significant others which is discrepant in content or structure from one's own reasoning.

Nurses can be encouraged and stimulated in their moral development through several mechanisms. Their working environment can embody a high level of moral reasoning, functioning, and expectations. Moral reasoning can be encouraged and supported through the recognition of conflicts and available avenues of resolution. Ethical rounds can stimulate cognitive development and provide forums for debates on conflicts.

Rights

Individuals struggling to clarify their values do not always identify human rights as a value. However, as values are peeled away to their basic layer, the rights of humans usually become clear.

Individuals have the human right to existence and therefore have the right to choose or make decisions concerning themselves as long as they are willing to accept the consequences. The concept of self in this respect refers to an individual's body, life, property, and privacy. Nevertheless, because individuals exist within societies, the actions associated with these choices cannot detract from another person's right. With the concept of human rights is the associated concept of duties and responsibilities. Rights equate with responsibilities. If one has a right to his existence, other persons and society have a duty or obligation not to kill him. Curtain (1982) also makes the point that health professionals, because of the roles they assume within society, assume additional duties toward others that other individuals do not assume.

The concept of rights generally includes the existence of five conditions that surround and expand the understanding of the concept (Bandman and Bandman, 1985). First, there is an accompanying condition of the freedom to exercise the right or not to exercise it if the individual so chooses. Second, rights are associated with duties for others to facilitate or at least not to interfere with the exercise of those rights. Third, rights are usually defined or defended in basic terms that equate with the principles of fairness, impartiality, and equality. A fourth condition is that a basic fundamental or significant right is considered enforceable by society. The final condition is also the result of societal maturation, because this condition concerns compensation due an individual whose right has been violated.

Leah Curtain (1982) provides a perspective on human rights with clarity and eloquence. She defines human rights as what a person is justly due. "Justly due" means that those rights are legitimate as a result of humanness. Human beings have rights because they are unique creatures that possess the ability to know and think. The source of human rights is what is known about oneself as a unique entity by himself. As a unique, self-contained human, an individual possesses certain needs in order for that existence to continue. Humans have a common origin, which results in having common needs and a resulting interdependence on one another. Because of these principles, human needs exist whether they are recognized or not.

Specifically defined sets of rights have developed in society as a result of the increased attention being devoted to the field of moral and ethical issues. Three sets of rights of particular relevance to nursing have been published and serve as examples of human rights. The rights proposed in these statements are not unique to the stated group. However, the inclusion of these rights for the stated group implies a particular relevance of that right for the group.

The first set of rights is referred to as the rights of elderly patients (Bandman and Bandman, 1985). Our elderly population is growing rapidly. By the year 2000, it is estimated that the elderly population will compose over 13% of the population. The health care needs of the elderly include more systemic and debilitating diseases than other age groups. The elderly use more health care resources than other segments of the population. Finally, the issues of death and dying are of greater significance to the elderly. This common set of moral principles developed for the elderly reflects the basic human right of self-determination as well as an inherent regard for the value and acceptance of the concept of individual rights.

The first elderly patient right is the right to respect. Within this right is the central issue of informed consent, as well as the simple dignity issue of addressing the elderly individual in a respectful manner. The importance of truth telling is relevant to this right. The second elderly patient right is the right to receive treatment. Within this right is the issue of allocation of resources. Does the ICU bed go to the 76-year-old with diabetes and congestive heart failure or to the 36-year-old man with a myocardial infarction? This then leads to the controversies between equality and fairness. Associated with this right is the issue of "added value." How much is a day of life worth? Is worth measured by quantity or quality? Complicating this question is the cost to other members of society when benefits are added to one individual. The third elderly patient right is the right to refuse treatment. This right most directly involves the right to self-determination. However, it also involves the conflict that occurs between the sanctity of life principle and the quality of life principle (Bandman and Bandman, 1985).

Another set of rights that many nurses are familiar with is the patient's bill of rights developed by the American Hospital Association (1974). What has disturbed professional nurses and others about this set of rights is the perception that these rights are being given to patients by the hospital. It is disturbing to think that the hospital has the authority and power to give and take at will. In reality, a patient already has these rights as an individual. The Hospital Association argues that this set of rights was a reaffirmation of human rights necessary after the dehumanization of the hospital care as a result of technological advances. Nevertheless, the patient's bill of rights also includes many of the same human rights found within the elderly patient's set of rights. These rights include (1) the right to respectful and considerate care and treatment, (2) the right to information about care treatment and costs, (3) informed consent about procedures and outcomes, (4) patient autonomy and the right to refuse treatment, and (5) the right to privacy and confidentiality (Davis and Aroskar, 1983).

The third set of rights of concern to nurses is the trilogy of a dying patient's rights (Bandman and Bandman, 1985). Again there is the right to treatment as well as the right to refuse treatment. These rights recognize the dignity and worth of an individual as being paramount. As a result, the dying patient has a right to the truth, to informed consent, and to respect. These rights are an obvious attempt to try and clarify the problems that surround dying patients. The President's Commission for Study of Ethical Problems has recognized how frequently providing care to dying patients creates a double bind situation and has also attempted to provide clarification.

An example of a double bind situation is the administration of increasing doses of morphine necessary to relieve pain, which also depresses a patient's respirations. The dilemma encountered with dying patients is largely a result of health care providers' long-standing ultimate goals of life preservation and restoration. It has only been within the last 15 years that dying has become an acceptable outcome by some health care providers. The assistance with dying now consists of relieving suffering and anxiety to make this final human experience as dignified and comfortable as possible (Bandman and Bandman, 1985).

This brief presentation of three sets of published rights has attempted to illustrate how concepts of human rights have been developed and expressed specifically within the health care setting. Other sets of rights have been developed for other types of settings and contain many of the same basic elements found in these three.

ETHICAL THEORIES

A brief summary of ethical theories has been included for several reasons. First, it will inform the reader of the magnitude and complexity of the available theoretical knowledge on ethics. Second, it will provide an introduction to specific theories in order that the reader may begin to inquire into his own value system. A particular theory may articulate what may previously have been only fuzzy thoughts in the reader's mind. Third, it is hoped that this summary will assist the reader to select one specific area to explore in more depth so that it will provide additional insight into his own ethical decision making processes.

Examination of societal values and moral issues has led to the study of ethics. Ethics is a branch of philosophy that deals with questions of human conduct, the values and beliefs that determine human conduct, and how these elements change over time. Metaethics concerns the study of moral judgments to determine if they are reasonable or in some way justifiable (Davis and Aroskar, 1983). As the study of ethics has developed, ethical theories have been proposed to identify, organize, and examine as well as justify human actions through the application of the concepts and principles of human rights and values. The ultimate goal of ethics is to be able to determine what is the right or good thing to do in a given situation. Ethical theory has been classified into normative ethics and non-normative ethics. Normative ethics is based on the acceptance of some universally acceptable principles or standards, such as human rights. Non-normative ethics, on the other hand, denies the existence of any universally accepted principles. It is apparent from these two dichotomous schools of thought that ethical theory has not yet developed any grand theories (Beckstrand, 1978; Curtain and Flaherty, 1982).

Within non-normative ethics there are three lines of reasoning. The first form of reasoning is called ethical emotivism. Ethical emotivism is concerned with the emotional response by an individual to a statement requiring a value judgment. The emotional response determines the rightness or wrongness of the statement. Ethical skepticism views humans as not knowing right from wrong. In this line of reasoning, there is no true right or wrong, just a difference of opinion. Recognizing this difference, weight is assigned to the argument in some objective manner to determine which argument carries more weight. In this manner, the correct or right decision is made. A third non-normative ethical line of reasoning is called ethical relativism. This reasoning perceives right and wrong as being relative to the three dimensions of the individual, the culture, and the situation (Curtain and Flaherty, 1982).

Normative ethical reasoning constitutes a much larger body of ethical literature and is based on universally applicable principles of right and wrong. There is an underlying assumption that these basic principles are rules that should not be broken. As a result, these rules or norms can assist individuals and societies in making the right decision in the majority of situations. It is recognized, however, that there are exceptions to these rules. Within the normative line of reasoning, two main categories, deontology and teleological theories, have evolved. Additionally, several more contemporary ethicists suggest theories evolving from these two categories.

The deontology theories take the perspective that existing human rights result in duties and obligations among individuals toward each other. Right and wrong is decided as a result of the congruency with those duties and obligations (Curtain, 1982, p. 48).

Immanuel Kant proposed three principles or standards to evaluate human conduct that have served as a large basis of much of the ethical literature. The first principle is that an individual must respect his own humanness and value his uniqueness. This then leads to the second principle of respecting all persons as individual and unique. The third principle states that individuals must always be treated as a means rather than as an end. Within the context of these three principles, the universalizability of the action is also considered. In other words, is it appropriate if all the other people in the world did the same thing (Kant, 1949)?

Another form of ethical deontology is the human nature perspective. The uniqueness of human nature is the ability to think, reason, and understand. Therefore, right and wrong are determined by rational thinking. This approach recognizes the complexities of human behavior and the existence of conflict between an individual's self-interests and the interests of others. It does not, however, apparently provide a satisfactory explanation for the use or place of human emotions in ethical decision making (Curtain, 1982, p. 50).

The third deontological set of theories deal with the law of God. Right and wrong are determined from the sacred writings inspired by God. These theories recognize that man may not know what is good for him. Unfortunately, interpretation of the Word of God by humans has led to actions that can never be considered good or right (Curtain, 1982, pp. 50–51).

W. K. Frankena's (1973) theory of obligation consists of two basic principles and is considered in the deontological vein. The first principle is the principle of beneficence. This principle demands the act of doing good, not the desirability of wanting good. Good encompasses more than just good actions. Good also includes not inflicting harm, preventing harm from occurring, and removing evil. The second principle is the principle of justice as equal treatment. Equal treatment involves the distribution of benefits and burdens equally. Equal distribution can be defined according to merit, according to equality, and according to need (Davis and Aroskar, 1983, pp. 32–33).

Another theory that reshapes the social obligation suggested by Kant is the justice as fairness theory proposed by J. Rawls. Rawls' position is that social and economic inequalities are to be arranged so that they are the greatest benefit to the least fortunate of society. More importantly, each person is to have equal right to the maximum liberty for all. Criteria for rightness include universality, or that everyone else can do the same thing in the same situation; generality; publicity; ordering, or the logic or reason to the enforcement of the principle; and finality, which places the principle over the demands of law and custom (Davis and Aroskar, 1983, p. 34).

The second category of ethical theories is called teleological theories. Basically, these theories define good or right with good or right consequences; wrong or evil with wrong or evil consequences. These theories raise several issues, however, that have not been satisfactorily resolved. Among these is the issue of the ends that may be good justifying wrong means. Another is a precise understanding of the concept of right or good. Within the teleological category there are three perspectives: utilitarianism, natural law, and scientism.

Utilitarianism defines right as that action that produces the greatest amount of good or the least amount of evil for the most people. Obviously, this approach would not be significantly concerned with the rights of minority groups of individuals such as the retarded or handicapped. Jeremy

Bentham, a well-known utilitarian, defined good as pleasure or happiness, and absence of pain (Bentham, 1983). Human nature is susceptible to the pleasures of sense, wealth, skill, amity, a good name, power, piety, benevolence, malevolence, imagination, memory, expectation, association, and the pleasure of relief (Bentham, 1969). John Stuart Mill, another well-known utilitarian, defined happiness on a broader level to mean social utility. Human actions contain a moral aspect, an aesthetic aspect, and a sympathetic aspect. All of these aspects contribute to the rightness or wrongness of an action and its ultimate worth to society (Mill, 1950).

Aristotle is an example of the natural law theorists in the second category of teleological ethics. The concept of an ideal human and the fullest potential for humanness is relevant for this group of theorists in determining right and wrong. These theories recognize the maturation of man and society, but there remain problems with the definitions of ideal and fullest potential (Curtain, 1982).

The third type of theory found within the teleological category is called scientism. This approach emphasizes the use of scientific data and objective knowledge in the determination of right and wrong. Right is that which conforms to fact and can be proved. Unfortunately, this approach does not deal satisfactorily with the issues of man's free will or spirit of humanism. Everything seems to be boiled down to chemical reactions (Curtain, 1982, pp. 52–53).

Firth (1970), a contemporary philosopher, can also be classified in the teleological category with his ideal observer theory that seems akin to Aristotle's way of thinking. In this theory, moral judgments are made by an ideal observer. This ideal observer possesses the qualities of consistency, disinterestedness, dispassionateness, omnipreciprence (all-knowing), and normality (Davis and Aroskar, 1983). Unfortunately, although Firth's theory provides us with insight as to how to work through an ethical decision, it provides no standards against which to evaluate the decision itself.

Vaux stated there are three dimensions of ethical insight. The first dimension of ethical insight is considered retrospective. Retrospective ethical considerations include biological, historical, religious, and philosophical perspectives and data. The second dimension of ethical insight is considered introspective. In this dimension, consideration would be given to the ethical situation in terms of its meaning to one's present life. Finally, the third dimension of ethical insight is called the prescriptive dimension. In this dimension, the ethical concern is considered in terms of the future and potential consequences (Davis and Aroskar, 1983). These dimensions are helpful to remember as this ethical discussion proceeds and ethical decisions in health care are specifically examined.

ETHICAL DILEMMAS

So far, there has been discussion of values, morality, and ethics somewhat generally. Before one can become more specific about the issues and strategies for dealing with health care ethics, it is necessary to become more specific about what is an ethical situation and what constitutes an ethical dilemma. An ethical dilemma always occurs within the context of an ethical situation, but an ethical situation does not automatically constitute an ethical dilemma.

Based on the discussion to this point, a clearer explanation of what constitutes an ethical situation is now necessary. An ethical situation may be regarded as broadly as an individual's perspective on a life-style, or as minor as how a nurse addresses an elderly patient. Likewise, an ethical situation may be as complex as in-vitro fertilization. Because ethics has to do with the determination of the right or goodness of human behavior, ethics involve all of human life. Although the philosophy of ethics may purport to address this grand perspective, in fact, ethics are studied in an effort not to address the daily ethical activities everyone finds themselves in but rather to deal with the ethical dilemmas faced.

Ethical dilemmas possess several characteristics that will quickly be recognized as familiar. Dilemmas are problems that usually cannot be resolved simply through the use of objective or empirical data. Usually a dilemma is perplexing because it involves a choice between two equal alternatives, such as two wrongs or two rights. The magnitude of the effect of an ethical dilemma is usually profound or far reaching in an area of significant concern. The effect may be within an individual by himself, between two individuals, or between an individual and society. A desired outcome of an ethical dilemma is to achieve either internal, individual peace of mind or external peace between individuals (Curtain, 1982).

Health care providers work in an environment oriented toward ethical situations. To ignore this is to ignore reality. The two main groups of health care professionals, physicians and nurses, have recognized the ethical essence of their work and have integrated ethical standards into their practice through the development of their professional codes of ethics.

The ANA Code for Nurses (1976) contains principles that are recognized from the earlier discussion on human rights. Within the Code, there are at least six ethical statements. First is the respect for human dignity. Privacy and confidentiality are two other principles. In addition to being responsible and accountable for her patients, the nurse also maintains competency in order to perform what is right, good, and beneficial to the patient. Besides the positive actions, she prevents harm from occurring through the safeguarding of the patient from incompetent providers. Honesty is another ethical principle embraced by the code for nurses.

The 1980 Judicial Council of the American Medical Association revised the AMA principles of medical ethics. These statements also include a respect for human dignity, promotion of the patient's best interest, confidentiality, informed consent, and honesty.

These statements are intended to serve daily practice as well as to provide a basis for dealing with the more complex ethical dilemmas. Within health care, ethical dilemmas occur in four general areas. These areas are health policy, allocation of resources, human experimentation, and clinical practice (Davis and Aroskar, 1983). Health policy creates ethical dilemmas because choices are made in regard to what kind of health services will be provided, how many services will be provided, and who will be the recipient of these services. What are the moral philosophies guiding these decisions? Will everyone receive equally, or should those that need the most receive? What is the greatest good for the majority—and how does that affect the health of the minority?

Within the area of health policy, several examples of ethical dilemmas can be identified. The determination of death is one example. Death determination is placed under the auspices of health policy ethical dilemmas because it has been addressed not only in the laboratory but also in the courts and in government halls. The heart-lung concept of death is no longer sufficient, and the concept of brain death is now the standard (Cowles, 1984). Yet, even the concept of brain death as defined by the various groups and scientific data at times seems inadequate for answering the ultimate question. Fletcher (1972), Veatch (1976), and Feinberg (1980) propose an essence of personhood that embraces the functioning of vital physical capacities, such as neocortical function, as well as the unique capacities of emotions, the soul, and actions.

Along the same lines, other examples of health policy ethical dilemmas are the policies and procedures associated with the "do not resuscitate" orders. Difficulty in determining what constitutes extraordinary means also enters into this situation. Pope Pius XII in 1957 defined extraordinary as that which would create a grave burden for anyone in any given circumstance, place, time, and culture (Bandman and Bandman, 1985). In a given time and place, heart-lung machines and ventilators may have become commonplace. However, the burden of using these resources could still be examined.

Resource allocation is probably receiving the most attention at this time because of the commonalities between economics and ethics. Both fields are concerned with promoting behaviors that yield well being; avoid dissipation of resources; and propose to establish, invest, and distribute value and worth (Curtain, 1982). Ethical dilemmas faced by the nursing leader in this area are frequent. The allocation of beds by critical care nursing administrators is not an infrequent dilemma. A decision to move a comatose ventilator-maintained, dialyzed, incontinent 75-year-old woman with CHF to a regular nursing unit in order to admit a 40-year-old man with an MI is a tough decision for many reasons. Likewise, the choice of sending the only available float RN to either the level-one nursery or the 40-bed oncology unit is a frequent dilemma experienced by nursing supervisors.

Within the area of human experimentation, there are many ethical dilemmas facing the nursing leader that encompass the entire continuum of the life cycle. In vitro fertilization, genetic manipulation, the transplantation of organs, and the use of artificial organs are just a few examples. Another type of ethical dilemma in this area is the use of humans in experiments and research protocols. Human rights are more carefully protected now than before. Nevertheless, it cannot be assumed that individuals are adequately protected. Utilization review boards or human use committees must use established guidelines in reviewing proposed projects for approval. Nurses within the clinical area must be aware of the mechanisms available to protect the rights of individuals in these circumstances and must be encouraged to ask questions and report concerns. The problems of informed consent apply to this area as well as to the clinical area in creating ethical dilemmas.

The clinical area provides fertile ground for ethical dilemmas because it is clearly an ethical situation. Health providers need to examine the way they perceive patients. Too often, patients are perceived as objects, not as individuals with basic human rights. When perceived as objects, providers and patients are in an "I-it" relationship. When perceived as individuals, providers and patients are in an "I-thou" relationship. In this latter relationship, the patient is more likely to be treated in a humane and ethical manner. Unfortunately, this does not always occur. The clinical situations that create ethical dilemmas for nurses have already been mentioned in earlier discussions. The conflict between life saving measures versus life support measures is one example. Another is the sanctity of life versus the quality of life. Each of these four issues are ethical dilemmas themselves. The issues raised by what constitutes informed consent frequently create ethical dilemmas in the clinical areas. Health providers with chemical dependency problems create another whole set of problems for the nursing leader and are addressed in a later chapter.

ETHICAL DECISION MAKING

How does one work through all these types of ethical situations and dilemmas? Socrates emphasized that reason, rather than emotions, should determine ethical decisions (Davis and Aroskar, 1983). Reasoning has been divided into deductive or inductive reasoning. Deductive reasoning involves basing a conclusion upon smaller premises or part to whole. The parts or premises are the known phenomena, and the conclusion naturally flows from the premises. In inductive reasoning, the whole or conclusions is the known phenomena and the parts that make up the whole are unknown. In ethical reasoning, an argument is considered logical and valid only if the stated outcome contains no more than is implicitly contained in the premises and would therefore be considered a form of deductive reasoning (Bandman and Bandman, 1985).

When involved in ethical decision making, it is helpful to remember that the outcome can take several forms. Human rights precede and preempt laws. Laws exist to enforce human rights and consequently have not kept pace with the development of society and the complex ethical dilemmas resulting from a technologically advanced civilization. Decisions that are made in these circumstances involving human rights and laws can be

TABLE 2–2
Process in Ethical Decision Making
1. Identify health problem 2. Clearly articulate ethical problem 3. Identify actors involved 4. Gather data 5. Identify alternative choices available 6. Consider consequences of each alternative 7. Choose an alternative 8. Examine consistency of decision with internal values 9. Monitor situation over time

considered both ethical and legal. An example might be the resuscitation of an 80-year-old man with cancer who is then maintained on a ventilator. A decision may be considered unethical yet legal, e.g., abortion. A decision may be ethical and yet illegal. This situation can be seen in a cancer patient receiving an unauthorized drug for therapy. Finally, a decision can be viewed as illegal and unethical. An example is a nurse who uses hospital narcotics to sustain her chemical dependency.

Now that the complexities associated with ethical decisions in health care have been presented, a process for making these difficult decisions is offered. There are nine steps in this decision making process: (1) identify the problem; (2) articulate the problem; (3) identify the players; (4) gather data; (5) identify alternatives; (6) identify short/long term consequences; (7) choose alternatives; (8) compare with values; and (9) monitor outcome (Table 2–2).

The first step is to identify the health problem. Although this may appear rather straightforward, in the clinical setting it is not always clear. For example, the comatose individual who has been unresponsive for weeks and whose diagnostic data indicate severe brain damage has on some occasions suddenly regained consciousness. The health problem, incorrectly identified, can result in an incorrect prognosis and treatment.

The second step is to clearly articulate the ethical problem. Unfortunately, there can be more than one ethical problem involved. It is necessary to define the ethical issues before proceeding. Identification of the actors involved is the third step. Who are the participants, what are their roles, who are the experts, and who are the observers are questions that may be asked.

Data gathering, the fourth step, is a significant step. One must include as many facts as possible. Observations and charting of nurses can be essential in determining an accurate picture of the situation. Data include both objective and subjective information. It is also important to recognize the emotional impact that ethical dilemmas have on the individuals involved. By putting all the cards on the table and recognizing the difficulty of the ethical problem, the emotions can be acknowledged and dealt with in some manner. It is not necessary to maintain roles with ineffective coping behaviors. Along with recognizing the emotional impact, consideration must also be given to the customs or rituals associated with those involved. One must consider the responsibilities attached to the assumed roles of the individuals involved. A physician may see his role only as a life saver and therefore may have difficulty dealing with a dying patient. An eldest son may have always made the decisions for the elderly patient involved, but in an ethical situation may be incapable of assuming that responsibility. It is equally important to identify the impact of actions on the individuals involved. Could these actions be regarded as extraordinary or ordinary? While gathering data, the knowledge and expertise of an expert or authority can be very beneficial. Finally, one must recognize what the institution's philosophy and/or politics contribute to the situation.

The fifth step involves the identification of all the alternative choices available. Consideration must then be given to the consequences of each alternative. In step six, short and long term consequences should be listed as well as possible and probable consequences. These consequences are identified in terms of the individual's right to respect, right to treatment, right to refuse treatment, and right to information. Is the action and its consequences an honest effort to be fair, and is it in the best interest of the individual? The action and consequences should not do harm, should prevent harm, and should in some manner promote good. In most situations, the individual involved is recognized as the ultimate decision maker. When the individual is not able to speak for himself, a surrogate should be appointed who knows him well enough to be able to speak for the individual. When no knowledgeable surrogate is available, a surrogate can be appointed to make a decision based on what he thinks and values as being in the individual's best interest.

Choosing an alternative is the seventh step. Once a decision is reached, it is helpful to examine how the decision rests with the decider's general set of values. This examination is the eighth step. The presence or absence of internal peace is of value to the decider. If the decider(s) is not the individual, the decision may be the best one for the individual but the decider may be in conflict.

The ninth and final step involves following or monitoring the situation over time. This helps to put the entire process into perspective and obtain feedback. As a result, this ethical dilemma can contribute to clarifying future situations.

TOMORROW'S ETHICAL STRATEGIES

Nursing leaders of tomorrow will face ethical decisions in four areas: professional, allocation of resources, human experimentation, and health policy. In order for nurses to be effective leaders, it will be necessary to identify carefully the moral and ethical basis for the individual's life. Once this grand philosophy is conceptualized, it naturally lends itself to the foundation of the individual's professional practice. The ethical basis of an individual's professional practice guides the individual in acting as a moral agent in these other areas as well. The importance of knowing one's personal, moral, and ethical base cannot be overemphasized. In a troubled, unclear world, this ethical base provides the anchor of stability and peace. This is important not only personally but also for nursing's clients and ultimately for society.

Professional ethical issues are several. The ethical basis of a nurse's practice is an elementary but essential one. As a result, there is order and meaning to the individual's practice. Issues concerning the preparation of professional nurses become tied to larger issues of society's ultimate welfare. Clinical issues as well as personnel issues are boiled down to the dignity and rights of human beings. The questions of quality of life and quantity of life will only become more complex in tomorrow's health care system. Nurses can understand their valuable contributions to this area through their careful observations and assessments. Nurses should assume a valuable place on panels and committees struggling with these issues. As technology dominates more and more of one's life, nursing can retain a clear picture of the human needs while not being intimidated by the data or the complexities of the equipment.

As moral agents, nurses will remain the primary patient advocates when resources are allocated. The historical size of the nursing service department will diminish to some extent. However, it will remain as the largest provider of services within the hospital setting. As such, the nursing department generates as well as controls patient information and patient outcome. Therefore, nursing leaders, armed with this power, will know what is ultimately the best use of these resources for the patients.

Experimentation and research will become more prevalent outside of university centers. As a result, nursing leaders will find more requests for access to patients. A strong ethical position can be very effective in these situations. As human use committees struggle with many complex issues, it will often be the nurse leader who is the best prepared to handle such situations.

Professional ethical decision making, as well as resource allocation and research, occur at the unit, department, or institutional level. The nursing leader's role in addition to direct involvement in these issues is to develop mechanisms within the patient care areas for staff to deal with them. Developing ethical rounds, policies, and procedures and providing the necessary education and support for staff are part of these responsibilities. The other main area in which nursing leaders should become high profile is in the area of health policy. As moral individuals practicing ethical nursing, nursing leaders are again in a uniquely qualified position to be directly involved in the development of health policy at the local or national level. Another favorable result would be the increased image of nursing's contribution to society.

Nurses are moral agents. As such, they are concerned with the values, choices, priorities, and duties related to the good of individuals, the nursing profession, and society (Davis and Aroskar, 1983). Because nurses are also human, it requires courage to make imperfect judgments about what is good. But it is only by asking the hard ethical questions that compose good and right that nurses as human individuals and as a society will ever come to understand and to know themselves.

References

AACN Task Force on Ethics in Critical Care Research (1985). Statement on ethics in critical care research (Part 1). *Focus 12*(3), 47–50.

Aroskar, M. A. (April 1977). Ethics in nursing curriculum. *Nursing Outlook, 25*, 260–264.

Aroskar, M. A. (March–April 1980). Ethics of nurse patient relationships. *Nurse Educator, 5*, 18–20.

Aroskar, M. A. (April 1980). Anatomy of an ethical dilemma: The practice. *American Journal of Nursing*, 661–663.

Bandman, E. L., and Bandman, B. (1985). *Nursing ethics in the life span.* East Norwalk, CT: Appleton-Century-Crofts.

Beauchamp, T. L., and Childress, J. F. (1979). *Principles of biomedical ethics.* New York: Oxford.

Beckstrand, J. (1978). The rotation of a practice theory and the relationship of scientific and ethical knowledge to practice. *Research in Nursing and Health, 1*(3), 131–136.

Bentham, J. (1948). *An introduction to the principles of morals and legislation.* New York: Hafner Press.

Bentham, J. (1969). *A Bentham reader*, M. P. Mack (ed.). New York: Pegasus.

Bentham, J. (1983). *Deontology, together with a table of the springs of action and article on utilitarianism: The collected works of Jeremy Bentham.* A. Goldworth (ed.). Oxford: Clarendon Press.

Brown, B. (ed.) (1986). Ethics and managerial decision making. *Nursing Administration Quarterly, 10*(3).

Callahan, D., and Bok, S. (1980). *Ethics Teaching* in Higher Education. New York: Plenum Press.

Cowles, K. V. (1984). Life, death and personhood. *Nursing Outlook, 32*(3), 169–172.

Creighton, H. (1984). Decisions on food and fluid in life-sustaining measures. *Nursing Management, 15*(6 and 7), (Part 1), 47–49, (Part 2), 54–56.

Curtain, L. L. (1978). A proposed model for critical ethical analysis. *Nursing Forum, 17*, 12–17.

Curtain, L. L. (1982). What are human rights. *In* Curtain, L. L., and Flaherty, M. J. (1982). *Nursing ethics: theories and pragmatics.* Bowie, MD: Robert J. Brady.

Curtain, L. L. and Flaherty, M. J. (1982). *Nursing ethics: theories and pragmatics.* Bowie, MD: Robert J. Brady.

Davis, A. J., and Aroskar, M. A. (1983). *Ethical Dilemmas and Nursing Practice* (2nd ed). East Norwalk, CT: Appleton-Century-Crofts.

Doudera, A. E., and Peters, J. D. (ed.) (1982). *Legal and ethical aspects of treating critically and terminally ill patients.* Michigan: AUPHA Press.

Feinberg, J. (1980). The problem of personhood. *In* Beauchamp, T. L., and Watley, L. (eds.). *Contemporary issues in bioethics.* Belmont, CA: Wadsworth.

Firth, R. (1970). Ethical absolution and the ideal observer. *In* Sellers, W., and Hospers, J. (eds.). *Readings in ethical theory.* Englewood Cliffs, NJ: Prentice-Hall.

Fletcher, J. (1972). Indicators of humanhood: A tentative profile of man. Hastings Center Report, Volume 2, November.

Fox, R. C., and Swazey, J. P. (1974). *The courage to fail—a social view of organ transplants and dialysis.* Chicago: University of Chicago Press.

Frankena, W. K. (1973). *Ethics* (2nd ed). Englewood Cliffs, NJ: Prentice-Hall.

Fromer, M. J. (1980). Teaching ethics by case analysis. *Nursing Outlook, 28*(10), 604–609.

Gilligan, C. (1982). *In a different voice: Psychological theory and women's development.* Cambridge, MA: Harvard U. Press.

Jameton, A. (1984). *Nursing practice: ethical Issues.* Englewood Cliffs, NJ: Prentice-Hall.

Jourard, S. (1964). *The transparent self.* New York: Van Nostrand Reinhold Co., p. 27.

Kant, I. (1949). *Fundamental principles of the metaphysics of morals*. The Little Library of Liberal Arts, O. Priest (ed.), No. 16, New York: Liberal Arts Press.

Kellmer, D. M. (1982). The teaching of ethical decision making in schools of nursing. *Nursing Leadership, 5*(2), 20–26.

Kohlberg, L. (1971). Stages of moral development as a basis for moral development. *In moral interdisciplinary approaches*. NJ: Newman, pp. 86–88.

Kohlberg, L. (1984). Essays on moral development, Vol. II. *The psychology of moral development: the nature and validity of moral stages*. San Franciso: Harper and Row.

Lewandowski, W., Daly, B., McClesh, D. K., Juknialis, B. W., and Younger, S. J. (1985). Treatment and care of "do not resuscitate" patients in a medical intensive care unit. *Heart and Lung, 14,* 175–181.

Lumpp, F. (1979). The role of the nurses in the bioethical decision-making process. *Nursing Clinics of North America, 14*, 13–21.

Marsden, C. (1979). Ethical issues in a heart transplant program. *Heart and Lung, 14*(5), 495–498.

McFarland, G. K., Leonard, H. S., and Morris, M. M. (1984). *Nursing leadership and management: contemporary strategies*. New York: John Wiley and Sons.

Mills, J. S. (1950). *On Bentham and Coleridge*. New York: Harper and Row.

Murphy, M. A., and Murphy, J. (1976). Making ethical decisions systematically. *Nursing 76*, May, 13–14.

Pense, T. (1983). Ethics in nursing, an annotated bibliography. *National Leagues for Nursing*, Pub. No. 20-1936, New York.

Probert, W. (1984). Ethics and the law of dying. *Death Education*, 70–76.

Rabb, J. D. (1976). Implications of moral and ethical issues for nurses. *Nursing Forum, 15*(2), 168–179.

Rachael, J. (1975). Active and passive euthanasia. *New England Journal of Medicine, 292*, 78–80.

Raths, L. E., Harmin, M., and Simon, S. B. (1966). Values and teaching. Westerville, OH: Charles E. Merrill Books, Inc.

Rawls, J. (1971). *A Theory of Justice*. Cambridge MA: Harvard University.

Robertson, J. A. (1983). The rights of the critically ill. *The basic American Civil Liberties Union guide to the rights of critically ill and dying patients*. Cambridge, MA: Ballinger Publishing Company.

Ryden, M. B. (November 1978). An approach to ethical decision making. *Nursing Outlook, 26*, 705–706.

Schnall, D. J., and Figliola, C. L. (eds.) (1984). *Contemporary issues in health care*. New York: Praeger.

Scott, R. S. (1985). When it isn't life or death. *AJN 85*, 19–20.

Simon, S. B., and Kirschenbaum, H. (1972). *Value clarification: A handbook of practical strategies for teachers and students*. New York: Hart Publishers.

Tucker, R. W. (1979). The value decisions we know as science. *Advances in Nursing Science, 1*(2), 1–12.

Uustal, D. B. (1977). Searching for values. *Image, 9*(1), 15–17.

Vaughan-Cole, B., and Kee, H. K. (1985). A heart decision. *AJN 85*, 535–553.

Veatch, R. M. (1976). *Death, dying, and the biological revolution: Our last quest for responsibility*. New Haven, CT: Yale University Press.

Veatch, R. (1984). Ethics and the dying. *In* Schnall, D. J., and Figliola, C. L. (eds). *Contemporary issues in health care*. New York: Praeger.

Walton, D. N. (1983). *Ethics of withdrawal of life-support systems: case studies on decision making in intensive care*. Westport, CT: Greenwood Press.

FOUNDATIONS OF NURSING LEADERSHIP

This section represents a major section of the conceptual framework. It presents the theoretical building blocks of nursing history, nursing theory, leadership theory, and nursing leadership theory. The large theoretical emphasis in this section helps to illustrate the need for research in these areas. As more knowledge is desired in these four areas, the need to conduct research becomes increasingly apparent. The lack of firmly established or grand theories in these areas indicates the lack of maturity in the development of these bodies of knowledge. At the same time, the emphasis on the available research is indicative of the importance of substantiating this important knowledge for practical use.

Our society is beginning to recognize the contributions of nursing to the development of society. As a result, more and different individuals and groups are examining the history of nursing. Looking at nursing in these different lights and perspectives can only give a fuller picture of itself. Nursing history is not usually found in specialty books such as this one. Rather, nursing history is self-contained in individual publications or merits a chapter in fundamental nursing texts. It is almost as though nursing history ceases to be of importance after an initial token review. This is indeed unfortunate, because nursing history is always with us, and we are constantly creating it. Understanding nursing in a larger social context can only be appreciated through the study of nursing history. If nursing is to learn from its previous behaviors, in order to avoid repeating mistakes and build on previous success, nurses must know nursing history. Nursing history is ultimately the affirmation of nursing's purpose, both in the past and now. For all of these reasons, and more, a chapter on nursing history is included in this section.

Chapter Three, Historical Perspective, is not just a history of nursing. Instead, this chapter briefly presents the history of nursing within the context of two other key forces: health care and women. The interrelationship of these three forces, nursing, women, and health care, remains even more relevant today.

Chapter Four, Theoretical Base for Nursing, is an overview of nursing theory. This chapter is not a substitute for the many excellent books dedicated to nursing theory. As with the chapter on nursing history, detail and comprehensiveness are not the objective. Rather, these chapters show the place, value, and contribution of their subject to both students and practitioners. Students will have other opportunities to explore these subjects in more depth. Practitioners will have an introduction to the main concepts and ideas and how they relate to practice. Further interest can be pursued through the reference list at the end of each chapter.

Chapter Five, Foundations for Leadership, presents the theoretical basis of leadership and management. The evolution of these theories has occurred to the point at which an eclectic approach is now being advocated. The tremendous organizational changes occurring within business as well as in health care are dictating new requirements for leaders and managers. The changing times, people, and goals can utilize aspects from much of this theoretical base.

Chapter Six, Nursing Leadership Theory, builds on the previous five chapters as it discusses nursing leadership in a related sense to the general body of leadership knowledge as well as specifically nursing leadership. The process of nursing behaviors is presented in a conceptual framework of nursing leadership behaviors at the executive, middle, and first line levels. Currently, many nursing organizations are composed of more than one level. The future indicates major revisions in organizational structures. This conceptual framework is general enough to be adapted to both current and future needs. In order for one to be an effective nursing leader, the knowledge and use of the concepts presented in this section are considered essential.

HISTORICAL PERSPECTIVE

INTRODUCTION

Nurses have always functioned as managers and leaders of resources and services of health care. A historical perspective is helpful because it serves to provide nurses with an enduring culture as well as with heroines, both of which contribute to the professional identity of a nurse. Historical references of the last ten years on nursing have assumed interesting variances from earlier investigations and analyses. These variations influencing the historiography of nursing have included two significant themes. The first major influence changing the way nursing history is viewed has been the effect of the women's movement. As a result, more non-nurses are investigating the history of nursing. Second, previous historical approaches centered on nurses who had been in the public eye. Because of interest in the meaning of feminism and gender differences, notoriety as defined in previous decades may no longer be sufficient to explain or describe the contributions of women and nurses adequately (Lagemann, 1983). Less rigid and less traditional explorations are being attempted. What these perspectives on the history of nursing can mean for the profession as well as for women remain yet to be seen. Caution should be exercised so that they do not serve only to polarize the genders but rather make an overall positive contribution to the civilization of society.

In addition to these influences, there has been an increased interest in defining the relationship and the impact of work groups and professions or transformations in our culture's politics and economy (Lagemann, 1983). Traditionally, historiography has approached the history of a group from the effects of society on the group rather than the group on society.

3

All of these influences have resulted in revision and publication of new stimulating historical perspectives on nursing. The reader is referred to Bullough (1984), Fitzpatrick (1983), Lagemann (1983), and Melosh (1982) as several excellent texts for more extensive reading.

THROUGH THE 1800's

Nursing as a profession struggled with its development in the new country of America. Early nurses in America were not formally trained or educated. Instead, individuals were attributed with a born gift for nursing, and learned from example. These nurses functioned primarily along the lines of public health nurses and midwives in that they ministered to the sick in their homes. Because their assistance was valued in these early years, these nurses probably possessed more power and authority than the average women of colonial America.

Health care in the U.S. progressed slowly during this period. The majority of health care was delivered in the home by either a rare doctor or a nurse, both of whom carried the extent of their repertoire in a bag.

The earliest hospitals in North America were built by Cortez in Mexico City in 1524 and in New Mexico (Donahue, 1985). Hospital development in Colonial America occurred in the form of infirmaries within poorhouses. One of the earliest infirmaries on record was located on Manhattan Island to care for sick soldiers and slaves arriving on ships. Records indicate the presence of infirmaries as early as 1612 in Virginia and several in the 1730's in Philadelphia, New Orleans, and New York City. Unfortunately, the care provided by the individuals in these infirmaries was often inhumane. The first voluntary hospital was Pennsylvania Hospital in Philadelphia, established in 1751. New York Hospital was established in 1769, and Massachusetts General was founded in 1811. The first mental asylum was established in Williamsburg, Virginia in 1773. By 1813, there were 178 hospitals in the United States. However, hospitalization was not the norm and the outcome usually fatal.

America did experience what could be considered a women's movement, which included the Women's Rights' Convention in Seneca Falls, New York in 1848. During this time, the majority of health care was still provided by women in homes or by physicians of variable qualifications that ranged from some formal education to apprenticeships (Donahue, 1985). Mary Wallstonecraft's book *A Vindication of the Rights of Women*, published in Britain, appeared to have little impact on the role of women in America during this period of time.

It was not socially acceptable for women to be involved in politics. However, issues associated with religious overtones were acceptable concerns for women, and it was under this pretext that women advocated health maintenance and disease prevention as well as anti-slavery. In the anti-slavery movement, one sees the situation in which women chose to align themselves with men who had power. In aligning themselves, women supported powerful men and gained these men's attention and respect. Thus, they were able to expose them to the women's concerns regarding health, children, and their own rights. Despite these efforts, however, many male abolitionists remained divided over whether women were truly their equal.

While nursing was just awakening to its own existence as a profession, the medical profession was undergoing tremendous changes that would significantly impact health care, physicians, and roles assumed by all other health care providers. It was in the 1850's that germ theory was discovered and medical schools were reorganized to include longer and more extensive education. As a result, physicians moved into an elitist role because of the control they engendered from this new-found knowledge.

The 1800's were a period of tremendous change and opportunity for women in general as well as for nurses. This was the age of such heroines as Dorothea Dix, who led the crusade to build mental hospitals. It was also during this time that Florence Nightingale's efforts became eminent in the history of nursing.

Nursing leadership during the Nightingale era was a position of dubious honor. Generally, nurses were untrained and were not held in much respect. As a woman with a certain amount of social status, it was acceptable for Florence Nightingale to become superintendent of Harley Street only because the owners/founders were respectable people and because it was an establishment for gentlewomen during illness (Kelly, 1985).

The dawn of modern nursing occurred as a result of Florence Nightingale's ability to organize and achieve positive effects for the soldier of the Crimean War in the mid-1800's, as well as her tremendous accomplishments within hospitals and the establishment of a training school (Donahue, 1985). Florence Nightingale's interest in caring for the sick as well as her determination to live her life the way she pleased was longstanding. Nightingale set goals for herself and discovered ways to achieve them. However, it was her friendship with Sidney Herbert, Secretary at War in the British Cabinet, that created the circumstances for Nightingale to be the first superintendent of nursing. Although this title gave Nightingale the responsibility and authority over the nurses, the relationship, leadership, and management exercised should be viewed within the context of the culture and times that she lived. Nightingale's relationship with Herbert could be interpreted as a collaborative effort between a politician and a professional to maximize the benefits to society. Nursing leaders and managers have found themselves in this situation many times since. Nightingale realized that as a woman and as a leader, she and her nurses would not be accepted by the military. In order to ensure her success, nursing was definitively placed under medical authority. Nightingale had power to select nurses and dismiss them. Everything else was subject to approval by the chief medical officers. As with Herbert, Nightingale aligned herself through diplomacy, tact, and ability with the groups who had real power and authority in order to achieve her mission.

In order for people in power and position to witness the effects of her efforts, it was necessary for Florence Nightingale to subjugate herself to military and medical officers. Although her opportunities to prove her abilities may have been begrudged by her and her nurses, Nightingale utilized each opportunity to demonstrate the effectiveness of the knowledge and skills of her nurses.

The selection and education of nurses was a different situation as far as Nightingale was concerned. This internal content and process of nursing was strictly the responsibility and domain of nursing. Nightingale's original school at St. Thomas was a financially independent, separate and distinct entity (Palmer, 1983). Because of her religious and altruistic philosophies, Nightingale's motives could be viewed as self-sacrificing and charitable. These philosophies as well as even earlier models of nursing are the influences that "Christianized" nursing. As a "Christianized" service to mankind, there was the expectation among both provider and client of self-sacrifice and charity. These influences plus the role and position of women have resulted in nursing, among other primarily female professions, not being considered as a primary leadership profession.

Nightingale was a prolific writer on the characteristics of a good nurse, the need for continuing education, and the need for sick nursing, as well as health nursing. Her writings reflected her extensive knowledge, still considered pertinent today, on such issues as hygiene, nutrition, environment, and the mental state of patients (Kelly, 1985). As a planner, administrator, educator, researcher, and reformer, Florence Nightingale serves as a leading role model for nursing and for women.

Tracing the history of nursing and the development of leaders and managers in nursing takes us back across the ocean to the time of the Civil War. What is considered to be a landmark in feminist literature was Dr. Elizabeth Blackwell's *Medicine as a Profession for Women*, which was published in 1860. During this time, women were beginning to think beyond their traditional roles, but the majority of women and nurses were still functioning as second class citizens. Women who broke out of the tradition were usually women who made the most of their opportunities. Therefore, it was women who possessed money from birth or marriage who were then able to develop and express themselves as individuals.

The Civil War provided examples of nursing visibility and impact. Many religious orders such as the Sisters of Charity, who possessed the most skill and experience in nursing, provided care to the soldiers (Donahue, 1985). Mary Bickerdyke traveled with General Sherman's army, supervising nursing, distributing supplies, and organizing diet kitchens, laundries, and ambulance services. Clara Barton worked to provide care for both the North and the South. Through her efforts and leadership, the American Red Cross was established in 1882. During the Civil War, nursing was frequently performed by convalescent infantrymen as well as by women, most of whom were uneducated and unskilled. As Superintendent of the Female Nurses of the Union Army, Dorothea Dix attempted to improve the quality of nurses by recruiting individuals with certain characteristics such as good character and superior education. One of the best known nurses of the Confederacy was Sally L. Tompkins, the only woman to hold a commission (Donahue, 1985). Kate Cummings was another Southern lady who gave distinguished service under severe conditions in Southern hospitals and who also recorded her experiences. Black nurses of the Civil War were also heroines. Harriet Tubman not only led slaves to freedom by way of the Underground Railroad but also nursed the wounded soldiers of the Union army. Sojourner Truth, an abolitionist speaker, also cared for the sick and wounded. Susie King Taylor, born a slave, served as a battlefront nurse for more than four years (Kelly, 1985).

The Sanitary Ideal was a concept that encouraged order and discipline by the direction of qualified people following clear lines of authority. The concept appealed to many people, including Dr. Elizabeth Blackwell, who helped organize the Sanitary Commission. The goal of the Sanitary Commission was to create the healthiest conditions possible in military camps, hospitals, and transports. To achieve this goal, the Sanitary Commission inspected facilities and then provided supplies, restructured facilities, improved sanitation and hygiene, tended the wounded, and attended to the dietary needs of the patients. A branch of the Sanitary Commission was the Women's Central Association for Relief. This group coordinated relief organizations throughout America, assisted in sending nurses to areas in need, and initiated preparatory programs for nurses in several hospitals in Boston and New York (Donahue, 1985).

In nineteenth century America, advanced education, except for rich women, was still considered a male privilege. Co-ed higher education did not begin until 1833 at Oberlin College. It was not until after the Civil War that higher education for women sought establishment and prestige with the opening of such institutions as Vassar in 1865, Smith and Wellesley in 1875, and Radcliffe in 1879. Therefore, nursing education, although hardly equated with the level of these colleges, was regarded as a real opportunity for many women. Although this period of time had a number of situations in which rich women and nurses collaborated, it is interesting to note the continued secondary status of nursing. This is illustrated by the fact that none of the prestigious women's colleges ever established a school of nursing except for Vassar, which had a preparatory course for nurses during World War I.

Dr. Valentine Seaman is credited with organizing the first regular training school for nurses at the New York Hospital in 1798. Dr. Joseph Warrington formed the Nurse Society of Philadelphia in 1839 to provide trained nurses for home maternity services. The Woman's Hospital of Philadelphia opened a nurses' training school in 1861, and the New England Hospital for Women and Children was involved in the teaching of nurses from 1860. These two programs were initiated and administered by female physicians (Donahue, 1985). Two graduates of the one-year program at the New England Hospital for Women and Children deserve mention. Melinda Ann (Linda) Richards was the first graduate of this program. She progressed to be a key figure in the development of nursing education. Another outstanding graduate was Mary Mahoney, the first trained black nurse (Kelly, 1985).

The second half of the 1800's saw the establishment of nursing schools in the United States. Although these schools claimed to be based on Nightingale's model, in fact none of them were independent institutions. Instead, these schools were based on the apprenticeship model. However, at that time, this model was not considered to be a bad model nor recognized as exploitive of women. Considering the culture and social situation of the vast majority of women, these nursing schools were considered opportunities. The establishment of Bellevue Hospital School of Nursing, Connecticut Training School, and Boston Training School at Massachusetts General Hospital occurred in 1873. By 1890, there were 15 schools of nursing, the majority of whose graduates went on to private duty nursing. The nursing leadership during this time was the product of the sexual roles, the effect of the sanitary ideal concept, and the order and discipline from the Nightingale model. As a result of these influences, the nursing leadership promoted and reinforced the model of a non-aggressive, mothering nurse, who was also self-sacrificing and obedient.

The Nightingale pledge, written in 1893 by Lystra E. Gretter, superintendent of the school at Harper Hospital in Detroit, is evidence of the principles of sacrifice, service, obedience to the physician, and ethical orientation of the emerging profession of nursing:

> I solemnly pledge myself before God and in the presence of this assembly;
> To pass my life in purity and to practice my profession faithfully;
> I will abstain from whatever is deleterious and mischievous and will not take or knowingly administer any harmful drug;
> I will do all in my power to maintain and elevate the standard of my profession; and will hold in confidence all personal matters committed to my keeping and all family affairs coming to my knowledge in the practice of my calling.
> With loyalty will I endeavor to aid the physician in his work, and devote myself to the welfare of those committed to my care (Kelly, 1985).

The settlement of the West contributed to the visibility of women and women's issues, because under the Homestead Act women could actually own their own land. Wyoming was the first state to give women the vote in 1869. Women and nurses united and were very visible under the Women's Temperance Union in the 1870's.

Leadership and organizing behavior was demonstrated by the training school's superintendents who established the Superintendents' Society in 1893 and the Nurses' Associated Alumnae in 1897. The purpose of these groups was to improve the quality of nurses and thereby improve the status of nurses and women. Through these groups, the training school superintendents strove to make the training schools' curriculums consistent, coordinate clinical and educational experiences, and restrict the admissions to the schools (Armeny, 1983, p. 18). The first president of the Nurses' Associated Alumnae was Isabel Adams Hampton Robb, considered to be one of the greatest leaders in American nursing because of her vision and administrative abilities. In addition to her own publications, *Nursing: Its Principles and Practice for Hospital and Private Use* (1984), *Nursing Ethics* (1900), and *Educational Standards for Nurses* (1907), Mrs. Robb was a member of the committee that founded the American Journal of Nursing (Donahue, 1985). The Society of Superintendents of Nursing Schools was also able to open the doors of Teachers College of New York in 1899 for nurses to take courses, which in turned opened the doors to higher education for many women. Mary Adelaide Nutting, the former superintendent of nurses and principal of the Training School for Nurses at Johns Hopkins Hospital, became the first nursing professor in the world at Teachers College in 1907 (Donahue, 1985). Teachers College was the first institution to provide education for nursing administrators. The required courses included psychology, ethics, psychology in teaching, physiology and hygiene, bacteriology, and chemistry. Management courses included hospital and training school management, home sanitation management, and social reform management (Erickson, 1983).

The Spanish-American War was a major influence on the collaboration between women of wealth and nurses. Yet simultaneously these two groups found themselves at odds with other members of their own sex. Although such conflicts frequently occurred among men, it did not appear to have the same disastrous effects as it did on nursing. Continuing with concepts from the sanitary ideal, some wealthy women and the Nurses' Associated Alumnae wanted to establish a war nursing system characterized by organization and efficiency. Their goals were to provide only well trained nurses for the war and provide administrative control over all nurses working in the war through the development of a hierarchy of nursing. Apparently, this collaborative effort between nurses and laywomen took time because the Daughters of the American Revolution preempted this plan and presented a functional system to Congress. Dr. Anita Newcomb McGee directed this Hospital Corps, which ascribed to many of the ideals and requirements espoused by the NAA group.

The goal of a homogeneous group of nurses under the control of a nurse executive was not realized during this war. Auxiliary No. 3 was another group of civilians interested in assisting the war effort. Lena Potter Cowdin, Elizabeth Mills Reid, and Anna Roosevelt Cowles of this organization were very effective in recruiting and placing well qualified nurses in military installations (Armeny, 1983). Clara Louise Maass, a graduate from the Christina Trefz Training School for Nurses of the Newark German Hospital, volunteered to nurse the victims of yellow fever in Havana. She died following an attack of yellow fever after submitting to a mosquito bite in an experiment to determine the cause of yellow fever. As the only woman to die during the yellow fever experiments, Clara Maass brought fame to

American nursing during the Spanish-American War because of her gallant efforts (Donahue, 1985).

In 1899, a bill was introduced in Washington that provided for a nurse to head the Army nursing service, a position held by Dita H. Kinney. Further illusions of power were to come in 1918, with approval of rank for nurses. Florence Blanchfield in 1947 became the first woman to be given a permanent commission of colonel in the regular Army.

1900 AND BEYOND

The industrial period in the early 1900's contributed to the promotion of women's issues and the development of nurses. By then, medical care had become much more complex and there were over 4300 hospitals providing services. The majority of these hospitals were concentrated in the heavily populated northeastern United States, where industry and immigrants were located. As a result of the increasing demand for health care, public health nursing assumed prominence and value. Instructive District Nursing Associations, as the visiting nurses' associations of this period were called, provided home care of the sick and education on the principles of hygiene, sanitation, health, and illness (Donahue, 1985). Nursing leadership in the public health movement was demonstrated by Lillian Wald, Margaret Sanger, and Mary Brewster.

The Henry Street Settlement is considered one of the first examples of nursing expanding into the public health nursing field. Established in 1893 as a cooperative and partially self-supporting neighborhood service, the Henry Street Settlement provided its founder, Lillian Wald, with a vehicle that impacted on society's health well beyond New York City. Together with a classmate, Mary Brewster, Lillian Wald founded public health nursing (Donahue, 1985).

Mary Beckinridge organized the Frontier Nursing Service in 1925, the first organized midwifery service in this country. The Frontier Nursing Service founded the Graduate School of Midwifery at Hyden, Kentucky in 1939 (Donahue, 1985).

Other examples of public health or early ambulatory care efforts are illustrated in the establishment of milk stations for babies of the poor in New York in 1893, the establishment of the Society for Social and Moral Prophylaxis in 1905, and the establishment of the Society for Mental Hygiene in 1908 (Jonas, 1981). Early forms of workman's compensation in such states as New York resulted in the establishment of industrial clinics, another form of ambulatory care and a situation requiring nurses to function independently (Jonas, 1981) because physicians could not meet this increased demand and because public health nursing was economical.

Lavinia Lloyd Dock is considered one of nursing's greatest leaders during this time. Dock's leadership was not limited to nursing, as she was also extremely active in women's rights and human rights movements. Lavinia Dock was the first secretary of the International Council of Nurses and was also active in the movement to implement legislative control of nursing practice (Donahue, 1985).

The American Nurses Association became the successor to the Nurses' Associated Alumnae in 1911, and within a year 39 state nurses' associations had been organized. However, the International Council of Nurses, established in 1899, remains the oldest of all international organizations of professional healthcare workers. In 1912, the American Society of Superintendents of Training Schools was renamed the National League of Nursing Education. The national honor society of nursing, Sigma Theta Tau, was founded in 1922 at Indiana University.

This period of time also began to see a growing awareness of the need to protect consumers from poor practitioners. Nursing leaders felt that registration would help develop more uniform intellectual and ethical codes, help to exclude competitors, and provide social and economic rewards (Tomes, 1983, p. 107). Initially, there were a number of training school superintendents who did not support the registration movement. However, this dissension within nursing could not stifle what Tomes felt was a pivotal and significant period in the professionalism of nurses. Taking an example from the medical model, regulation of nurses became a priority during the early 1900's. New York State's 1903 registration act was considered to be the most restrictive and served as a model for many other states. By 1923, 48 states had registration laws. These registration laws were unlike those of medicine in that unregistered individuals could still practice nursing but could not use the designation R.N. Many private duty agencies did not require registration, but most forms of institutional nursing did require registration (Tomes, 1983).

Legislation requiring mandatory registration and licensure did not occur until 1920. Unfortunately, by that time, hospital administrators and physicians were more aware of the potential outcome of such legal monopoly and power of self-regulation. As a result, these two groups successfully lobbied for the membership of the board of nursing to include a physician and hospital administrator. This involvement of non-nurses working to protect their interest resulted in ultimate loss of power by nurses, who again did not control their own destiny.

The year 1910 saw the Army Nurses Corp and Red Cross Reserve organized and presenting opportunities for nurses. The union movement also demonstrated examples of female leadership that was not always appreciated by nursing for their own working situation. Also in 1910, what was referred to as the Great Uprising made the International Ladies Garment Worker's Union a force not to be ignored. Likewise, politics also contributed to the status of women's suffrage and resulted in a reform platform of the Progressive party that improved labor laws. The nineteenth Amendment was also introduced but was not passed at this time.

In 1914, World War I found nurses aligning themselves differently than in earlier years. In an effort to promote and improve their identity as professionals, nurses turned to politicians and physicians rather than to female or religious groups. The leadership of Annie Goodrich and Frances Payne Bolton led to the establishment of the Army School of Nursing in 1918, which developed an outstanding reputation among both the military and civilian world. The American Red Cross Nursing Service, under the administrative leadership of Jane Delano, recruited and assigned over 20,000 nurses to military service. The critical shortage of nurses created a public and political movement to waive various admission and graduation require-ments as well as licensing requirements in order to increase the supply of nurses. M. Adelaide Nutting, Annie Goodrich, and Lillian Wald formed the National Emergency Committee on Nursing to counteract this movement and to provide alternative solutions for the nursing shortage. One alternative was the development of preparatory courses for college graduates seeking admission to schools of nursing. The first of these preparatory courses was the Vassar Training Camp; other colleges with similar programs were Western Reserve, University of Cincinnati, University of Iowa, University of Colorado, and the University of California. These training camps at such prestigious colleges brought college recognition to nursing by the public and introduced nursing to well-educated, affluent women (Donahue, 1985).

Edith Cavell was an English nurse in World War I who became a heroine as a result of her leadership. In addition to establishing a school of nursing in Brussels, Belgium in 1909, Miss Cavell assisted in the escape of Allied soldiers. Charged with harboring and assisting the enemy, Miss Cavell was executed by a German firing squad in 1915 (Donahue, 1985).

The Goldmark Report: Nursing and Nursing Education in the United States, published in 1923, was a landmark document that emphasized the need for quality nursing education (Kalisch and Kalisch, 1978). Yale University, Western Reserve University, and Vanderbilt University developed collegiate schools of nursing as a result of this report.

The Great Depression in 1929 had a tremendous impact on the status of women and nurses. During the Depression, 26 states had laws forbidding the employment of married women. It is estimated that as many as 10,000 graduate nurses were unemployed. The number of nursing schools declined from 2286 in 1927 to 1472 in 1936 (Kalisch and Kalisch, 1978). Hospitals found themselves with empty beds because people did not have the money to pay for hospital care. As a result, hospitals began selling insurance for medical care. Up until then, insurance was practically unheard of except in isolated industries. From such humble beginnings, we have the start of one of the largest social forces ever experienced by our society.

From the ruins of the Great Depression, there occurred explosive and phenomenal social and economic changes. Shifting morbidity patterns, the decline in the types of illnesses that required private duty nursing care, and the improved reputation of hospitals changed the status, importance, and contribution of public health nursing. This fall from grace of public health nursing has lasted until current times, which are now witnessing the move to alternative health care methodologies. The new reimbursement mechanisms for hospital care and a capital intensive support of medicine resulted in the United States spending 3.5% of its Gross National Product on health care. The majority of the money used to pay for health care was still that from private sources. Only about 20% was paid for by the government, insurance, or charities (Roemer, 1982, p. 5; Reverby, 1983, p. 134).

The medical profession made a significant change during this period as a result of Abraham Flexner's report. Flexner predicted dire consequences for both society and medicine if higher standards and better and longer education were not embraced by physicians. Up until that time, medical schools had variable entrance requirements and inconsistent programs of studies. In 1938, Johns Hopkins Medical School was established at the graduate level, and thus medicine moved to become an even more elitist and monopolistic profession. Almost 50 years later, nursing is still struggling to resolve this same issue of basic educational preparation.

Archer and Goehner (1982) point out that leadership in nursing until World War I consisted of the leadership of very few nurses from a very small segment of nursing. When the biographies of nursing leaders during this time are surveyed, it is seen that the dominant features that characterized these individuals indicated the narrow segment of the nursing population they represented. The majority of these nursing leaders were unmarried; lived in the Northeast; and had educational, not hospital or registry backgrounds (p. 44). It was these nurses who attempted to overcome the restrictive gender roles that were the prescription of their time. Despite their limited and narrow perspective of nursing and the resistance they encountered, it is truly amazing that the profession made any progress at all. The fact that significant changes and growth *did* occur is truly commendable for these early farsighted nursing leaders.

Until the 1960's, specialization in nursing administration prevailed at the baccalaureate level, owing largely to the status of formal education for nurses as well as the influence of the Goldmark Study of 1923. Programs at the masters level that prepared nursing administrators were initiated by the University of Chicago in 1934 and Northwestern's School of Commerce in 1943.

Examples of nursing leadership during World War II can be seen in the formation of the Nursing Council of National Defense, an umbrella organization of all the professional nursing associations. Initiated by Isabel Stewart, the Nursing Council for National Defense was to formulate plans to inventory registered nurses, determine the role of nurses and nursing schools in the defense program, and expand nursing school facilities. Major Julia Stinson of the Army Nurse Corps was the Council's first chairwoman (Donahue, 1985). Outstanding nursing leadership was provided during World War II by Lucille Petry, Director of the United States Cadet Nurse Corps; Captain Sue S. Dauser, Superintendent of the Navy Nurse Corps; and Colonel Florence A. Blanchfield, Superintendent of the Army Nurse Corps. The importance of nurses was also illustrated by the introduction of a bill in 1945

CAROLE B. MERHOFF

by President Roosevelt for the conscription of women nurses (Kalisch and Kalisch, 1978). Nurses have continued to demonstrate courage, leadership, and sacrifice throughout every military conflict since World War II, including the Korean War and the Vietnam War.

Lagemann (1983) identified another significant period of growth for the nursing profession after the 1940's. The tremendous growth in medicine and technology expanded the use of nurses because of the need for their specialized skills and observations. Because medicine was no longer palliative but interactive, physicians needed nurses at the bedside, where physicians could not be for long periods of time. The short supply of nurses increased their value to society. However, Lagemann notes, "as nurses claimed more control and assumed command of imposing technology their work jarred cultural prescriptions for women's place." Because the post-war society called for return to domesticity, nursing's expanding role was contested and challenged (Melosh, 1982). Although the majority of women who had supported the war effort by working willingly left the factory to return home, nurses found themselves in different situations. Nurses were not really aware of the significant opportunities afforded to them by being alongside of the "revered" physicians. As a result, nursing did not fully take advantage of this situation. Nurses who did not assert themselves or who by chance were given responsibility and vestiges of power were the exception and became characters illustrative of women's abusive power over men. Nursing characters dramatized in *One Flew Over The Cuckoo's Nest* or by Hot Lips in *MASH* were not known for their intelligence or professional abilities. Neither of these extreme images of nursing were images to be proud of or to be advocated.

Recommendations for schools of nursing to be in the mainstream of the collegiate setting as well as the need for nursing schools to be accredited were made in Dr. Esther Lucille Brown's 1948 book, *Nursing for the Future*, and were widely advocated by nursing leaders. Standards of nursing education were also improved by the development of the State Board Test Pool, which was utilized in all 48 states by 1950. Nursing was "the first profession for which a common licensing examination was used throughout the nation" (Kalisch and Kalisch, 1978, p. 549).

The education of nursing service administrators finally received some concentrated attention in 1951 with the initiation of a major grant from the W. K. Kellogg Foundation. Subsequently, 14 universities developed proposals to prepare nurses for nursing administration. The Kellogg curriculum proposed during development of the project included content on philosophy of nursing, knowledge of health care in society, trends in administration, knowledge of administrative theory, interpersonal relationships, leadership, research, and evaluation. However, not all schools endorsed the entire proposed curriculum (Erickson, 1983). By 1960, there were seven schools offering administration/supervision as a functional focus; four schools had a joint focus with clinical practice; and 13 other schools included or offered administration in minor capacities (Erickson, 1983).

As humanism became a cultural trend, society began to recognize the physical intimacy associated with health care. Health care was being experienced by a significantly large percentage of the population and no longer was provided in the privacy of the home. As a result, there was concern about subjecting body, mind, and soul to the mysteries of medical science. Exposure of people's inner most person resulted in extreme responses. Since nurses provided a majority of care within this intimate area, they were conceptualized as either saints or sinners.

Feminists were not very active in the period from 1940 to about the 1960's. This lack of assertion by women was also evidenced by a decline in the percentage of women enrolled in universities, a decrease in the marriage age from the twenties to the teens, and a decline in the number of women in occupations traditionally associated with women, namely teaching and social work (Melosh, 1982, p. 37).

The 1960's were a landmark time for women and nursing. Tremendous leadership was demonstrated in both segments. The civil rights movement helped to give momentum to a growing consciousness of women and nursing issues as well as to concerns for individuals' right to health care. As feminism developed, the movement looked for heroines. Unfortunately, the feminists did not readily or eagerly look to the nursing profession for its role models. As an organized group of women, nursing can be credited with the first major professional association for women, the Nurses' Associated Alumnae of the United States and Canada, publication of the first professional magazine for women, *The American Journal of Nursing*, and the first major professional group to integrate their black and white members. Female deans of university schools of nursing and high ranking female military officers were probably some of the most visible professional women to achieve acknowledged status in the professional world (Archer and Goehner, 1982, pp. 41–42). Despite all of these accomplishments, nursing was not considered by feminists to be aggressive enough in promoting their issues and not really in the mainstream of the true male professional world. Apparently, a women's world was considered second class by even women and therefore not worthy of emulation.

The 1960's experienced President Kennedy's Commission on the Status of Women; Betty Friedan's *The Feminine Mystique*; the Equal Pay Act, the Civil Rights Act, the establishment of the National Organization for Women; Medicare; the Surgeon General's Consultant Group on Nursing report, *Toward Quality in Nursing*; and the Nurse Training Act of 1964. Concurrently with this tremendous outsurge of social consciousness raising, health care was experiencing its own quantum leap in progress. The shortage of physicians lent support to the development and utilization of nurse practitioners and midwives. Apparently, nursing was again considered insufficient or inadequate to meet this need, and another group of male dominated physician extenders was created in the form of physicians' or surgeons' assistants. Frequently, these individuals, despite their substantially lesser education, were more readily accepted by physicians, hospitals, clients, and nurses than the advanced prepared nurses.

The increasing financial support of health care from government sources, primarily the result of such legislation as Medicare and Medicaid, contributed significantly to the rapid proliferation of health services and their utilization. Within this rapidly growing system, as long as nurses acted within the boundaries of their occupation they were acknowledged, supported, and encouraged. If nurses attempted to move outside of this boundary, they were quickly sanctioned. Despite tremendous shortages and difficult working conditions, the nation's sick and suffering were cared for and cured. Again nurses served their country in times of war. During the Vietnam conflict, nurses cared for the wounded stateside as well as in field hospitals and MASH units. Ten nurses (eight women and two men) were killed. Nine were members of the U.S. Army Nurse Corps; one was an Air Force nurse (Spelts, 1986).

Nursing's leadership was increasingly aware of forces within and without nursing and were farsighted in realizing that nurses needed to be active participants in their own future. The American Nurses Association position paper in 1964 was a turning point for nursing's visibility and professionalism. Archer and Goehner (1982) point out that every major development in nursing is demarcated by a change in the education of nurses. The ANA position paper was no exception. Despite the recognition by nursing leadership for the need to cement the education of professional nurses with the collegiate status of a baccalaureate degree, there was little support for this commitment to excellence. The idea was very threatening to nursing's own ranks. Hospital administrators and physicians were not motivated to support the idea. Even the Surgeon General's Office promoted the idea that "a nurse is a nurse is a nurse." This resulted in not an increase in the number of BSN graduates, but rather the development and full scale support of community and junior colleges of nursing (Lysaught, 1981, p. 44). Imagine where nursing might be today if these resources and energies had been directed at the full scale implementation of the ANA position paper.

The decade of the 1970's was composed of many significant occurrences for and to nursing. The expansion of voluntary health insurance has led to the growth of health industry to rank as the third largest industry in the United States. This growth placed a tremendous demand on nursing. The Nurse Training Act enacted in 1971 provided funds to help ease the shortage of nurses. The American Association of Colleges of Nursing in 1969 was created to provide deans and administrators of baccalaureate and graduate degree nursing programs with a vehicle to review developments in the field of health (Donahue, 1985). The final report of the National Commission for the Study of Nursing in the United States directed future concerns and solutions for nursing. As a result of such efforts, nursing leadership had identified several areas on which to focus its attention. These areas are both internal and external to nursing.

Internally, there is an increasing effort and attention being directed at developing a science of nursing. Associated with this is the ongoing effort to enhance the educational preparation of nurses. Diploma programs are closing down, and associate degree program admissions are leveling off. There are now over 150 graduate programs, and enrollment has increased dramatically, from 2800 students in 1964 to 17,000 students in 1983 (NLN, 1984). Programs leading to a doctoral degree in nursing began in the early 1960's. In 1962, there were four doctoral programs, which enrolled 144 students. Graduates numbered less than 20. In 1982, there were 25 doctoral programs, enrolling over 1300 students and graduating over 125 individuals (NLN, 1983). Even the public no longer appears confused over a nurse who is addressed as Dr. Smith.

The decade of the 1980's has witnessed the escalation of issues and trends, many of which were initiated in the 1970's as a result of the women's movement and the growing health industry. The title of the 1980 American Nurses Association Convention, *The 80's: Decade for Decision*, appropriately described the significance of this decade. Many decisions about the profession have occurred in the 1980's.

The issue of comparable worth has been of prime concern to both the women's movement and to nursing. Resistance and denial of the comparable worth issue by industry and government indicate the magnitude of this issue. Although some gains have been made, discrimination remains widespread as an ongoing indication of the second class status of women in our society. Nursing has provided leadership in this area through testimony before government groups. The U.S. Supreme Court refused to review a discrimination case by a group of Denver nurses. This case was considered a key test case on the issue of comparable worth.

Associated with the issue of comparable worth have been the economic and general welfare issues for nurses. As more and more women entered the work force, economic and general welfare issues were on the forefront of nursing concerns in the early 1980's. Union activity was very strong. Although union activity leveled off in the mid–1980's, it is predicted to resume in intensity in the late 1980's.

Nursing education has experienced major change during this decade. A new licensing examination that focused on behaviors nurses need to know was initiated in 1982. Mandatory continuing education for re-licensure had become mandatory in over 14 states. At the 1985 ANA convention, the association voted to accept the title of professional nurse for the BSN graduate and the title of associate nurse for the technical nurse. This statement was also endorsed by the National League for Nursing. Since that time, many states have moved in the direction of implementation of these two levels. Over twenty years have passed since the ANA's 1964 position statement delineated the basic educational level of professional nursing to be the BSN. It now appears that the 1980's may witness the beginning of the culmination of this ideal. This decision has also been supported by activities of the Western Interstate Commission for Higher Education (WICHE). Funded by the W. K. Kellogg Foundation, the WICHE has prepared two sets of competencies: one for new associate graduate nurses, and one for new BSN graduate nurses. Although the Institute of Medicine study (1983) was not supportive on continuing funding of undergraduate nursing education, funding has continued at a reduced level. Other changes in the national health and government scene have had an impact on nursing education. The scare of the budget deficit enabled the Gramm-Rudman law to be passed in 1985. Prospective payment for Medicare patients reduced the amount of money hospitals were reimbursed for diploma education and impacted attractiveness of nursing as a profession. Enrollments in schools of nursing dropped in 1984–1986, anywhere from 5 to 14%, raising concerns of what now has become a new shortage of nurses.

In 1981, the ANA issued a landmark policy statement on the scope of nursing. Nursing was defined as the diagnosis and treatment of human responses to actual or potential health problems. As such, this definition sets the scene for nursing. This *Scope of Nursing Policy Statement* delineates the four defining characteristics of nursing: phenomena, theory application, nursing action, and evaluation. This definition and the characteristics are reflective of nursing's responsiveness to a changing society and a changing concept of health.

Another major decision, in 1982, altered the organizational structure of the professional nurses association. The American Nurses Association became a federation of state nurses associations. This organizational change was initiated in an effort to be more responsive and accessible to individual nurses.

The 1980's witnessed nursing again aligning itself with powerful groups and politicians. In 1981, nursing representatives were named to the board of a new coalition on pay equity. Consisting of representatives from labor, women's groups, and civil rights organizations, this coalition provides testimony and information on comparable worth and equitable pay issues. As a result of intense lobbying efforts from nursing groups, the House and Senate overrode a December 1985 presidential veto and approved reauthorization of a National Institute of Health bill. This National Institute of Health bill established a National Center for Nursing Research at the National Institute of Health, which opened April 18, 1986.

Nursing continued to change during the 1980's in an effort to be responsive to the changing health and nursing needs of society. This is reflective of the emphasis placed on nursing being knowledgeable about new technologies. These new technologies include laser treatment; hyperbaric oxygen therapy; advances in drug administration, such as insulin pumps; indwelling catheters; and synthetic blood. Home dialysis, ventilators, and organ transplants are not unusual health care events requiring nursing practice in the 1980's. The computerization of health care has required that nurses also become computer literate.

The health care concerns of society are also reflected in nursing's concerns with health promotion and disease prevention. The appearance of new health concerns such as toxic shock syndrome, legionnaires' disease, and AIDS has overpowered previous concerns about cardiovascular, cerebral, diabetic, and cancerous threats to society's health. Ongoing battles with chemical dependencies on drugs and alcohol have provided opportunities for nursing to demonstrate the efficiencies and effectiveness of its services.

Nursing leadership in the 1980's continues to evolve from earlier decades, in the sense that leadership by nurses is not confined to a small segment of nurses leading nursing. Nursing leadership is being demonstrated both within nursing and outside of nursing. Within nursing, Barbara Nichols has provided visionary leadership of the professional organization. She has served as president of the ANA from 1978 to 1982, during a turbulent time of debate and decision making. Additionally, Ms. Nichols also served as director of the International Council of Nurses. Lulu Hassenplug has contributed to the interdependence of nursing practice, nursing education, and nursing research. Advocates such as Ada Jacox have testified before legislative bodies and groups such as the Equal Employment Opportunity Commission to promote the value of nursing.

Minority nurses have a heroine in Mary Carnegie, the former editor of Nursing Research, who facilitated the integration of minority groups into nursing. Another nursing minority advocate, Doris Schwartz, has facilitated nursing's work with the Navajo Indians.

Public health and community nursing can look to the efforts of several nursing leaders over the last ten years. Marion S. Bailey, initially involved with the New York City Henry Street Settlement, has made a major contribution to the development of practice and educational standards for community-based nursing. Role models are provided by Sister Bernadette Mullin and four other RNs in establishing a private shelter in Manhattan called "Dwelling Place" to meet the needs of the homeless.

Anne Zimmerman, a nursing leader for many years, has worked arduously for the profession of nursing. In addition to being president of ANA, she has been an active proponent of the ANA's economic and general welfare program.

Nurses have also been demonstrating leadership outside of nursing as well. Faye G. Abdellah was the first nurse and first woman to hold the rank of Deputy Surgeon General of the U.S. Public Health Service. Her activities in developing intensive care units, self-care units, and the federal nurse scientist program are only some of her major accomplishments. Other contemporary names of nursing leaders include Rozella Schlotfeldt, Vernice Ferguson, and Sister Rosemary Donnley, the Dean of Catholic University of America.

Less well known but still significant is Mary E. Kelly, the first nurse attorney to make an appearance before the U.S. Supreme Court. In 1986, Connie Curran became the first Vice President of Nursing of the American Hospital Association, a newly created position.

Nursing activities within the political arena are also noteworthy. Rhetaugh Dumas, a psychiatric nurse, has served as deputy director of the

National Institute of Health. Marilyn Goldwater, a delegate of the Maryland House of Delegates from 1974 to 1980, is an example of one of several elected nurses in government. Cheryl Beversdorf has served on the Senate Committee on Veterans Affairs. Sheila Burke has achieved prominence as Senator Robert Dole's deputy chief of staff.

One of the most prominent nurses in the 1980's was Carolyn K. Davis, who was Associate Vice President for Academic Affairs at the University of Michigan. In 1981, she was appointedthe administrator of the Health Care Financing Agency, the federal agency responsible for the administration of Medicare funds. In this powerful and highly visible position, Ms. Davis brought about major changes in health care through the institution of Diagnostic Related Groups and prospective payment. Ms. Davis resigned under pressure in September 1985. The shadow cast by the conditions of her resignation, believed by some to be the result of unpopular promotion of further reduction in health care spending, cannot lessen the impact of her administration.

As the role of the nursing administrator has continued to evolve, so have the educational preparation requirements changed also. Since 1972, employers have been requiring more advanced degrees from individuals seeking head nurse, clinical director, assistant director, supervisory, and director of nursing positions. In 1983, the National Commission on Nursing called for nurse executives and managers to be qualified by education as well as experience (Butts et al, 1986). The Institute of Medicine (1983) also recommended that more nurses be prepared with masters and doctoral degrees to fill positions in administration and management. As a result, there has been an increase in the number of nursing service administration programs at the graduate level. In 1974 there were 24 university schools of nursing that offered a major in nursing administration. In 1983, there were 53 nursing administration programs (Erickson, 1983). The Council for Graduate Education for Administration in Nursing (CGEN) has drafted guidelines for the educational preparation of nursing administrators (1986) that demonstrate the complexities of the current nursing administrator's role.

The fragmentation within the profession remains the heaviest burden that nursing will carry from its past into its future. Membership of speciality organizations is growing, but not membership in the ANA. However, leadership within the speciality groups seems to be recognizing the needs and benefits of a cohesive voice for nursing. Evidence of this concern can be seen in the growth and activities of the National Federation of Nursing Specialty Organizations. Perhaps it will be through this mechanism that finally each group of nurses will feel they have a voice.

Nursing has interacted with society, changed as society has changed, and shaped its decisions and actions in light of or in reaction to the beliefs and values prevailing in each American era. Sometimes nursing was a little ahead, often several steps behind, but rarely has nursing been in direct conflict with the dominant culture (Sheahan, 1978, p. 33).

Externally, nursing remains committed to caring for human beings in need. The needs have not changed remarkably since the 1700's. Although the society and environment have changed dramatically, nurses will continue to work with and for people of all ages, to achieve the highest level of total health and well being society can attain.

Since the 1970's, our society has become preoccupied with the issues of poverty, health, and a safe environment. Nursing has a great deal to do with these issues, and therefore nursing has been actively involved and visible and changing along with these issues. As rights of consumers and their activism have increased, an increased awareness of the role and value of nurses has also changed, generally for the better. Recognition of the need to protect clients through credentials has added prestige to nursing, which has long been active in this area through such organizations as the American Academy of Nursing. The Year of the Nurse in 1977 also provided an opportunity to enhance the understanding and image of nursing. As a result of successful collective bargaining efforts, nurses tapped their strength in numbers. Learning from their successes, the political arm of the ANA was organized in 1974. Nurse Coalition for Action in Politics (NCAP) is an excellent example of nurses who fortified themselves and who have ventured outside of the world of nursing to make changes in social policy for social good.

The changing health science in the United States has created havoc with the long term plans of most occupations and professions. Our society has gone from spending 3.5% of the GNP on health in 1929 to 9.4% in 1980. This increase has been attributed to the changes in the nature of our population, their diseases, advances in medical and related technologies, and modified methods of financial support (Roemer, 1982, p. 5). There are now over seven million health personnel, resulting in approximately one physician for every 700 people and one RN for every 380 people. Our health care system is composed of a combination of public and private structures that include hospitals, nursing homes, pharmacies, health care product suppliers, laboratories, ambulatory health care centers, and physicians' offices or clinics. A major assumption that has underlined much of the health care policy in the U.S. is that health will be improved by increasing the quantity of health resources available to a population. This assumption is being challenged in this decade. Studies now suggest that health may be most effectively impacted by affecting educational, occupational, and income variables (Miller and Stokes, 1978). Good health, equality, accessibility, and the larger concern of environmental health are assuming roles in health care policy formation in this period of history. Increased organization and regulation of health care is changing the patterns of health care utilization. Professions such as medicine and nursing are scrambling to adapt and prepare for current and anticipated changes, and the history of nursing in this decade will be written by the readers of this text, the doers and the risk takers.

SUMMARY

Throughout history, the history of nursing and the history of nursing leadership are not perceived at a prominent level. This is due to several reasons. Certainly, one of the most prevailing reasons has to do with the low place of women in society. In a male dominated society, a female leader advocating more female action is considered an aberrancy who has little chance of success. As an alternative strategy, nursing leadership aligned itself with male dominated or supported causes and thereby made gains for itself and for society. With the rise of the women's movement in the late twentieth century, this strategy has been severely criticized by liberal women. Evaluation of the use of this strategy in current times depends on motives and ultimate outcomes and therefore should not really be debased for this decade. Evaluation of the use of this strategy repeated over the last two centuries using the same criteria of motives and outcomes of benefit to society indicates a successful strategy for nursing. This strategy, however, is not without its drawbacks and disadvantages for the future.

Our culture and society have changed drastically in the last ten years. These changes provide opportunities not possible before and offer potentials worth exploring. However, tradition and role expectations have a way of being firmly embedded in a culture and society. Nursing needs to be cognizant of its history and make conscious decisions about how, when, and why it may want to change its roles. To expect changes without careful planning and effort is foolhardy and doomed to failure for both nursing and society. It is relevant for nurses to decide how the advantages and disadvantages of their role affect the motives and ultimate goals of the profession. If the advantages outweigh the disadvantages, there may not be a reason to change such strategies as alliances with powerful groups, but rather to concentrate on them. Efforts might be better directed toward minimizing the disadvantages of nursing's position and power in our society, not necessarily changing them.

Nursing's quest for independence and autonomy may not, in fact, be the most effective way to achieve its goals. These conditions should not be advocated until all alternatives are objectively evaluated. Alternative choices are a product of the society, culture, times, and people. History cannot change, but nursing can, in order to create its history for this century.

References

American Association of Colleges of Nursing, and American Organization of Nurse Executives (1986). Joint position statement on graduate education in nursing administration. *AANC Newsletter, 12*(1), 3.

Archer, S.E., and Goehner, P.A. (eds.) (1982). *Nurses, a political force.* Belmont, CA: Wadsworth Health Sciences Division.

Armeny, S. (1983). Organized nurses, women philanthropists, and the intellectual bases for cooperation among women, 1893–1920. In Lagemann, E.C. (ed.). *Nursing history: New perspectives, new possibilities*. New York: Teachers College Press.

Bullough, L. (1984). *History, trends, and politics of nursing*. East Norwalk, CT: Appleton-Century-Crofts.

Butts, P.A., Berger, B.A., and Brooten, D.A. (1986). Tracking down the right degree for the job. *Nursing and Health Care, 1*(2), 90–95.

Dolan, J.A., Fitzpatrick, M.L., and Hermann, E.K. (1983). *Nursing in society: A historical perspective*. Philadelphia: W.B. Saunders Co.

Donahue, M.P. (1985). *Nursing: The finest art*. St. Louis: C.V. Mosby.

Erickson, E.H. (1980). The nursing service director, 1880–1980. *The Journal of Nursing Administration, 10*(4), 6–13.

Erickson, E.H. (1983). *The historical evolution of nursing administration education*. Paper presented at the Council for Graduate Education for Administration in Nursing. Philadelphia, Pennsylvania.

Fitzpatrick, M.L. (ed.) (1983). *Prologue to professionalism: A history of nursing*. Bowie, MD: R.J. Brady Company.

Institute of Medicine (1983). *Nursing and nursing education: Public policies and private action*.

Jonas, S. (1981). *Health care delivery in the United States* (2nd ed.). New York: Springer.

Kalisch, B.J., and Kalisch, P.A. (1978). *The advance of American nursing*. Boston: Little, Brown.

Kelly, L.Y. (1985). *Dimensions of professional nursing* (5th ed.). New York: MacMillan.

Lagemann, E.C. (ed.) (1983). *Nursing history, new perspectives, new possibilities*. New York: Teachers College Press.

Lysaught, J.P. (1981). *Action in affirmation: Toward an unambiguous profession of nursing*. New York: McGraw-Hill.

Melosh, B. (1982). *"The physician's hand": Work, culture, and conflict in American nursing*. Philadelphia: Temple Press.

Miller, M.K., and Stokes, C.S. (1978). Health status, health resources, and consolidated structural parameters: Implications for public health care policy. *Journal of health and social behavior, 19*, 263–279.

National League for Nursing (NLN) (1984). NLN Nursing Data Book. 1983–84. (Pub. No. 19–1954). New York: NLN.

One Strong Voice: The Story of the American Nurses Association, compiled by L. Flanagan. Kansas City, MO: ANA.

Palmer, I. From whence we came. *In* Chaska, N.L. (ed.) (1983). *The nursing profession: A time to speak*. New York: McGraw-Hill.

Reverby, S. (1983). "Something besides waiting": The politics of private duty nursing reform in the Depression. (pp. 18–26). In Lagemann, E.C. (ed.). *Nursing history: New perspectives, new possibilities*. New York: Teachers College Press.

Reverby, S., and Rosner, D. (eds.) (1979). *Healthcare in America: Essays in social history*. Philadelphia: Temple Press.

Roemer, J.I. (1982). *An introduction to the U.S. health care system*. New York: Springer.

Sheahan, Sr. D. (1978). Scanning the Seventies. *Nursing Outlook, 26*, pp. 33–37.

Spelts, D. (1986). Nurses who served — and did not return. *American Journal of Nursing, 86*(9), 1037–1039.

Tomes, N. (1983). The silent battle: Nurse registration in New York State, 1903–1920 (pp. 107–118). In Lagemann, E.C. (ed.). *Nursing history: New perspectives, new possibilities*. New York: Teachers College Press.

THEORETICAL BASE FOR NURSING

INTRODUCTION

The conceptual framework presented in Chapter 1 identified nursing theory as a fundamental element that contributes to the concept of nursing leadership and management. It does so because of the elements included in this concept, which are theory, research, and practice. The discussion of nursing theory and its function in regard to nursing leadership and management must begin with a discussion of the meaning of theory. What a theory is and what it purports to accomplish have important ramifications for the reader's ultimate understanding and use of nursing theory. Significance and relevance are based on an individual's or a profession's set of values. The relevance of theory in nursing has not always been well understood. As nursing has struggled to establish its professional standing, various factions within nursing, primarily in the academic settings, have developed a commitment to theory. It cannot be assumed, however, that knowledge, appreciation, or application of theory is inherent in any faction of nursing.

What theory is, what it does, and why it is relevant to professional development is presented in the first section of this chapter. The development of nursing theory composes the second section. The third section reviews the most widely known nursing theories. The fourth section discusses the relationship of nursing theory to nursing leaders and managers. Finally, issues in nursing theory are presented. These five sections provide an overview of the status of theory development of nursing. The intent of

4

this chapter is not to be an exhaustive analysis of nursing theory, but rather to indicate the nature of the concept and its relationship to nursing administration. Students will have opportunities to examine these concepts in greater detail. Practicing administrators can benefit from the overview.

THEORY

In a selective review of the literature on theory (Chinn and Jacobs, 1983; Dickoff and James, 1968; Duffy and Meulenkamp, 1974; Ellis, 1968; Jacox, 1974), it becomes apparent that there is no one definition of theory that is universally accepted. Rather, arbitrary definitions are proposed, defined, and then utilized within the context of the discussion. Chinn and Jacobs (1983) proposed a definition of theory that represents many of the basic concepts and propositions used in theory literature. A theory is defined as "a set of concepts, definitions, and propositions that projects a systematic view of phenomena by designating specific interrelationships among concepts for the purpose of describing, explaining, predicting, and/or controlling phenomena" (Chinn and Jacobs, 1983, p. 206). A theory contributes to understanding one's world because it provides a framework for analyzing the phenomena that compose that world. Scientific disciplines such as chemistry, physics, and microbiology explain, predict, and control much of their knowledge through the use of theories.

Dickoff and James (1968) identify four levels of theory that parallel the description, explanation, prediction, and controlling functions of Chinn and Jacobs (1983). The first level of theory is termed "factor-isolating theory" and corresponds to the description function of theory in Chinn and Jacobs' definition. The second level of theory in Dickoff and James is "factor-relating," which relates to explanatory theory. "Situation-relating theories" relate to predictive theory and compose the third level of theory. The fourth level is the "situation-producing theory" and is also known as prescriptive theory (Dickoff and James, 1968). All levels of theory are essential to the ultimate development of knowledge and understanding. Generally, theories can begin as basic descriptors. Likewise, "theory is structuring proposed as a guide, control or shaper of reality, and is not itself reality . . . [it is] an entity of the conceptual level" (Dickoff and James, 1968, p. 198).

A theory then attempts to describe, explain, predict, or control phenomena and thus contribute to knowledge and understanding. Theories can be applied to phenomena through the use of research. Research results contribute to knowledge and understanding whether or not the results agree with the description offered by the theory. Theories are then adjusted/changed/modified to account for the information obtained through research. Theories are conceptual entities with a purpose. This purpose is to describe, explain, predict, or control. Research is then conducted with the intent either to support or to reject the hypothesis that has been developed as a result of the theory. The relationship between theory and research is a reciprocal one.

Theories are developed for four very practical purposes. The initial purpose is simply to help distinguish facts from fiction. A second purpose is to help converge facts from a number of related or non-related fields for use by yet another field. The third purpose is to provide direction in practice. Theory is also useful as a systematic way to store and retrieve data (Ellis, 1968).

Both the development and use of theories are relevant to the development of a profession. Professions are characterized by several generally accepted qualities. These characteristics include (1) a long, disciplined educational process; (2) authority and autonomy over practice; (3) a value to society; (4) a professional organization; and (5) a defined, systematic body of knowledge. It is in the describing, explaining, predicting, and controlling of the professions' body of knowledge that theory development and use are essential. As an occupation becomes a profession, theories are developed to define the occupation's body of knowledge. Maturation of a profession is the result of the application of those theories in research and practice. Without the conceptual framework or system that theories provide, professions have no systematic body of knowledge and therefore are not truly professional. Instead, these occupations possess an assortment of facts and ideas without a method to pull the facts and ideas into a context, category, or relationship that has meaning or purpose. Without meaning or purpose there is no social value, which is another essential characteristic of a profession.

NURSING THEORY DEVELOPMENT

If "the development of theory is the most crucial task facing nursing today" (Chinn and Jacobs, 1978, p. 1), what did nursing accomplish prior to 1978 or, for that matter, since? Nursing developed an interest in theory because it was considered a legitimate way of establishing nursing as a profession through the establishment of nursing's unique body of knowledge. Professional status was perhaps the prime motivator for theory development. Other benefits of theory development have succeeded in motivating efforts independent of the first. These benefits include practice based theory and the discovery of new knowledge useful for nursing practice.

Walker and Avant (1983) trace the development of nursing theory in *Strategies for Theory Construction in Nursing*. These authors divide literature on nursing theory into four groups and propose a model that illustrates the linkages among levels of theory development (Fig. 4–1).

The first level of theory development is called meta-theory and is concerned with the who, what, and why of theory in and for nursing. The literature included in this level began with R.P. McKay's (1965) doctoral

FIGURE 4–1. Linkages among levels of theory development. (Reprinted with permission from Walker, L. O., and Avant, K. C.: Strategies for Theory Construction in Nursing. Appleton-Century-Crofts, 1983.)

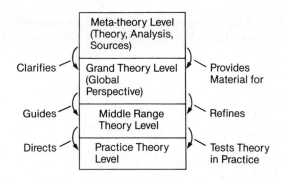

dissertation, *The Process of Theory Development in Nursing,* and included the proceedings from the conferences on The Nature of Science and Nursing held in 1968 and 1969. The First Nursing Theory Conference was held in 1969, followed by the Second and Third Nursing Theory Conferences in 1970 and 1971. Dickoff, James, and Wiedenback published what is considered by some to be classic articles on "Theory in a Practice Discipline" in *Nursing Research* in 1968. In 1978, the National League for Nursing discussed theory in the publication "Theory Development: What, Why, How?" B.J. Stevens published her well-used reference on nursing theory in 1979. Impacted in part by the increase in doctoral education for nursing, there has been an outpouring of nursing literature concerning theory in the last five years. Publications include a number of books, as well as an abundance of journal articles. The references at the end of this chapter include journal listings. It is important to remember that controversy continues over the labeling of these works as theories or models. Many experts disagree on terminology and definition of the terms theory, model, and framework. Some would argue that the lack of development and research renders the majority of these nursing works to the level of models or frameworks. Other experts view theory development differently and argue for the label of theory. Since there is no agreement or consistency, readers will find titles that utilize all three terms in their literature search.

The next level or group of theory work organized by Walker and Avant (1983) is referred to as grand nursing theory. This grouping intended to include theories developed on a large scale that apply to all of nursing and all of humanity. These global theories for the most part are oriented toward the culture and societies found in the United States and are inappropriate for use outside of the U.S. The grand theories have several common themes. These themes include a similar definition of nursing, a basic valuing of man, a value of health, and the relationship between man and nurse. Since these definitions and values are not consistently held by other countries, a major gap exists in the development of grand nursing theories. It is obvious to say that man exists throughout this world as does health, illness, and nursing, the latter three with varying definitions. However, there is no one nursing theory that contributes to the understanding or knowledge on this larger scale.

Early grand nursing theories surfaced in the 1950's and 1960's. These works included the efforts of Peplau (1952), Orlando (1961), Wedenbach (1964), Henderson (1966), Levine (1967), and Ujhely (1968) (Walker and Avant, 1983). But it was in the 1970's that a number of theories were presented to the nursing world at a time when nursing seemed most receptive. As a result, these theorists have developed individual followings to the point of religious fervor in some cases. In rapid succession, Rogers (1970), King (1971), Orem (1971), Travelbee (1971), Newman (1974), Roy (1976), and Auger (1976) presented their work with nursing theory. Walker and Avant (1983) argue that these grand theories are of little practical use for nursing because they are too general and cannot be applied at a precise level. However, there appears to be growing interest in the use of these theories in specific nursing situations (Derdiarian, 1983). In reviewing the literature, it is apparent that these theories are generating scholarly activities in a variety of situations.

The two remaining levels of theory as identified by Walker and Avant (1983) constitute middle range theories and practice theories. These two lower types of theory are much more specific and limited in their focus. As a result, they are more testable. It is not unusual to discover a grand theory that has been down-scaled to consider a smaller segment of the universe. Since this grouping of theories is somewhat arbitrary, it is not essential to classify specific theories further. What *is* significant is the amount of work currently being done in the area of theory development for and of nursing.

There are several groups that are making significant contributions in the area of nursing theory. ANA's Council of Nurse Researchers promotes a variety of mechanisms to develop and explore nursing theory. Efforts to apply different theories in a multitude of practice settings have secured funding and should be an exciting source of new information even as this book goes to press. The collaboration of nursing theorists in support of this research effort is an indication of the potential significance of the results to the profession of nursing.

NURSING THEORIES

Berthold (1968) defines nursing theories as a conceptual structure of knowledge, useful and necessary to attain the goals established by nurses. The purpose of this section is not to present a synopsis of the major theories and models available in the nursing literature. The reader is referred to the references at the end of the chapter for a list of excellent sources that either present one theory or review several theories together. The purpose of this section is to identify commonalities as well as unique aspects of the structures in order to introduce and perhaps raise the curiosity of the reader to read further. It is only through research, investigation, and an examination of philosophies of practice that a defined conceptual structure can be useful in helping to attain the nursing goals that have been established. In other words, one must clarify for oneself those concepts essential to one's practice and identify what they mean. Then one can examine available resources for a conceptual structure that conforms to beliefs and try it on for size through research and practice. Additionally, one should examine applications of the various theories to a particular practice setting in clinical nursing, nursing education, or nursing management. This will provide valuable insight and clarification. If there are no theories that meet one's expectations, it may be necessary to hypothesize or synthesize one's own. Stevens' (1984) chapter on common themes in nursing theory is an excellent summary of this topic. As she points out, the basic subject matter of nursing theory has concerned itself with man, the nurse, and health. Many theories do not limit themselves just to these three basic subjects. Additionally, definitions and interpretations of these three subjects are quite extensive and varied. That is one of the exciting aspects of nursing theory development. Nursing theories do not appear to be cloned out of the same mold. Instead, there is a great deal of variety and diversification, which suggests unlimited opportunity for research, healthy discussion, and implications for change.

Using these three subjects of man, nurse, and health, theorists approach them in different but systematic ways. There are interactive theories that emphasize one or more interactions among the three subjects. The Newman Health Care System Model is an example. There are developmental theories that see man on a developmental or growth continuum. Peplau is the author of a developmental model. Systems theory has also had a significant impact on all nursing theories, and it is not practical to delineate which theories use a strictly systems model because although some theories are more systems oriented than others, they also emphasize developmental or interactive principles. Stevens (1984) classifies the approaches into intervention, conservation, substitution, sustenance, or enhancement but recognizes that there are still theories that do not easily fall into one of these categories. (A summary of the major theories has been reprinted in Table 4–1 from Fordyce, 1982.)

RELATIONSHIP TO RESEARCH, EDUCATION, AND PRACTICE

In order for nursing to develop and grow as a profession, the relationship among theory, research, and practice must be understood, explored, and supported. Before the relationship can be discussed, it is necessary to examine the concept of research in more depth. So far in this chapter, the necessity for the identification of the unique body of knowledge that constitutes the science of nursing has been proposed. Nursing science can be viewed as both a process and a product. Inherent in the process of

(Text continued on page 66)

TABLE 4-1
A Comparison of Selected Nurse Author/Theories

Major Origin(s) of Thought or Influences on Author/Theorist	Applicability of Theory/Model	Other	View of Nursing Process	Key Terminology
V. Henderson 1939, 1955, 1964/66 F. Nightingale, Annie Goodrich Need Theory (Thorndike) Rehabilitation Experts, Yale Nursing Colleagues	Cites implications for Practice, Research and Education based on her concept of nursing	Informational Nurse leader Set trend in Nursing Research—influenced by her wise foresight Presents personal memoirs and historical perspective	Individualized care planning with continual analysis to meet the patient's needs	The Nurse is Primary Rehabilitation Agent Patient–centered Care Independent Role and Function of Nurse
H. Peplau 1952 Harry Stack Sullivan Erich Fromm Staff of Chestnut Lodge and Wm. Alanson White Institute of Psychiatry	Views of Practice, Research and Education are presented	The kind of person the nurse becomes makes a difference to the patient and nursing care given Multiple roles of nurse(s) are identified as occur in phases of the nurse-patient relationship	The phases of nurse-patient relationship: four interlocking phases—Orientation, Identification, Exploitation, Resolution Nursing Process is educative and therapeutic	Psychodynamic Nursing
I. Orlando (Pelletier) 1961, 1980 Personal findings from study of verbatim nursing notes	Focus in on Practice Research—Publications are findings of her personal study, other possibilities Education—content of instruction	Observe, state perceptions and associated thoughts/feelings (validation with patient is essential), then do disciplined nursing response—deliberative nursing process is presented	Process occurs with the Nurse Nursing process is tool to do what nurse is to do, the process the nurse follows to get an outcome Nurses' perceptions of the patient's behavior, reaction of the nurse, nursing action (say and do)	Nursing activities as deliberative or automatic
E. Wiedenbach 1963, 1964, 1968, 1970 V. Henderson I. Orlando Needs Theory Dickoff and James	Focus is on Practice Suggests types of Research States view of Education	Emphasis on Philosophy of the individual nurse Principles of helping are identified Presents a tool for analyzing nursing incidents	The helping process: identification of help needed Ministration of help Validation that help was given Coordination of resources for help and of help provided	Rational, Reactionary or Deliberative nursing action
D. Johnson 1959, 1961, 1980 General Systems Theory Needs Theory	Education—the foundation in the science of nursing Research—must provide the base for nursing Practice—is the focus of concern for use and source of knowledge	Seven behavioral subsystems constitute a behavioral system	Nursing Process—for essential stages: Asessment—1st and 2nd level Diagnosis Intervention—four modes: restrict, defend, inhibit, facilitate Evaluation	Components of each subsystem: goal, action, set, choice. The nurse is an external regulator of the environment Sustenal imperatives

Reprinted with permission from Fordyce, E.M. In Flynn, J., McCann, B., and Heffron, P.B. (1984). *Nursing: From concept to practice.* Bowie, MD: Brady Communications.

TABLE 4–1
A Comparison of Selected Nurse Author/Theories

Definition/View of Nursing	View of the Human Person	Central Theme
"The unique function of the nurse is to assist the individual, sick or well. In the performance of those activities contributing to health or its recovery (or to peaceful death) that he would perform unaided if he had the necessary strength, will or knowledge. And to do this in such a way as to help him gain independence as rapidly as possible." (1964, 63) Viewed the nurse as the authority on nursing care Aim of nursing to promote normalcy and independence Nurse is a substitute for what the patient lacks	Personhood—Mind and Body are Inseparable	Unique and Independent function of the nurse
"Nursing is a significant therapeutic, interpersonal process. It functions cooperatively with other human processes that make health possible for individuals in communities . . . Nursing is an educative instrument, a maturing force, that aims to promote forward movement of personality in the direction of creative, constructive, personal, and community living." (1952, 16) Nursing is psychodynamic, an applied science, a function Nursing is an interpersonal process Nursing is a human relationship between a patient and a nurse who is able to respond to the need for help Assist patients to meet human problems of everyday life Tasks and performances of the nurse-patient relationship	Each Person is an individual with the potential for growth, whose personality is developed by the interaction of cultural forces and biological constitutions	Nurse Patient Relationship in Nursing or Interpersonal Relations in Nursing and The Personal Growth and Development of the Nurse
The purpose of nursing is to supply the help a patient requires in order for his needs to be met (1961, 8) To find and meet the patient's immediate needs for help directly or indirectly (the nurse's responsibility) is the practice of professional nursing		The Dynamic, Interpersonal Nurse-Patient Relationship: Identification of principles to guide nursing practice and a theory of effective nursing practice for nursing students
Nursing is a service, a helping art—a goal-directed activity The purpose for clinical nursing is "to facilitate the efforts of the individual to overcome the obstacles which currently interfere with his ability to respond capably to demands made of him by his condition, environment, situation and time." (1964, 14–15) "To meet the need the individual is experiencing as a need-for-help." (1964, 15) Clinical nursing has four interlocking components: Philosophy, Purpose, Practice, Art 　　Why—Purpose 　　Way—Philosophy 　　What—Practice 　　How—Art Nursing action is deliberative action	Four assumptions about human nature are described (1964, 17)	The nurse, elements of practice and process which determines its Philosophy, Purpose, Practice, Art of Nursing
Nursing is a science and an art Nursing Care—a direct service to people "The achievement and maintenance of a stable state is nursing's distinctive contribution to patient welfare and the specific purpose of nursing care." (1961, 64) Activities of nursing are centered on human needs Nursing Action—supply of sustenal imperatives: Nurturance, Protection, Stimulation	Person—Bio-psycho-social being Human organism is a complex set of behavioral subsystems and boundaries Further assumptions see (Riehl and Roy, 1980, 208)	Behavioral systems and subsystems of Man

Table continued on following page

TABLE 4–1
A Comparison of Selected Nurse Author/Theories Continued

Major Origin(s) of Thought or Influences on Author/Theorist	Applicability of Theory/Model	Other	View of Nursing Process	Key Terminology
I. King 1968, 1971, 1973, 1981 V. Henderson H. Peplau, I. Orlando General Systems Theory Numerous sources associated with the identified concepts	Theory derived from her personal research Views her framework as Practice Education—concepts as basis of learning the practice of nursing	Presents a Goal-Oriented Nursing Record Concepts of framework are presented according to the three interacting systems: Personal—Interpersonal—Social	Human process, an interpersonal process—a process of action, reaction, interaction, transaction between individuals and groups in social systems. Illustrated by interlocking circles, a methodology for study of nursing process (1973, 515)	Major concepts are interaction, perception, communication, transaction, self, role, stress, growth and development, time and space (1981, 145)
D. Orem 1971, 1980 V. Henderson General System Theory	A basis for Practice Education—used as curriculum model Suggests Research possibilities	Design of Nursing Systems Partly Compensatory-Wholly Compensatory Supportive-Educative (developmental) Systems Development of new language about nursing Man's need for self-care is emphasized	Nursing an interpersonal process Deliberative action Step one—nursing diagnosis Initial determination of need for care Step two—designing and planning a system of nursing Step three—actions of nurse A cycle of assisting, checking, adjusting and readjusting activities	Self-Care Agency Self-Care Deficit Self-Care requirements and Demands
M. Rogers 1970, 1980 Physics (Einstein) Systems Theory Field Theory Evolutionary Theory Paranormal Psychology	Provides a conceptual framework for Practice Education—used as curriculum base Has been basis for Research studies	Life process and homeodynamics and continuous interaction between man and environment are emphasized A mild extender	Setting for nursing is life process and human field Nursing diagnosis intervention Evaluation of intervention	Helicy and Resonancy (nature and direction of change)
J. Travelbee 1963, 1964, 1966, 1969 Karl Jaspers V. Frankl Yale Nursing Colleagues (Orlando)	Basis for Practice of Nursing Education—model for teaching interpersonal relationships Research—possibilities are inherent	Focus on existential aspects of life For the nurse "to care for and to care about"	An Interpersonal Process Phases of a nurse-patient relationship: Original Encounter, Emerging Identities, Empathy, Sympathy, Rapport (1966) Utilization of Observation, Interpretation, Decision Making, Action, Evaluation	Coping, Meaning, Caring, Empathy, Sympathy
Sr. Callisia Roy 1970, 1971, 1973, 1974, 1975, 1976, 1980 Adaptation theory of Helson Dorothy Johnson	Roy suggests her mode, offers possibilities for providing "a scientific basis, a body of knowledge for education, and an area of practice" (1970, 44)	Modification of Johnson Model, based on Helson's Adaptation-Level Theory	Problem-solving process: Six step Nursing Process Assessment —1st level —2nd level Problem Identification Goal Setting Intervention Selection of approaches Evaluation	Man has four modes of adaptation: Physiological Needs, Self Concept, Role Function, Interdependence Man has two types of adaptive mechanisms: Cognator, Regulator

| TABLE 4–1 | | |
| A Comparison of Selected Nurse Author/Theories Continued | | |

Definition/View of Nursing	View of the Human Person	Central Theme
"Nursing is a process of human interactions between nurse and client whereby each perceives the other and the situation, and through communication, they set goals, explore means, and agree on means to achieve goals." (1981, 144) "The goal of nursing is to help individuals and groups attain, maintain, and restore health." (1981, 13) ". . . help individuals die with dignity." The focus of nursing is on human beings The domain of nursing—Personal, Interpersonal and Social systems Identifies factors in nursing that have persisted through time (1971)	Persons are open systems (1981, 20) Specific assumptions about human beings are identified (1981, 143)	Conceptual nursing framework for a theory for nursing A theory of goal attainment. Interrelationships of concepts and the process of human interactions
Nursing—a helping service, human service Technology and Art "A creative effort of one human being to help another human being." (1971, 69) "Nursing is a personal, family and community service within the health field. Its dimension of concern for human life and well-being is shared with other health services. Nursing differs from these services because of the nature of its contributed effort. Provisions for making nursing available in a social group should consider both its shared and its unique dimension." (1971, 41) Goal of nursing—the health and well-being of the individual Focus of nursing—helping the individual to achieve health results	Person is Unique Man is an integrated whole	Self-care—Universal and Health derivations
Nursing a Science and an Art "Professional Practice in nursing seeks to promote symphonic interaction between man and environment, to strenghten the adherence and integrity of the human field, and to direct and redirect patterning of the human and environmental fields for realization of maximum health potential." (1970, 122) Homeodynamics are Principles of Nursing Science Patterning and Organization define field People at center of Nursing Purpose Responsibility to Society	Synergistic Man— Four dimensional, negentropic, unified whole Conceptual boundaries of an energy field	Unitary Man and his life processes Nursing Science
"Nursing is an interpersonal process whereby the professional nurse practitioner assists an individual or family to prevent, cope with, the experience of illness and suffering and, if necessary, assists the individual or family to find meaning in these experiences." (1966, 5–6) Functions of nursing are derived from the definitions and purpose of nursing Views nurse as supporter, sustainer and change agent	Uniqueness of man	Interpersonal relationship, nature and uniqueness of professional nursing practice
Nursing is a scientific discipline, is practice oriented "Nursing is concerned with man as a total being at some point along the health-illness continuum." (1970, 43) Goal of nursing—to bring about an adaptive state in the four adaptive modes	Biopsychosocial being Eight assumptions about man, also see (1974, 136–138; 1980, 180–182)	Adaptation and 8 assumptions about Man

Table continued on following page

TABLE 4–1
A Comparison of Selected Nurse Author/Theories Continued

Major Origin(s) of Thought or Influences on Author/Theorist	Applicability of Theory/Model	Other	View of Nursing Process	Key Terminology
Josephine G. Peterson, Loretta T. Zderad 1976				
Buber Marcel de Chardin Numerous other scholarly works	Developed and used in clinical situation Education—focus of a course Humanistic Nursing taught by the authors Research—presents possibilities to be explored	Methodology for studying nursing— phases of phenomenologic nursology 1) experiencing 2) reflecting 3) describing	"Stuff of nursing includes all possible responses of man; man needing and man helping a clinical process—an experience lived between human beings an active presence—personal and/or professional	Nursology, reobjectification, active presence, all-at-once, witness, "thing itself" "the between" "the stuff of nursing"
Myra E. Levine 1966, 1967, 1971, 1973, 1978				
Paul Tillich Walter Cannon René Dubos Hans Selye Others	Practice centered 1973 text was prepared for an introductory nursing course Many possibilities for research are inherent in this nursing approach	Precise use of vocabulary and origin of words defined and described Focus of concern on the individual Therapeutic and Supportive intervention defined	Not specifically defined Patient-centered nursing care plans "The substance of nursing science" (1967, 47) is the identifying of specific patterns of adaptation of each individual patient and accurately responding	Conservation Wholeness Health Integrity Adaptation Integration
Betty M. Neuman 1972, 1974, 1980				
Gestalt Theory Field theories Hans Selye	Developed and utilized as a conceptual model for a graduate nursing course Presents a framework for health care providers including nursing and other disciplines Many research possibilities	Man and his environment is the basic phenomenon An individual's reaction to stress and factors that begin reconstitution Utilizes Primary, Secondary, and Tertiary prevention levels	An assessment/intervention tool provides for obtaining: Biographical data of the client Stressors as perceived by the client Stressors as perceived by the care givers Identifying of intra-, inter-, and extra-personal factors (Model diagram) Statement of the problem Summary of goals Intervention plan	Stressors Flexible line of defense Formal line of defense Lines of resistance Reconstitution

nursing science is the process of nursing research. Nursing science is the body of knowledge that is the product of that process. Scientific investigation or research is a controlled, organized attempt to think through or examine events and processes. Theories provide the framework for conducting the scientific process and research. As stated earlier, the relationship of theory to research is a reciprocal one. Theory directs research because it provides the question as well as the structure for research. Research directly relates to theory development in four distinct ways. Through research, a theory can be confirmed. As confirmation is substantiated through replication, a theory can develop and expand to serve more areas. Theory can also be modified through research to become more specific or more general. On the other hand, research can disprove theory, which is also valuable information as it prevents false direction. Finally, research can provide information for the development of completely new theories.

Dickoff and colleagues (1968) stated, "theory is born in practice, is refined in research and must and can return to practice" (p. 145). Unfortu-

		TABLE 4–1		
		A Comparison of Selected Nurse Author/Theories Continued		

Definition/View of Nursing	View of the Human Person	Central Theme
Always an interhuman act, a living human act "an experience lived between human beings" a transactional relationship—an inter-subjective transaction	Unique, wholistic, intellectual ever evolving person	Humanistic Nursing The existentially experienced nursing situation Individuals—knowing and becoming
Nursing is a keeping together function—the wholeness of the patient Nursing care is "focused on man and the complexity of his relationships with his enviroment" (1973, 46) "Nursing intervention is, . . . a conservation of wholeness." (1971, 258) Nursing can fulfill its conservation function in four major areas of care: Conservation of Patient Energy Conservation of Structural Integrity Conservation of Personal Integrity Conservation of Social Integrity (1967, 47–59)	Unity of mind and body A living being who responds to change, continually interacting with his environments and adapting to change Wholeness—holism	Conservation Holistic Nursing
Nursing is ". . . a unique profession . . . concerned with all the variables affecting an individual's response to stressors." (1980, 121)	Every individual is unique with a composite of characteristics within a normal range Man is an open system who interacts with his environment	A Health Care Systems model for a total person approach to patient problems

nately, the relationship of theory to practice is usually a point of disagreement among various nursing groups. Sometimes it appears that nurses would rather spend time talking about the disagreements than examining the alleged disagreements and discovering ways to reduce them. Theory is viewed by some nurses as being impractical, whereas practice is viewed as being practical. For the purposes of this discussion, practice includes the three areas of clinical nursing, education, and management.

If nursing is to practice beyond folklore, intuition, and tradition, the conduct of practice requires the knowledge of science, ethics, and logic (Beckstrand, 1978). The purpose of nursing theory is to describe, explain, predict, and control real events and processes. These events and processes occur in nursing practice. Without them, theory is of no purpose. Likewise, nursing practice provides a testing ground for theory as well as its application. Practice utilizes theory and generates new questions to be answered by theory through the process of additional research. In the clinical setting, a professional nurse theorizes about her practice, recognizing when the theories she learned describe or explain what she is actually observing as well as when they do not. In nursing education, theory is the subject matter in a curriculum because education teaches the body of knowledge that is nursing. Theory also helps design and organize the curriculum of the school, provides the framework that determines evaluation criteria, and defines areas requiring research.

The nursing administrator utilizes theory in organizing the purpose, structure, and functions of her nursing service department. A nursing service administrator who utilizes a theoretical framework for her practice translates this into a framework of philosophy and operations within her department. A theoretical or conceptual basis for nursing administration defines the values of the actors within the setting as well as the boundaries of practice. The goals and objectives of the nursing department are determined by the theoretical basis. For example, if Orem's self care is the basis, the goals and objectives will be directed at reducing self care deficits and improving nursing agency. The nursing service administrator who utilizes Neuman's model will develop the department's goals and objectives aimed at reducing negative forces and building up stabilizing forces. The application of theoretical models is actualized down to the unit level, where the nursing process utilizes it as a framework in direct patient care. A common theoretical basis for a nursing department can help to unify it and improve communication at all levels.

There is a major relationship between research and practice. Research develops and defines the boundaries of the discipline. As a result of research, nursing practice has expanded into new areas and has also become more independent. Research identifies the uniqueness of nursing as well as clarifies common elements and goals. These efforts help to give nurses more control over their own practice as well as to provide a basis for debate, communication, and further research, not only within nursing but also with other disciplines (Jacobs and Hutcher, 1978).

The nurse administrator utilizes research in her practice in several ways. Research provides the opportunity to validate the theoretical or conceptual basis for her practice. In doing so, the research contributes to the body of knowledge supported by that particular theory or framework. Additionally, the nurse administrator can utilize his framework when clinical problems are identified. The framework utilized can facilitate the design of effective research and methodologies to help solve the problem. As a result of this theoretically based research, nurses will have a more concrete basis for their practice. This in turn can lead to both greater patient success and staff satisfaction.

The essential relationship of theory research and practice has been illustrated in the conceptual framework for nursing leaderships and management presented in Chapter 1. As such, nursing theory, founded in research and affirmed in practice, provides basic structure and perspectives to guide the practice of nursing administration within the unique field that is nursing. Likewise, the nursing administrator utilizes research and theory from business management and other relevant fields to assist him in his practice. Application of theories and research from other disciplines can result in new opportunities to substantiate the research findings and theories.

Continued efforts by nurses are being made to clarify the essential relationships between theory, research, and practice. In addition to graduate research requirements, undergraduate course work now frequently includes a research component. As a result, more staff nurses will be comfortable in not only the reading, understanding, and application of nursing research, but also in the participation in research. The increase in the number of doctorally prepared nurses will also support and enhance these relationships. As better educated nurses move into the three practice settings, communication and cooperation will be enhanced. Concern over reduced funding for nursing research must become more widespread. The creation of a Center for Nursing within the National Institute of Health in 1986 had its followers as well as its dissenters. Whatever the reasons for their stands, the dissension cannot be viewed by politicians as lack of interest among nurses in pursuing nursing research. There are some pessimists who predict the extinction of nursing. The optimists see the opportunities provided by the triad of research, theory, and practice and will seize them.

CURRENT ISSUES

There are several issues in the area of nursing theory that promise to impact significantly each nurse directly. For purposes of discussion, the issues have been grouped into internal and external issues. Realistically, however, there are areas of overlap, and interactions will be numerous and probably also significant.

A major external impact on nursing theory and the science of nursing are the major trends occurring in society. These trends as identified by Naisbitt (1982) include moving from an industrial to an information society; from forced technology to high tech/high touch; from a national economy to a world economy; from short term to long term thinking; from centralization to decentralization; from institutional help to self-help; from representative democracy to participatory democracy; from hierarchies to networking; from north to south; and from either/or to multiple options. Another trend that has reached almost fever pitch is the emphasis on health promotion, prevention, and maintenance. This is accompanied by a personal sense of responsibility for these matters, a great emphasis on self-care. Along with this is an increasing awareness of the importance of the environment on human health and well-being.

Inherent within all these trends is the rapidity of change that is ever present, which makes it difficult to plan and predict. That is why the emphasis on prevention is so important. These trends have obvious implications for the profession of nursing. It will be essential for nursing to expand and define its boundaries in light of these trends in order to be responsive to the needs of individual man, families, and societies. Nursing needs to anticipate the impact these trends will have and be willing to experiment and change as necessary. In order to control and predict these trends, tremendous work in the area of nursing theory and research will be required. Visintainer (1986) has conceptualized theory as a road map. The theory or map of a discipline provides a framework for selecting and organizing information. In this, the information age, it becomes increasingly more difficult to acquire and maintain current data concerning a given phenomenon. Because there is too much to know, maps or theories, whether nursing related or borrowed from other disciplines, provide an efficient method of using unfamiliar data. The use of theory enables the nursing administrator to react more quickly. Because of theory's function in controlling and predicting phenomena, the use of theory enables the nursing administrator to forecast and plan proactive responses to the changing health care environment.

Yet another external issue in society facing nursing is the change from a goal driven model of nursing to a resource driven model of nursing. Historically, nursing set goals for or with patients and then determined what kinds of resources were necessary to achieve them. Society supported this model, as evidenced by the percentage of the Gross National Product spent on health care. It is now becoming unacceptable for illness to receive carte blanche resources as society recognizes that resources are not unlimited and that there are too many individuals going without basic health care. Changes in values are resulting in changes in priorities and ultimately changes in allocation of resources. Consequently, nurses are first having to identify resources available to determine which goals can realistically be sought. Hospital days, type and number of supplies used, and assistance from significant others now directly impact on the the quantity and quality of patient care services that are rendered. Nurses should not have too much difficulty with this situation, however, because they are well-known for their ability to conserve, improvise, and stretch resources. Nursing research can contribute to streamlining the delivery of health care by studies that evaluate traditional policies and procedures as well as the cost effectiveness of nursing services.

Internally, issues concerning nursing theory are in several cases carried forward from the past. As nursing progresses as a profession, nurses will be expected to find themselves functioning more independently and utilizing cognitive processes more extensively. It will be difficult for many nurses to consider giving up the familiar, comfortable, safe, traditional practices. Some will be successful; others will not, and unless they can find havens in which to practice, these nurses will undoubtedly leave the profession. Higher education of nurses is an integral part of changing with the times, and nurses have generally come to recognize this as fact. At the same time, it must be noted that the use of better educated nurses and the justification for the use of more expensive labor to health administrators may be more difficult than ever before. The prospective payment environment mandates a demonstrable difference in performance that impacts favorably on cost/benefit ratios in order to justify a more expensive professional labor force. Nursing theory and research are the ways and means to demonstrate the efficiency and value of professional nursing.

Research and theory development in both management and nursing administration is sorely needed. McFarland (1986) stated that management theory, if it exists, is in a rudimentary, fragmented condition and must be credited mainly to researchers in disciplines other than management. The reasons for this confusion in management theory development are several, not the least of which is the interdisciplinary nature of management. As in nursing, management benefits from advances in other disciplines, but must uniquely apply this knowledge to managements' own domain. Management theory has been described as a jungle (Koontz, 1961, 1980) that reflects the different disciplinary, methodological, and philosophical aims occurring within management theory development. McFarland states, "Management, like most social sciences, is in the preparadigm or paradigm development stage" (1986, p. 19). Arguments abound for and against a unification of management theory through synthesis of contributions from areas such as business theory, organization theory, administrative science, and decision making theory. Contingency models for general management theory are beginning to appear and reflect the contribution of the behavioral and quantitative approaches to theory. These contingency models emphasize the impact of situational variables and the use of open and closed system models. Unlike nursing theory developments, however, management theory currently emphasizes applied research and de-emphasizes theoretical developments. To this end, McFarland (1986) urged the evolution of management theory to a level called macromanagement. This evolution in management theory is in keeping with today's increasing emphasis on the management of organizations with regard to the organization's role as a component of social institutions and society. Nursing theory development in general possesses many of the same characteristics as management theory. Research and theory development in nursing administration is in worse shape than management theory. There has been minimal research and theory development in nursing to contribute to the nursing service administrator's body of knowledge. Loomis (1985) looked at emerging content in dissertation abstracts and titles from 1976 to 1982. Of the 319 dissertation abstracts and titles analyzed, less than 10 involved the administrative area. Deficits were reported in such administrative areas as nursing economics and politics. Research concerning the educational preparation of nursing service administrators indicated confusion and disagreement over required course work, perceived ability to perform, and expected level of performance by employees (Grossman, 1972; McLane, 1978; Freund, 1985; Simms, Price, and Pfoutz, 1985; Price, 1984). Changing economic forces within health care have initiated a greater interest in determining the cost of nursing care. Numerous studies have been conducted or are in progress. However, the majority of these studies have no theoretical base.

Ongoing issues internal to nursing directly involve theory development. The question of having a mega-theory or many theories is still very much subject to debate. Are theories "for" nursing or "of" nursing, and what exactly is the difference? Should nursing borrow theories from other disciplines or develop unique theories? Do theories from other disciplines become unique when modified for use by and for nursing? Resolution of these questions is not really essential because they promote and encourage scholarly endeavors by nurses seeking knowledge to answer these questions. And it is only through these investigations, inquiries, and research that the body of knowledge that is and for nursing will become established.

References

Aiken, L.H. (ed.) (1982). *Nursing in the 1980's: Crisis, opportunities, challenges.* Philadelphia: J.B. Lippincott.

Beckstrand, J. (1978). The rotation of a practice theory and the relationship of scientific and ethical knowledge to practice. *Research in Nursing and Health, 1*(3), 131.

Berthold, J.S. (1968). Prologue. *Nursing Research, 17*(3), 196–197.

Chaska, N.L. (1978). *The nursing profession: View through the mist.* New York: McGraw-Hill.

Chaska, N.L. (1983) *The nursing profession: A time to speak.* New York: McGraw-Hill.

Chinn, P.L., and Jacobs, M.K. (1978). A model for theory development in nursing. *Advances in Nursing Science, 1*(1), 1–11.

Chinn, P.L., and Jacobs, M.K. (1983). *Theory and nursing: A systematic approach.* St. Louis: C. V. Mosby.

Crawford, G., Default, Sister K., and Rudy, E. (1979). Evolving issues on theory development. *Nursing Outlook,* May, 346–351.

Derdiarian, A.K. (1983). An instrument for theory and research development using the behavioral system model for nursing: The cancer patient. Part I. *Nursing Research, 32*(4), 196–201.

Dickoff, J., and James, P. (1968). A theory of theories: A position paper. *Nursing Research, 17,* 197–203.

Dickoff, J., James, P., and Weidenback, E. (1968). Theory in a practice discipline. *Nursing Research, 17,* 415–435, 545–554.

Duffey, M., and Meulenkamp, A.F. (1974). A framework for theory analysis. *Nursing Outlook, 22,* 570–574.

Ellis, R. (1968). Characteristics of significant theories. *Nursing Research, 17*(3), 217–222.

Ellis, R. (1982). Conceptual issues in nursing. *Nursing Outlook, 30*(7), 406–410.

Fawcett, J. (1978). The relationship between theory and research: A double helix. *Advances in Nursing Science, 1*(1), 49–61.

Fawcett, J. (1984). Another look at utilization of nursing research. *Image, 16*(2), 59–64.

Freund, C.M. (1985). Director of nursing effectiveness: DON and CEO perspectives and implications for education. *The Journal of Nursing Administration, 15*(6), 25–30.

Gortner, S.R. (1980). Nursing research: Out of the past and into the future. *Nursing Research, 29*(4), 204–207.

Greenfield, E. (1985). Orem's self-care theory of nursing: Practical application to the end stage renal disease patient. *Journal of Nephrology Nursing, 2*(4), 187–193.

Grossman, H.T. (1972). The diversity within graduate nursing education. *Nursing Outlook, 20*(7), 464–467.

Hardy, M.E. (1973). *Theoretical foundations for nursing.* New York: MSS.

Harper, D.C. (1984). Application of Orem's theoretical constructs to self-care medication behaviors with elderly. *Advances in Nursing Science, 6*(3), 29–46.

Jacobs, M.K., and Hutcher, S.F. (1978). Nursing science: The theory practice linkage. *Advances in Nursing Science, 1*(1), 63–73.

Jacox, A. (1974). Theory construction in nursing: An overview. *Nursing Research, 23*(1), 4–13.

Koontz, H. (1961). The management theory jungle. *Journal of the Academy of Management, 4*(12), 174–188.

Koontz, H. (1980). The management theory jungle revisited. *Academy of Management Review, 5*(3), 175–187.

Leddy, S., and Pepper, J.M. (1984). *Conceptual bases of professional nursing.* Philadelphia: J.B. Lippincott.

Loomis, M.E. (1985). Emerging content in nursing: An analvsis of dissertation abstracts and titles, 1976–1982. *Nursing Research, 34*(2), 113–119.

McClosky, J.C., and Grace, H.K. (1983). *Current issues of nursing.* Boston: Blackwell Scientific Publications.

McFarland, D.E. (1986). *The managerial imperative: The age of macromanagement.* Cambridge, MA: Ballinger.

McFarlene, E.A. (1980). Nursing theory: The comparison of four theoretical proposals. *Journal of Advanced Nursing, 5*, 3–19.

McLane, A.M. (1978). Core competencies of master's prepared nurses. *Nursing Research, 27*(1), 48–53.

Meleis, A.I. (1984). *Theoretical nursing: Development and progress.* Philadelphia: J.B. Lippincott.

Mosconitz, A.O. (1984). Orem's theory as applied to psychiatric nursing. *Perspectives in Psychiatric Care, 22*(1), 36–38.

Naisbitt, J. (1982). *Megatrends.* New York: Warner Books.

Nicoll, L.H. (ed.) (1986). *Perspectives on nursing theory.* Boston: Little, Brown.

Norris, C.M. (ed.) (1982). *Concept clarification in nursing.* Rockwell, MD: Aspen.

Nursing Development Conference Group (1979). *Concept formalization in nursing.* Boston: Little, Brown.

Nursing Theories Conference Group (1980). *Nursing theories.* Englewood Cliffs, NJ: Prentice-Hall.

Price, S.A. (1984). Master's programs preparing nursing administrators: What are the essential components? *The Journal of Nursing Administration, 14*, 11–17.

Riehl, J.P., and Roy, C. (1980). *Conceptual models for nursing practice,* (2nd ed.) New York: Appleton-Century-Crofts.

Ross, M.M. (1985). The Betty Neuman systems model in nursing practice: A case study approach. *Journal of Advanced Nursing, 10*(3), 199–207.

Silva, M.J. (1984). Philosophy, science, theory: Interrelationships and implications for nursing research. *Image, 9*, 59–63.

Simms, L.M., Price, S.A., and Pfoutz, S.K. (1985). Nurse executive: Functions and priorities. *Nursing Economics, 3*(4), 238–244.

Smith, M.J. (1984). Transformation: A key to shaping nursing. *Image, 16*(1), 28–30.

Stevens, B.J. (1984). *Nursing theory: Analysis, application, evaluation.* Boston: Little, Brown.

Visintainer, M.A. (1986). The nature of knowledge and theory in nursing. *Image, 18*(2), 32–38.

Walker, L.O., and Avant, K.C. (1983). *Strategies for theory construction in nursing.* East Norwalk, CT: Appleton-Century-Crofts.

Whelan, E.G. (1984). Analysis and application of Dorothea Orem's self-care practical model. *Journal of Nursing Education, 23*(8), 342–345.

FOUNDATIONS FOR LEADERSHIP

INTRODUCTION

Much has been written and continues to be written about leadership. Of this literature, some is research; much is not. As a result, no compendium

5

or consensus exists on leadership. This lack of consensus results in a wide latitude permitted to anyone bold enough to examine leadership. The purpose of this chapter is to provide a brief overview of the evolution of the more well-known leadership theories. It is these authors' perspective that leadership theory has evolved in response to changes in our societies and cultures. Since man's society and culture are ever-evolving, even the most recent interactionist leadership theories will probably be insufficient to describe, explain, or predict leadership behavior in the twenty-first century. However, these theories do provide a basis for further research, as well as a springboard for action by nursing leaders. As a result, nursing leaders could contribute to leadership theory development for the next century.

Following the presentation of leadership theories is the presentation of several key concepts inherently associated with leadership: power, communication, motivation, decision making, and groups and organizations. These concepts are also subject to wide variation. The next chapter presents a conceptual framework, based on the work of Yura, Ozimek, and Walsh (1981) and of Epstein (1982), for discussing nursing leadership at the executive, middle, and first line levels within an organization.

THEORY DEVELOPMENT

The literature abounds with information on leadership, management, and executive characteristics. Nursing is turning more and more frequently to the leadership literature that is found outside of nursing and in the areas of business and management. There are several well-known theories that have provided the basis for much of the leadership research that has been conducted. These theories are also illustrative of the evolution of leadership. Early theories were limited to descriptions or lists of characteristics or behaviors of people identified as leaders. Also known as trait theories, these theories subscribed to the saying, "leaders are born, not made." Research has shown that such traits as intelligence are associated with leadership but are insufficient for defining effective leadership.

Another category of leadership theories is the behavioral theories. These theories concentrated on the leader's action, not on the traits of the leader, with limited attention to the followers. The research of Lewin, Lippitt, and White in 1930 identified the leadership style patterns as authoritarian, democratic, and laissez-faire. This first level of leadership theory development included the establishment by Halpin and Winer of two categories of leadership behavior known as initiating structure and consideration. Initiating structure includes task-related functions, whereas consideration behaviors are relationship-oriented. Blake and Mouton (1964) have developed these concepts in a management grid theory that attempts to explain the various combinations of high and low emphasis on tasks and on people.

Motivational leadership theories began examining the make-up of the followers in addition to the leader. This group of theories is frequently based on Maslow's theory of motivation and on a humanistic philosophy that values the individual. McGregor's (1960) Theory X and Theory Y are two such theories. Herzberg (1966) enlarged upon McGregor's Theory Y and divided the needs that affected a person's motivation into hygiene factors or motivational factors. Hygiene factors include factors that provide security and basic needs. Motivational factors are needed for an individual to grow spiritually and psychologically. Theory Z (Ouchi, 1981) was developed from a study of successful Japanese organizations. Elements within this theory are collective decision making, long term employment, slower promotions, indirect supervision, and a holistic concern for employees.

A third group of theories resulted from the failure of the other types of theories to address the significance of the environment, organization, goal, or situation on leadership. This group of theories is referred to as situational theories. Fiedler's contingency theory is one such situational theory. Research based on this theory indicates that the most effective leaders are those who can adapt their particular style to the situation. Georgopoulas, Vroom, and House (1970) are credited with the development of the path-goal theory. This situational theory addresses the scope of the task to be done, role ambiguity, the employee's expectations and perceptions of the task, and ways in which the leader influences these expectations (Tappen, 1983, p. 58). Situational research has continued to examine a large number of other variables that affect leadership. Tappen (1983) provided an incomplete list of these variables: position in group, group size, communication networks, social status, interpersonal stress, designation of leadership, and organization structure (p. 59).

Interactional theories can be viewed as the compilation of everything that has gone before in an attempt to pull together the three elements of leader, follower, and environment. Schein (1970) proposed a complex man and open systems framework in an attempt to synthesize trait, behavioral, motivational, and situational theories. Hollander's (1978) elements of a leader situation are composed of the basic three elements, but the interrelationship and interdependence of them places his work into this group of interactionist theories. Schreisheim, Mowday, and Stogdill (1977) also emphasize the interdependence between the leader and group in any given complex situation as determining the leadership process.

Prentice (1983) stated that a leader's ability to understand and relate to individuals as complex and unique beings was a major factor in the leader's effectiveness. This interpersonal activity resulted in a leader being able to marshal individual collaboration toward goal achievement successfully (p. 141). The leader is cognizant of his own contribution to the effectiveness of the organization, but in his interpersonal relationships he focuses on the unique contribution his individual staff members can make (Tramel and Reynold, 1981, p. 67).

Tannenbaum and Schmidt (1983) summarized the synthesis of personality and interpersonal relationships in leaders that result in success as follows:

The successful leader is one who is keenly aware of those forces which are most relevant to behavior at any given time...(Secondly) The successful leader is the one who is able to behave appropriately in the light of these perceptions (p. 163).

Styles of leadership have been classified into many types. Tramel and Reynolds (1981) identified three general categories as tight, team, or loose rein, whereas Likert delineated four leadership styles. The exploitive or authoritative style appears synonymous with the autocratic style espoused in the early 1970's. There is also the benevolent-authoritative style, which is less autocratic. A third leadership style is a consultative style. A fourth style is a participative leadership style.

Leadership style comes from a variety of factors. Individual personality, life philosophy, and socialization in early life have a significant impact on the leadership style developed. External factors also contribute to the leadership style. These factors include the characteristics of the group, the leader-group relations, and the requirements of the organization. An organization in which the product is the result of a group effort demands a leadership style different from an organization in which individuals are responsible for separate products. The type of leadership valued by the organization and society also affects the style. As leadership theories have evolved, it has become more popular to emphasize a blending of styles by any one leader, depending on the time, place, people, and product (Baird, 1982).

Tannenbaum and Schmidt (1983) emphasized that there are three sets of forces that determine the leadership pattern that will be most successful. The set of forces found within the leader, such as personality, knowledge, and background, is a primary determinant of leadership style because it is the closest force to the leader. The second set of forces has to do with the individuals involved within the relationship. These forces include motivation, knowledge, and understanding. The third set of forces that determines the style of leadership that will be successful is composed of forces within the environment. These are the organizational and societal forces mentioned previously.

Baird (1982) identified three other factors that affect the leadership style used. Assumptions that a leader makes about people is one factor. Within this factor is the use of Theory X versus Theory Y (McGregor, 1957). Theory X states that people are by nature lazy, lack ambition, and are self-centered. Additionally, people are resistant to change, dislike responsibility, and must be led. Theory Y states that people have the potential for development and responsibility. These capabilities are present in all people, and leaders are the catalyst to bring them out. Another assumption about people is called the self-fulfilling prophecy. These leaders believe that people become what others expect them to become (Baird, 1982, pp. 5–9).

A second assumption that Baird (1982) proposed is the way a leader uses or shares power. He states that there are four basic ways to use or share power. The autocratic leader shares no power. This is not necessarily bad and can be very efficient, especially in emergency or crisis situations. It is also effective when the leader is working with a group of inexperienced managers or subordinates. A second use of power is the democratic use of power. A democratic leader shares power, usually with experienced, qualified subordinates. It can be less efficient because it is more time consuming. In this situation, the leader may only be able to exert power in a consultative manner, which may not be effective in situations such as an emergency. Laissez-faire, according to Baird, is essentially no power for the leader. This leadership style may occur as the result of subordinates having more expertise than the leader. The final use of power is situational, in which the leader varies the use of power among the first three ways.

The third force that Baird (1982) stated determined the style of leadership pertained to the way in which the leader communicated. A leader may choose to keep his head buried in the sand like an ostrich. Another way is seen in the leader who avoids conflict and attempts to be friends with everyone. The hard nosed leader emphasizes productivity at all costs and is strictly business. The mainstay of most organizations is the middle of the road leader who does neither a good nor bad job of communicating. The most successful leader communicates by emphasizing both the interpersonal relationship and the productivity (pp. 15–17).

Fiedler's (1967) research on contingency theory identified three major factors that influenced the leader's effectiveness. The relationship between the leader and individuals involved is very important. The nature of the task or goal also determines the effectiveness of the leader. This includes the clarity of the goal, the actual goal or task, as well as the potential for completion. The third factor deals with the leader's ability to punish or reward group members. The coalignment theory (Kotter and Lawrence, 1979) suggested that contextual or structural variables and process variables interact to determine a leader's effectiveness.

Leadership is composed of a group of individual characteristics and behaviors that utilize a wide compendium of human relation abilities, management techniques, and power. The unique blend of these actions results in the movement of individuals toward goal setting and goal achievement. A successful leader is one who maintains a high batting average in accurately assessing the forces that determine what his most appropriate behavior at any given time should be and actually being able to behave accordingly while getting the individuals involved to participate (Tannenbaum and Schmidt, 1983).

POWER

Basic Concepts

Claus and Bailey (1977) offered a succinct definition of power when they defined power as "the ability and willingness to affect the behavior of others" (p. 17). This definition allows for a consideration of the variable theoretical bases of power. The above definition of power presumes a relationship of two or more people. Weber (1947), Dahn (1957), and Emerson (1962) describe this relationship as one party being dependent on another. Kotter's (1983) description of organizations being composed of dependent relationships promotes this theoretical framework. Another theoretical base of power emphasizes the individual who seeks power. McClelland and Burnham (1983) conducted research that categorized individual characteristics of managers. Those individuals with a strong desire to make an impact, be influential, and be willing to perform accordingly were more effective leaders than others. This theoretical base identified the significance of the individual characteristics important for power; i.e., the individual must have the internal capacity, intention, or willingness to engage in a relationship that involves power.

A collaborative approach to power developed by Craig and Craig (1974) promotes an "I'm ok—you're ok" or "win-win" conceptual approach to power. Synergistic power is cooperative action of independent persons "to increase the satisfaction of all participants" (Claus and Bailey, 1977, p. 17). This approach is limited, however, because it does not encompass the entire spectrum of power, including the direct and frequently negative connotations associated with power.

Within a power relationship there are three elements identified in the proposed definition. These three elements are strength or ability, energy, and action (Claus and Bailey, 1977). Proposed as a can → will → do pyramid, this is a useful conceptual framework for nursing leaders to remember when examining their own power relationships. Strength or ability includes the internal resources of a strong self-concept and an awareness of reality. But strength also consists of more tangible assets such as resources and information. Energy is composed of both internal and external energy. Most leaders possess high energy levels that are expressed as positivism, optimism, and enthusiasm. The energy element is also composed of the ability to harness the energy of others. This ability to get the cooperation of others in the relationship then leads to the final activity in the power relationship, the act. Power is frequently discussed in terms of results. It is the action occurring within the power relationship that determines these results. Power differs from influence and authority, although they are closely related. Power is a source of influence (Claus and Bailey, 1977). Influence cannot occur without the presence of a power relationship. However, influence emphasizes the ability and energy elements more so than the action element of the power relationship. Authority is usually considered a specific type of power.

French and Raven (1960) are credited with identifying currently well-known types of power such as reward, coercive, referent, legitimate, expert, and informational power. Reward power describes a relationship in which one agent possesses a resource that is essential in maintaining the dependency of the other agent. Coercive power emphasizes the influencing agent's ability to apply negative sanctions. Referent power describes a power relationship in which the dependency consists of a close identified relationship with the influencing agent. Legitimate power is based on an accepted value or social standard. Expert power describes the influencing agent as possessing superior knowledge or skills. Informational power identifies the dependency on the need for information as the fulcrum of the power relationship. This categorization, although interesting, does not significantly contribute to the more practical issues of who are powerful, how do they become that way, and how do they use that power within the health care systems in which nursing leaders function.

Power in Health Care Organizations

The next discussion of power occurs within the context of a hospital or health care organization. Who are the powerful people in the health care organization? Research suggests that power within organizations is significantly related to formal authority positions. This is not to minimize the existence and impact of informal power that does occur, but this impact of informal power and the significant power related to formal authority positions will be elaborated upon as the discussion progresses. The concept of an organization includes order and lines of responsibility and authority. Positions are then an integral component of organizations. Individuals who occupy positions that are considered central within an organization are frequently individuals who possess power. For example, a research chemist who works independently on projects is not in a central position within an organization. As such, he possesses very little power, other than perhaps expert power. Positions that have many rules associated with them, are highly technical in nature, or are limited to affecting only the immediate work area are not powerful. Individuals in positions within organizations that are allowed flexibility, don't need approval for a majority of their decisions, have a great deal of contact with people from all levels of the organization, and focus on more general goals are individuals with power potential. Although the scientist may have internal desire, will, and ability to possess power, he does not possess all the strength and energy resources necessary for a power relationship to exist because of his position within the organization. The individual in a central position, on the other hand, has access to acquiring the external elements of strength and energy if he also possesses the internal strength and energy.

According to Kanter (1983), it is these individuals in central positions who can access the three basic sources of power. The first source of power deals with the lines of supply. Of these, financial resources are the best. Other resources include materials, man-hours, and time. The second source of power is the line of information. Information comes in all forms, and none can be disregarded as insignificant. Verbal information, as well as formal or informal written information, contributes significantly to the strength of the powerful individual. The third source of power is the line of support or cooperation from above, below, and around this individual in a central position. Close contact with sponsors or mentors as well as a firmly established network of peers and subordinates provides the powerful individual with the energy to complete the power relationship.

A strategic contingencies theory model of organizational power expands on this concept of individual position centrality to consider nursing as an organization. In this model, organizations are composed of subunits. Within the subunits, there are three variables that govern the subunit's power. The first variable is the subunit's degree of centrality. Centrality in this model refers to the extent of the subunit's interdependence with other subunits. Effective strategies within this variable include ways for a nursing subunit to increase its connection and involvements with other subunits. The second variable relates to the degree of substitutability. The less likely a subunit is able to be replaced by other substitutes, the more powerful it is. Maintaining control over areas and functions legally defined as nursing is the main strategy in this variable. Other strategies include the graduation of fewer nurses and not assuming responsibilities for non-nursing tasks. The third variable is the ability to cope with uncertainty. Through the processes of prevention, information control, or assimilation, nursing units can demonstrate their ability to handle problems and make a positive contribution to the organization (Stuart, 1986).

There are a number of other situations or occurrences that contribute to an individual's perceived power that can be used effectively in a power relationship. Frequently, a leader is perceived as a parental figure by his subordinates. Not all individuals desire power, and many welcome remaining in the child role. For these individuals, the person possessing power can reinforce his position by meeting this role expectation. These statements will not meet with total approval and acceptance by everyone who reads them. Some will insist that adults need to be treated as adults, if they are to act like adults. Ideally, this happens when mature individuals make up the relationship. In reality, however, not all individuals or professionals are mature. A leader works with the individuals he has inherited, regardless of their level of maturity. Maturation can be encouraged, however, through a nurturing environment established by a parental figure. This approach recognizes the value of all individuals no matter what their stage of growth and development. A leader maximizes the contribution of everyone by the correct assessment of the needs of each individual and the application of the appropriate style of management.

Another situation that contributes to an individual's power is a crisis situation. When an individual handles a crisis quickly and effectively, and the crisis as well as the intervention is publicized, the individual acquires power. A crisis no one knows about is not a crisis. Efficient and effective handling of a long term situation, as opposed to a crisis that is short term, is not as effective in contributing to an individual's power.

Another condition that contributes to an individual's power is the amount of paranoid thinking that occurs within an organization. The less secure and stable an organization (which is highly characteristic of all health organizations today), the greater the amount of paranoid thinking that occurs. The individual who is perceived as not succumbing to this dread disease is perceived as being powerful. Likewise, the individual who contributes to reducing paranoia among others is perceived as powerful.

Ritual or ceremonial situations can also contribute to an individual's perceived power. This may be due to the employees' increased identification with the organization for the source of their significant relationship, since families, friends, and neighbors are increasingly fragmented. Consider the popularity of a president who restores glamour and ceremony to the Executive Office. Although there are always employees who critically examine the Chief Executive's clothes, car, and home, people do expect to look up to their leaders. Therefore, a CEO who looks like a leader is perceived as being more successful and therefore more powerful than the CEO who wears jeans and rides a motorbike (Zaleznik, 1983).

Strategies for Acquiring Power

Assuming that an individual has the desire, ability, and will to be powerful, and occupies a central position within an organization, and given these other conditions and situations, what are some of the other strategies for acquiring power? Tramel and Reynolds (1981) present several strategies designed to increase an individual's power. Creating a good first impression can be very helpful. This is accomplished in a number of ways. Appearing confident in oneself and being creative are two such ways to create a good first impression. Having a caring and considerate attitude toward others that is reinforced through considerate behaviors is another strategy.

There are several nonverbal power tools that are helpful at any time. Acceptance and wise use of one's sexuality is one example. This means, for females, finding a comfortable ground that entails being feminine without being sexual or helpless, professional without being hard or neuter. The advantages of being female are communicated differently than being a superior sex. This is a difficult self-concept to establish, but it contributes to one's power. A part of physical make-up includes posture and body language. Standing straight, not folding one's arms or legs, and not sitting while others stand are examples. It is important to recognize others even if only with a nod, smile, or eye contact. The handshake may also be important. It does not have to be a bone crusher, but it should be better than a limp rag. Obviously, dress is important for both males and females; however, women may be subjected to closer evaluation in this area. Fashion designers are finally recognizing the need for attractive clothing for women in leadership positions. Tailored suits are always in good taste. Power dressing, on the other hand, indicates that a woman is not afraid to recognize the uniqueness of her femininity. Attractive clothing that is softer yet in good taste is now available in better clothing lines. This type of dressing sets one apart from the men but in a non-offensive and often appreciated manner. Research indicates that attractive people are perceived as being more powerful than others. Investment in a good wardrobe and well-manicured hair and nails can make a significant difference in how one is perceived. Maximizing one's assets with the right colors is yet another tool to improve one's perceived power.

In addition to the nonverbal power tools, there are verbal power tools that a nursing leader can utilize. Rational thinking is a basis for using these tools. By thinking before speaking, one can edit comments, clearly identify the purpose of those comments, and choose the proper timing. As a result, one will be more tactful and will be free to perceive the other person correctly. At the same time remaining conscious of the message being sent, one can quickly assert oneself to question who "they" are and cut off gossip. Other verbal power tools will be presented in the communication section.

Benziger (1982) suggested four basic strategies that enable an individual to add to the power base. It is imperative that a potentially powerful leader learn and use the organization's language and symbols. For nursing, that means knowing more than just nursing. A powerful nursing leader has to be able to be conversant with individuals from a large number of disciplines, health related or not. Chief among these groups are the financial and marketing staff and the planners of the organization. Of similar importance is understanding the organization's priorities and incorporating their ultimate goal achievement into all activities. It is essential to know the other power positions in the organization, know the individuals in these positions, and establish a working relationship with them. It is important to determine how decisions are made, who is reputed to have power, what are considered symbols of power, and who possesses them. Committees can occasionally possess significant organizational power. Identification of the powerful committees and attainment of an appointment to these committees could be helpful in building power. Avoidance of the albatross committees is equally important. The other strategy has to do with maintenance. In order to remain powerful, one must continue to develop knowledge and skills so that one can retain expert power.

Utilizing the four strategies just described as a springboard, the following behaviors can contribute to power strength, energy, and action. A true nursing leader is not just active but is also proactive. In this respect, he is involved in planning for the future, not just acting in the present or reacting to the past. The nurse leader does not ask for authority but assumes it. This entails risk taking. If the leader utilizes the principles of education (for himself, his subordinates, etc.), rational thinking, and communication, he will minimize his chance of error and maximize his potential for success. Following this success, it is vital that the good news of success be publicized so that others may feel good about it. The unique needs of one's superior must be identified as well and integrated into daily activities. In the final analysis, however, successful outcomes are dependent on an individual taking care of himself. Ultimately, no one else will. In doing so, nothing should be taken too seriously. The ability to laugh is an effective tool not just for an individual's mental health, but for the organization as well. Likewise, it is best to leave work problems at the office at the end of a reasonable work day.

Is a discussion of power realistic for nurse leaders? Sometimes it seems easier to talk about sex or religion to nurses than power. Yet in every nursing publication, the lack of qualified nursing leaders is lamented. If in fact Stevens (1983) is correct in her statement that nursing is the epitome of women's traditional powerless role and that the health care system is characteristically paternalistic, why bother to try? These questions only seem to emphasize the negative aspect of power. We are past the point of debating the pros and cons of nurses using power. Nurses are using power and being successful. This is the foundation on which nursing must build to carry it into the future. Nurse leaders can develop these power tools and actualize their power potential. Once nurse leaders come to terms with their own power, they can rid themselves of the guilt and worry they have carried around with them. It will then be possible to share these skills eagerly with other nurses and broaden the power base of nurses all the way down to the staff nurse level. That is the strategy that will ultimately carry nursing successfully into the future.

DECISION MAKING

The purpose of this section is to discuss the elements and processes involved in decisions made by nursing leaders. The skill of decision making can be acquired through practice and conscious effort. It is necessary for the nurse leader to be knowledgeable and skillful in these techniques in order to be effective. Additionally, it is the nurse leader's responsibility to educate new nurse leaders and managers in these techniques so that they in turn can acquire these skills and increase their effectiveness. The economy of health care is that there are a limited amount of resources available to meet the health requirements of society. This reality mandates that choices will be made by nurses. Skillful decision making maximizes the best utilization of these health resources for the individual and collective patient needs.

Problems arise for a variety of reasons, and no one would dispute their existence. Nevertheless, ownership of a problem is a question that is seldom even considered, let alone answered. Too often, unfortunately, nurses too easily pick up and carry unnecessary anxiety and guilt for problems that are not relevant to nursing. A "fix-it" and martyr complex held by many nurses encourage this attitude toward problems and obviously are not always in nursing's or the patient's best interest. Unfortunately, there are others who would take advantage of these complexes and assign problems to nursing that are not truly nursing's.

Choices and decisions are made numerous times throughout the day by every nurse leader at all levels of the organization. Frequently, the situations are complex; hysteria and crises orientation can appear to be the norm; and there remains the urgent desire by administrators, medical staff, as well as nurse administrators to put out fires in order to get some temporary relief. As skill in decision making develops, the process can become more automatic and sometimes less time consuming. The optimal time for decision making never occurs. Nevertheless, the nurse leader is comfortable with making decisions and would rather make them than not.

The decision making process is the basis upon which the nursing process is built. Therefore the sequence and elements of the decision making process are very familar to most nurses. As a model for many, the nursing process' success is an indication of the value of its usage. As a process, it also represents a continuum that allows for forward, backward, and circular movement. It is a process that also involves an attitude and ultimately a solution. The attitude exists prior to and during the decision making process. The nurse leader's attitude is that of a willingness to give fair consideration to all data and individuals involved in the process. An open mind that includes a combination of involvement as well as detachment enables the leader to get inside the problem actively as well as to step back from the situation and consider the process as a stranger might view it.

Because problems create discomfort, the degree, scope, nature, and intimacy of the discomfort motivate the nurse leader into the decision making process. The first step in the decision making process is the data collection or assessment phase. Data collection needs to be as objective, relevant, and valid as possible. This is very often not the case, and subjective and/or incomplete data may be the only available data. This makes verification of the data extremely difficult. Subjective data frequently consist of cliches, stereotypes, and emotional or biased information. This information needs to be labeled as such and ultimately discarded. During data collection, it is also extremely helpful to define key terms, as this will assist in the decision making process.

When as much data as possible has been gathered, it is then necessary to define the problem clearly. This step is also frequently overlooked because nurses want to get to the "fix-it" or solution part of the process. The nurse leader must avoid the tendency to jump to a solution. Whether the nurse leader is making a solitary decision or a decision in concert with a group, validation of the specific problem with those involved is necessary. One must be sure that the problem is labeled clearly and correctly. When the problem is clearly identified, the nurse leader must uncover any basic underlying assumptions that contribute to the problem. These assumptions must be ultimately taken into account.

The planning or strategizing step is the next process in decision making. First, all of the possible alternative solutions to the specific problem must be identified. This can be accomplished utilizing several different techniques, depending on the circumstances and number of individuals involved.

The brainstorming technique (Osborn, 1979) is a very popular technique usually employed in group decision making. It can be used by a solitary nurse leader as well. This technique involves four basic steps to which have been added follow-through procedures. The first step is to list every possible solution exactly as it first comes to mind. While this is occurring, it is important not to judge the suggestions. Following the initial quick response, additional solutions can be generated by examining the initial responses and looking for associated or related solutions. The use of each solution is then described, again without judgment or critique. Then the solutions are rated, and discussion proceeds from there. Following the discussion, the solutions are rated again.

Another technique is known as the Nominal Group Technique (NGT), developed by Delbecq and Van de Ven (1971). Brainstorming occurs, but on paper rather than verbally. This encourages a more complete participation from all involved and prevents domination by a few. These ideas are then tabulated visibly for all parties. Following a discussion of each alternative, the solutions are rated and decision making proceeds from that point. A solitary nurse leader can utilize this technique by writing down his alternatives rather than just listing them mentally.

A third technique developed by Kalkey (1967, 1969) at the Rand Corporation is a systematic but time-consuming process that does not require the involved individuals to be physically present as a group. The Delphi Technique involves the solicitation and collection of information or alternatives from individuals through a series of questionnaires. Each successive questionnaire summarizes information obtained and feeds it back to the group while simultaneously requesting additional information.

Regardless of how the alternatives are generated, it is important to canvass a wide range of alternatives thoroughly. Each alternative must then be examined for how completely it solves the problem. Usually a problem has several objectives, and each alternative should be identified as to how completely it meets all of the objectives. Then the positive and negative consequences of each alternative are listed. The costs and risks associated with each of the consequences are then examined. Additionally, the values associated with each alternative should be explicitly defined. Before a choice is made, it is helpful to look for any new information that may have since become available. This last-minute information needs to be taken into consideration even if it isn't compatible with the direction the decision seems to be taking.

The alternatives are then rated or valued, based on several factors. More than one solution or alternative can be chosen. But regardless of how many solutions, the same considerations must be made. The best decisions are those that are the most acceptable to those that implement it and are affected by it. The decision must accurately solve the problem and be realistically applied. The right decision will also usually be the decision that generates the least amount of conflict with individual values. Finally, the decision cannot unduly tax the resources of the system correcting the problem.

The best decision is not a successful or effective decision until it has been implemented and the problem solved. It is then necessary to develop a schedule of time, tasks, and responsibilities. All of the steps involved in implementing the system are listed. The total amount of time available is identified. This total time is allocated to the individual tasks. Responsibility is assigned to each task. This task can take many forms, including a Gantt chart (Fig. 5–1). The Gantt chart illustrates the time frame and relationship of steps to achieve stated objectives. In crisis situations, it may exist only in the nurse leader's head. Then implementation begins. Drucker (1983) stated that the effective decision "is based on the highest level of conceptual understanding but the action commitment should be as close as possible to the capacities of the people who have to carry it out." A good decision is only as good as its implementation. Implementation is usually the longest and hardest part of the process.

Implementation and evaluation, the last part of the decision making process, really occur simultaneously. Etizoni (1967) encouraged a scanning process. This involves a review of the situation early in the implementation phase to allow for feedback, alterations, or modification in the schedule for implementation of the decision, or decision itself. Concurrent monitoring ultimately provides more data, which is used in the final evaluation process. Depending on the situation, this data may not be communicated to the nurse executive but rather delegated to the implementers for their use. The nurse executive may only want the final evaluation.

Evaluation is considered from the very beginning of the decision making process. The how and when of evaluation is an integral part of the decision. This makes evaluation a relative and valued process. Evaluation examines both objective and subjective results. Were the results the ones expected, and were they the positive results desired or negative results? In addition to evaluation in context of the unique problem, evaluation can occur in relation to application for future problems. Evaluation can occur in terms of the entire decision making process incurred for this particular situation. Which steps were performed adequately or inadequately? What did the nurse leader or leadership group learn as a result of the process? Finally, evaluation allows for the identification of serendipitous findings.

Decision making in leadership and management literature has trended toward the quantitative, operations-research, and management-science approaches. These trends are the result of efforts to improve the decision making process through the improvement of the preciseness of data measurement or improvement in the confidence of the validity of the involved relationships. Several concepts that are applicable to any decision making theory or model have evolved that enable a nursing leader to assimilate this knowledge more easily.

All decision making models and processes are based on some form of systems model or systems analysis. This common denominator to decision making theories or models can provide the nursing leader with a basic

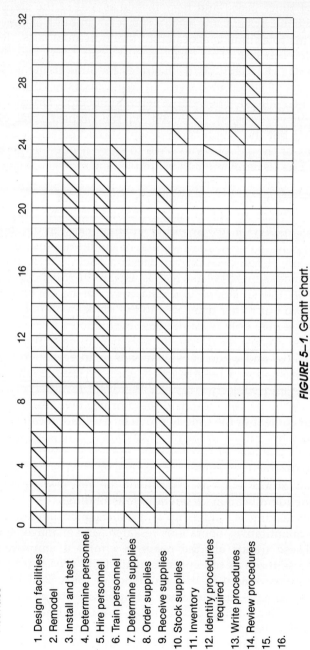

FIGURE 5–1. Gantt chart.

TABLE 5-1
Illustrative Applications of Formal Analysis

Quantitative Techniques
Simulation
Queuing theory
Network analysis
Inventory models
Linear programming
Nonlinear programming
Goal programming

framework for understanding these theories and models. The second commonality among decision making theories and models is the essential nature of information. Communication of information via either a computer decision system or through an organization's behaviors is an inevitable component in decisions that are made. This implies the essential need of an organized management information system involving all types of information. Logic is another basic concept of any decision making theory. Finally, the contribution of the subdecisions that occur during the decision making process has been recognized as an integral, basic, and essential component of all decision making theory.

The chief contribution of modern decision theory has been the systematic employment of probabilities, either Bayesian or objective, to describe the pattern of future events (Hough, 1970, p. 59). Bayesian probability theory emphasizes the careful subjective estimates of probability. The objective or mathematical models have emphasized economic estimates of the future from each choice and estimates of the probability of specific future influences on each alternative choice. Both of these approaches illustrate the basic principles of probability and statistical inference that underlie decision making theories (Jedamus and Frame, 1969, p. 5).

Formal analysis using complex mathematical computations has been developed in operations research to assist in decision making. Application of these decision making models has occurred in a variety of settings, mostly industrial and technological. Application within service industries such as health care is occurring. Therefore, the nurse leader should be cognizant of these models' purpose and potential function. Table 5-1 lists several examples of these models. Of these models, linear programming has become a popular management tool in constructing plans, schedules, allocations, and assignments. However, Hough (1970) cautions against blindly attempting to transfer these models for use with complex relationships or with behavioral or special systems without adequate sampling and use of past experience.

Decision making occurs frequently in the complex world of nursing leaders. Decisions are made in isolation as well as within the context of various groups. As a result, the nurse leader develops skill in a variety of decision making techniques and processes, which enables her to make the right, effective, successful decision.

MOTIVATION

Basic Concepts

As our society has become more industrialized and also more humanistic, the concept of motivation has assumed an increased amount of attention
by behaviorists and others. Motivation is concerned with the individual's
stimulus or reason for behavior. Motivation is considered as the key to
productivity in this era of diminishing resources and cost containment
(Timmreck and Randall, 1981). It is not, however, the complete answer for
a nursing leader at this time or in the future, for several reasons. Motivation
does not address the many other variables contained in the environment or
situation affecting goal achievement. But because health care is labor intensive and nurse intensive, motivation does significantly contribute to goal
achievement. Industrialized society created a fertile ground for research on
motivation of individuals within an organized system. As a result, there are
several theoretical formulations of motivation that describe, explain, and
attempt to predict people's reasons for their behavior as well as the behavior
itself. Because of the organizational situation, these theories usually extensively refer to job satisfaction. As such, they are applicable for the nurse
leader.

McFarland, Leonard, and Morris (1984) classified organizational theories
of motivation into aspects involving the job (Hoppock, 1935, 1967; Smith,
Kendall, and Hulin, 1967; Vroom, 1967), aspects involving the individual
(Super, 1953, 1957, 1969; Maslow, 1954; Super and Bohn, 1970; Kormon,
1966, 1970), and the interaction of individual and job aspects (Herzberg,
1971; Lofquiat and Davis, 1969; Holland, 1959, 1966). Of all of these theories,
those of Maslow and Herzberg are very popular. Maslow's hierarchy of
needs is used by many disciplines to explain an individual's behavior inside
or outside of an organized system. It is a straightforward structure, and an
easy to understand theory that can be applied to any individual at any stage
of his or her life. It involves the necessity of first and foremost meeting the
basic physical needs of sleep, food, water, and air. Once these needs are
satisfied or as long as these needs are satisfied, they cease to be motivators.
These needs also overlap to some extent, and there are degrees of satisfaction.
Safety and security needs are the second level of Maslow's hierarchy. These
involve needs for protection against danger, threat, deprivation, or retalia-
tion. Social needs, which are the next level of needs that stimulate behavior,
are involved with love, affection, and affiliation. Following the social needs
are self-esteem and achievement. The ultimate needs that are not ever
achieved by some individuals, who get hung up on meeting the needs of
lower levels, are the needs of self-actualization. The term self-actualization
is "loosely described as the full use and exploitations of talents, capacities,
potentialities, etc." (Maslow, 1968). Maslow developed his hierarchy further,
but these additional propositions are rarely discussed in motivational pres-

entations. The hierarchy was expanded to encompass the complex concepts of B values, or being values; curiosity or the need to know; and aesthetic needs, such as the need for beauty. The concept of altruism enters Maslow's motivation theory at this point (Monte, 1977, p. 491). Maslow's ultimate interest was in the healthy growth of the total individual and that of society. This perception parallels leadership in several ways. The leader is motivated to achieve self-actualization and ultimately does so. The leader then is freed from the demands of meeting lower level needs and can expand outside of self to become altruistic toward others.

Despite the popularity of Maslow's theory of human motivation, the proposition of a progressive hierarchy created unresolved problems. Additionally, Maslow's work has not been well substantiated with empirical data. Clayton Alderfer (1972) proposed an ERG theory to explain basic human needs and their interrelationship. ERG theory draws heavily from Maslow's work and refers to three basic categories of human needs: existence needs, relatedness needs, and growth needs. These three categories of needs are considered innate or primary needs, but not necessarily biological needs. As innate needs, these three categories of needs are not learned, although a need may be strengthened through the learning process. As a motivational theory, ERG theory examines the two human subjective states of satisfaction and desire. Within the context of the three needs categories, there are dimensions of satisfaction and desire. Satisfaction is considered an internal subjective state resulting from an event occurring between a person and the environment. Alderfer stated that satisfaction is synonymous with getting and fulfilling. Frustration is the opposite of satisfaction. Unlike satisfaction, desire as a subjective need state has no external reference; it is entirely internal. An individual possesses satisfaction and desires concerning all three categories of needs in varying intensities. The three categories of needs contain the five levels identified by Maslow. Existence needs encompass the physiological and safety needs suggested by Maslow. A person's requirements for any material or energy exchange, as well as the need to reach and maintain a homeostatic equilibrium, compose the existence needs. The relatedness needs concern the transactions with other humans and encompass Maslow's safety, interpersonal love, and interpersonal esteem needs. Growth needs are related to an individual experiencing a state of wholeness or fullness and encompass Maslow's self-esteem needs and need for self-actualization.

Maslow's theory consists of a strictly ordered hierarchy, whereas Alderfer's ERG theory lacks a strict hierarchy. Substitution of one need for another unsatisfied need is a frequent occurrence, according to ERG theory. Alderfer's theory also differs from Maslow's theory in suggesting how frustration of higher-order needs affects lower level desires and how chronic desires relate to satisfaction. As such, ERG theory offers the nursing service administrator another theoretical framework for analyzing and dealing with human behavior.

Approaches to motivation have also been classified according to the mechanistic approach or the cognitive approach. The mechanistic approach identifies need and drive as the sources of motivation. Mechanistic approaches would include the work of Freud (1947), Hull (1943), Maslow (1948), and Alderfer (1972). The cognitive approach identifies mastery, understanding, and information seeking as the sources of motivation. Cognitive theorists are divided into cognitive-consistency theorists, such as Heider (1958) and Festinger (1962); attribution theorists, such as Jones and Davis (1965), Kelly (1967), and Weiner (l974); and expectancy-value theorists Lewin (195l), Rotter (1954), and Atkinson (1966).

The cognitive model of motivation preceded the attribution theory. According to the cognitive model, a stimulus leads to cognition, which leads to response. The incoming stimulus is translated by a belief system that gives it meaning or assigns a value. Cognitive operations such as information processing, judgment, and decision making determine and direct the response, which includes affect and behavior. Tolman (1932) and Lewin (1938) were among the early advocates of cognitive theories of behavior. These theorists conceptualized the organism as possessing beliefs, opinions, or expectations concerning the world around him. Learning was the result of changes in beliefs, and behavior was goal directed to attain valent objects or events and to avoid negative ones (Vroom, 1982).

Vroom (1982) proposed another model of motivation that stated that the choices made by a person among alternative courses of action are related to psychological events occurring contemporaneously with the behavior. According to the concept of valence, at any given point in time a person has preferences among possible outcomes. Using the concept of valence as the main proposition of his theory, Vroom explained occupational preference, morale, need achievement, group cohesiveness, job satisfaction, and motivation for effective performance. As a result, Vroom's work has relevance to individuals in supervisory positions.

Heider (1958) is considered the founder of attribution theory, which was derived from Lewin's (1951) field theory. Attributions are the causes a person attributes to an event. The focus of this theory is on the perceived causation of motivation, not the actual causation of behaviors. The individual explains his world by attributing causes of behaviors, events, and circumstances to those factors the individual believes to be the cause. Heider's (1958) attributional theory uses the terms can and try in describing the two components, power and motivation, which compose personal causality. Power is determined by the ability or "can" component. Motivation is the "try" component. Motivation, according to Heider, consists of two elements, intention and exertion. Intention is what the individual is going to do. Exertion refers to the effort of the individual to do the behavior.

Heider's (1958) theory included the environmental variables of task difficulty and luck. The outcome of any behavior is attributable to the four factors of ability, effort, task difficulty, and luck. Basic assumptions of attribution theory are (1) individuals are motivated to attain cognitive mastery, and (2) actions are related to attributions. Empirical support for the role attributions play in the motivation of behavior was reported by Storms and Nisbett (1970) and by Aronson and Carlsmith (1962).

In addition to the relationship of attributions on behavior, there are expectancy-value theorists who believe that it is the expectation that the response will lead to the goal and the value of that goal that determine the intensity of the motivation (Becker and McClintoch, 1967; Hollon and Garber, 1980). Expectancy is a central concept in achievement motivation theory. Research demonstrates that following success, expectancy generally rises; after failure, it falls. Expectancies for success and failure are based in part on past experiences and outcomes. Other research within the realm of these cognitive reinforcement—motivational theories includes looking at locus of control and the impact of personality variables such as self-esteem.

It can be understood from the previous discussion that motivational theories attempt to account for a myriad of internal and external determinants. Another method of classifying motivational theories uses the external versus internal determinants framework. External determinants of motivation include the effect of reinforcement and incentives. These external determinants provide satisfaction independent of the activity itself and are controlled by someone other than the subject. Deci (1975) proposed that intrinsic motivation occurred when the activity itself was the only reward. Despite the apparent distinctness between internal and external motivation, there is a reciprocal relationship that Deci conceptualized between external and internal determinants. Eysenck (1982) promotes "the effects of incentives on task performance can usually be regarded as depending on four classes of variables: the nature of the incentive; the processes required by the task; the aspects of performance selected for measurement; and individual differences in mood or state and in semi-permanent personality characteristics" (p. 87).

According to Eysenck (1982):

1. Incentive changes the priorities accorded to environmental events, producing increased attentional selectivity.
2. Incentive characteristically speeds up the internal processing and external response rate, but does so at the cost of reduced performance quality.
3. Incentive usually affects an internal motivational state, but can also produce frustration and/or anxiety.
4. Incentive often has adverse long-term effect on performance because it reduces . . . intrinsic motivation.
5. Powerful incentive reduces parallel or shared processing.
6. Incentive increases arousal.
7. Incentive is related to performance by means of a curvilinear relationship.
8. Incentive may increase distractibility (p. 94).

These general understandings concerning the incentive determinant on motivation have evolved from the research done using the external and internal reward framework. There remains at this date, however, little investigation into how the different variables, ascribed as being either intrinsic or extrinsic, interact with one another and what kind of effect this interaction has on motivation and ultimately on performance. Nursing leaders can assimilate this general knowledge concerning incentives in developing their motivational strategies.

Another mechanistic theory that has been applied directly to the health care environment is Herzberg's (1959) motivation-hygiene theory. This theory has achieved popularity for several reasons. Its specificity for the work world is one reason for its popularity. This theory also accounts for many of the variables identified as effectors of behavior and does so in an organized manner. That is very comforting to the manager who has had to switch from a product orientation to a people orientation.

Beginning with the premise that individuals are oriented to think of themselves as either happy or unhappy, satisfied or dissatisfied, Herzberg incorporated this premise as essential for positive motivation to occur. Variables that determine happiness are called hygiene or maintenance variables and are very similar to the physical, safety, security, and social needs in Maslow's theory. These hygiene variables include supervision, interpersonal relations, working conditions, salary, administrative policy, benefits, security, and status. These variables must be attended to in order to establish the climate for motivation. When hygiene variables are not accounted for, dissatisfaction and unhappiness exist. Only when these variables are controlled for can the group of individuals involved move on to the next step, which is being motivated.

"To experience personal growth, one has to be allowed to achieve through tasks that are individually meaningful" (Timmreck and Randall, 1981). Motivation occurs within individuals when their hygiene variables are satisfactory and they are involved in activities that enable them to feel personal, social, or psychological growth. This growth can occur as a result of goal achievement, recognition, responsibility, and advancement. Timmreck and Randall (1981) have adapted Herzberg's theory for the health care setting, and it is presented in Figure 5–2. Scanlon (1976) summarized motivation occurring as a result of six internal and external conditions. The internal conditions are the individual's need for achievement, the belief that one is adequately compensated, that the job requires skills and abilities that are possessed, and that there is an opportunity to participate. The external conditions are that the organization values the contributions and skills of the individual and the individual is provided with feedback, and that there is a mechanism to effectively evaluate the individual.

These theories are certainly not all inclusive of the variables that affect individual motivation. McFarland, Leonard, and Morris (1984) conducted nursing research using the theory of work adjustment by Dawis, Lofquist, and Weiss. This theory examines the "fit" between individual desires and abilities and the requirements of the job. An interactionist theory, the work adjustment theory examines the impact of job requirements more so than Herzberg's theory.

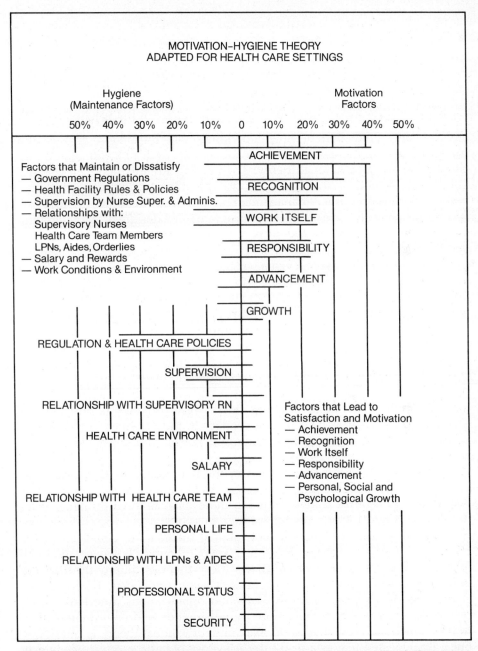

FIGURE 5–2. Motivation-hygiene theory adapted for health care settings. (Reprinted with permission from Timmreck, T., and Randall, P. J.: Motivation, Management and the Supervisory Nurse. Supervisor Nurse, March, 1981.)

Tomorrow's Motivational Strategies

The use of these motivational theories, whether a specific theory or a composite by the nurse leader, is an essential practice. These motivational theories provide a solid framework to examine the status of the nursing organization, whether it consists of a group of nursing personnel or a specific shift or the entire nursing service department.

Motivational theory provides a basis for examining the behavior of staff and for describing the relationship between individuals and their working environment. Prediction of how individuals will respond to factors and changes affecting them can also be made as the result of a nursing administrator's use of motivational theory. The nursing administrator can also use knowledge of motivational theory to evaluate departmental or institutional policies and procedures, management styles, the environment, and the reward systems that exist. As new programs are designed, consideration should also be given to the impact of these programs on employees' performance.

For example, the last few years wrecked havoc with what are considered by Herzberg as hygiene variables for most individuals in the nursing organization: supervision, interpersonal relations, salary, benefits, and working conditions. As a result, employees are demoralized, insecure, threatened, frightened, and unmotivated. The solutions for creating a positive and satisfying work environment in the late 1970's and early 1980's will not work in the late 1980's, for several reasons. The first reason is that many of these solutions were aimed strictly at hygiene factors and never progressed beyond them. As a result, there is little available knowledge about what works to motivate health care employees. The closest documentation is probably the Magnet Hospital Report (1983). The changes in the priorities of health care and resource allocation are two significant reasons for the need for new solutions.

Nevertheless, within the context of the here and now these variables can be systematically identified, assessed, and examined for the individuals responsible to a nurse leader. Utilizing these data, rational thinking, communication, and problem solving are then possible.

The knowledge and use of motivational theories are beneficial to the nurse leader of the future. She must keep in mind, however, that the information age we are now in affects these theories differently than the period of time when most of the theories were formulated. Likewise, the coming age will impact on individuals and organizations differently. As a result, the emphasis may shift more to the situation and environment than to the individual. How this will impact on motivational theory is unknown, but it is suggested that as a result the relevancy of basic survival needs may assume a higher significance than previously. Therefore, the nursing leader of tomorrow must command as much control of the environment and situation as possible in order to affect motivation. These actions by themselves will not be sufficiently effective, however, without mastery of the personal component. The nurse leader will have to be competent in the area of situational and environmental motivational factors in order to concentrate on identifying and assessing the status of individuals' basic needs. In a labor intensive department such as nursing, this is no small task. Delineating how the goals of the institution and department are relevant to numerous nursing service employees' basic needs will be a difficult and time consuming process. However, this is the key for successful motivation in the coming decade.

COMMUNICATION

Introduction

This section discusses the concept of communication. Communication constitutes the foundation of interaction among human beings. Although a complex concept, communication can basically be defined as the process of sharing a message with another person. Yet the significant magnitude of this concept on one's existence deserves closer scrutiny. Researchers have found that supervisors and managers spend as much as 70% of their waking hours in communication activities (Goble, 1972). This is an indication of the significance of communication for nursing leaders. Of all leadership activities, it is the most important. Understanding communication, how and when it occurs, barriers to it, as well as how it contributes to leadership effectiveness should be a top priority.

Research supports the crucial contribution positively perceived communication makes to both nurses' morale and their productivity. In a field study of 327 nurses, Pincus (1986) explored the relationship between different types of organizational communication and job satisfaction and job performance among hospital nurses. Results showed that three types of communication were strongly correlated with job satisfaction. Communication with the immediate supervisor, personal feedback, and the communication climate were significantly correlated with job satisfaction. Less strongly correlated, but significant, were communication with top management, horizontal communication, organizational integration, media quality, and organizational perspective. The findings of this study are comparable with results from Thiry's (1977) study of the relationship of communication satisfaction to need fulfillment among Kansas nurses. A relationship between communication and job performance was demonstrated, but it was not as strongly correlated as communication and job satisfaction. Pincus (1986) pointed out that these results were not congruent with Herzberg's theory, which categorizes interpersonal relationships as a hygiene factor directly related to job dissatisfaction. The results of these studies are significant when coupled with other research (Baird and Baird, 1985), which indicated that communication breakdowns in nursing organizations are not unusual. When combined with contemporary administration literature and human relations theories, there is little room for doubt concerning the relevancy and significance of effective communication on personal and organizational success (Wolf, 1986).

Communication theory describes communication as consisting of a minimum of three elements. These elements are the sender of the message, the message, and the receiver of the message. In addition to these three basic elements, some theorists include a coding process of the message by the sender and a decoding process by the receiver. Another conceptual approach to communication builds on these three elements but emphasizes the message. The message consists of two parts. The first part is the actual content of the message. The second part is the relationship that exists between the sender and receiver (Tappen, 1983). There are several other elements that compose most communication theories. Communication is subject to interference. This interference can be human or material. It can be external to the sender, message, or receiver, or internal to one or to all of them. The tendency to judge, evaluate, approve, or disapprove is considered the main barrier to communication (Roger and Roethlisberger, 1985). This form of interference is even greater when feelings and emotions are deeply involved. Such interference would be an internal form of interference found within the receiver. Another name used for interference is noise. Internal noise could include the frame of reference used; the selective perception of the receiver, which can serve as a filter to the message; or the attitude of either the sender or the receiver. The message may be in the form of inappropriate language. External noise or interference includes distractions and the environment, such as the cultural background of the participants and the situation where the communication is occurring.

Another element identified in communication is the channel the sender uses to send his message. The channel may be sound or ink on paper. The channel may contribute to the interference. For example, a letter of apology may take four or five days to get to the receiver, whereas a telephone call delivers the message sooner and with less possibility of internal or external interference.

Communication Channels

In a discussion of channels used in communication, the choice of channel as well as the vehicle of communication warrants attention. The choice of communication channel and vehicle can be related to brain research on the function of specific areas within the brain. Initiated with Paul Broca's work in the 1800's on isolating the speech area, research has become more highly technical and sophisticated. It has also evolved from an emphasis on one particular hemisphere to a more "whole brain" approach. The important contribution of brain research to communication is the knowledge that every person's brain is different in the way in which it prefers to process and interpret information, messages, and experiences. Brain research has identified those traits and abilities unique to the various parts of the brain.

TABLE 5–2
Whole Brain Communication Processing Preference

Cerebral Left
Present logical, rational information
Emphasize facts and details
Present in concrete format
Outline
Allow for analytical discussion

Limbic Left
Are very organized
Reference authority
Emphasize order and clarity
Use role models as examples

Limbic Right
Use case studies of role playing
Prepare to debate and/or negotiate
Emphasize interpersonal nature of information
Seek emotional involvement

Cerebral Right
Use pictures or models
Present on conceptual or abstract level
Acknowledge value of intuition
Emphasize creativity

Individuals vary in their use of these areas. Some individuals have developed one part of their brain, whereas other individuals use various parts of their brain to process messages. For the majority of people, the left brain is better at performing logical, analytic, mathematical tasks. The right brain is better at nonverbal ideation, intuition, holism, and synthesizing activities. Each hemisphere has been distinguished further into characteristics of the right cerebral and right limbic components and the left cerebral and left limbic components.

In determining which communication channel or vehicle to use for a message, the sender can utilize this research. If the receiver preference or hemisphere for processing messages can be identified, the channel and vehicle can be appropriately chosen. If the receiver's preference is unknown or if there are a number of receivers for the message, a whole brain approach to communication may be used. A whole brain approach utilizes a combination of approaches to meet the needs of all hemisphere components. In order to communicate effectively with a cerebral left receiver, the message should be clear, concise, and full of facts and details. The more technical and concrete the message, the more clear it is to a cerebral left receiver. The limbic left receiver processes messages that are written down and itemized, as opposed to verbal messages. The cerebral right receiver understands pictures and visual images best. These receivers do not process tables or numbers well. The limbic right receiver will respond best to the subjective, emotional, spiritual, or interpersonal parts of the message. Table 5–2 categorizes preference by brain dominance. The perceptive leader will plan her message channel(s) and vehicles accordingly and thereby maximize the reception and processing of her message.

Direction and Feedback

Anytime an individual wants to send a message to another individual, communication occurs. It is also proposed that all behavior is motivated; is the result of interaction with our environment; and therefore has meaning, which is a message or form of communication. Although it may sound somewhat extreme to state that all behavior has meaning and all behavior is a form of communication, it may help to increase our awareness of the amount of communication that is actually occurring.

At the same time, this discussion of behavior as communication brings out two other points to be considered in our discussion: one/two way communication and feedback. The first point concerns the direction of communication. Communication is viewed as being either one way or two way. One way communication is the sender directing the message to the receiver and there is no response or return message. Examples of one way communication are the newspaper, memos, policies, or even TV and radio. Two way communication includes the receiver sending back a message to the original sender. When the returning message is related to the first message, this is referred to as feedback, another concept relevant to communication. If one subscribes to the belief that all behavior means something, one way communication is exceedingly rare. Consider the examples of one way communication stated earlier. Receivers of messages via the newspaper, radio, TV, memos, etc., do respond. The message they send back may not be directly to the original sender but to another receiver. This then is really a form of two way communication, but not feedback because the original sender is not involved in the reception of the second message.

Feedback is the receiver sending the same message back to the sender or sending a message related to the original message back to the sender. In sending the original message back to the first sender, the receiver is validating the message because of concern for interference. This enables the first sender to know that the message was sent and received correctly. It provides the receiver with clarification that the message is the one intended.

Feedback consisting of a message related to the original message attempts to do more of the same but is not always as effective. In this situation, feedback may consist of primarily a reaction or response to the original message. Although this is usually of prime interest to the sender, it is subject to interpretation based on the assumption that the initial message was correctly received. With all of the possibilities for interference, it is highly possible that the message was distorted. Therefore, whenever possible it can be extremely beneficial to the parties involved for the sender to get feedback on the original message before proceeding further.

Feedback that does not consist of validation of the original message can be categorized into five types of responses (Rogers, 1965). The most frequent response is the evaluative or judgmental type of feedback, which is not considered beneficial to either the sender or receiver. Interpretative feedback attempts to state the message in a different way or to explain the message.

Another response is a supportive response that encourages additional messages from the original sender. Probing feedback seeks more information about the message. Finally, understanding feedback usually indicates approval or identification with the original sender or message.

Nonverbal Communication

Based on our discussion so far, it becomes apparent that communication can be both verbal and nonverbal. Verbal communication includes tone and emphasis. Nonverbal communication includes behaviors other than speech, such as gestures, body stance, position, eye contact, and facial expression. It has been suggested that 65 to 70% of a person's meaning is associated with his or her nonverbal activities. Even the distance between people communicates something. If indeed a part of the message is dependent on the relationship between sender and receiver, how close they are can communicate this relationship.

Cringle (1984) lists Hall's spatial relationships. Intimate or caring relationships are communicated by a distance of 18 inches or less, including direct body contact such as hand holding, hugging, etc. A personal relationship is expressed at a distance of 18 inches to four feet. Social distance is from four to twelve feet. A public relationship is expressed at a distance of twelve feet or more. These spatial relationships can also be used to explain the use of space in confrontation and other communication techniques. By placing oneself directly in front of and within 18 inches to four feet of an individual, one will be demanding attention. In placing a desk or table that averages three feet between two people, the communication that occurs will have to overcome this significant barrier. Additionally, the person behind the desk is communicating a message about the relationship.

Lamar (1985) emphasized the potential of communicating individual personal power through the use of nonverbal behavior. Included in nonverbal behavior is what is referred to as the management of impression. Through the use of nonverbal behavior, individuals determine to a large extent the impression made on other individuals or groups. Impressions are the result of eye contact. Frequent uninterrupted eye contact conveys the message of confidence and honesty. Impressions are also communicated nonverbally by appearance and means of adornment, such as jewelry and make-up.

An individual's posture can also communicate conditions that may influence an initial impression. Posture communicates an attitude toward people or objects. During interaction with an individual who may be regarded as a superior, an individual's posture may be more erect, even to the point of standing or sitting upright. Likewise, among peers or subordinates, an individual's posture may be more relaxed and include sitting or leaning back. Posture can also communicate the emotional state of the individual. The appearance of being tense can be communicated by rigidity in standing or being poised in a fixed position, or by sitting with arms and legs crossed.

Obviously, then, communication constitutes a significant portion of our existence within society. Communication enables us to learn or teach; to influence or to be influenced; to express feelings; explain or clarify; relate; accomplish a goal; reduce tension or conflict; or solve a problem (LaMonica, 1983). Through communication, we can dispense information, initiate requests, and advise or consent. In order to accomplish all these great and wonderful things, the nursing leader must possess communication skills. Sheridan, Bronstein, and Walker (1984) identify communication skills as encompassing a broad range of understanding, interpersonal relations, group dynamics, and organizational systems. Additionally, communication skills consist of mastery of the concrete aspects of communication: speaking, writing, listening, and all the other medias used in communication.

Effective Communication

Claus and Bailey (1977) stated that effective communication is based on three things. The credibility of the individual sending the message, the ability to send a clear message, and trust by the receiver are those things that contribute to effective communication. The enhancement of effective communication occurs as the result of a conscious effort to increase one's credibility, improving one's ability to send a clear message, and the development of trust. Leaders have high credibility with other people because their motives are clear. Role expectations for all parties in the relationship, including the leader's role, are clearly defined. Leaders are dependable in the sense that they stand their ground concerning basic issues and values. Leaders are effective communicators because of their ability to send clear messages. Frequently, leaders use more than one channel to communicate a message. The messages sent by leaders are usually complete and specific. The leader clearly assumes responsibility for the content of the message, which provides meaning and depth to the message. A leader develops trust in her relationships in a number of ways. Not the least of these is the use of feedback both to the leader and to the receiver. The leader also earns trust through her genuine concern for the welfare of the individual.

Tramel and Reynolds (1981, p. 186) identified four types of "I" messages that influence the effectiveness of the communication. All of these "I" messages communicate a more personal relationship because they disclose how the sender feels personally and imply a trust relationship with the receiver. An appreciative "I" message could be "I am glad" or "I'm happy...." Disclosing statements include "I value..., I feel..., or I think...." Information messages identify a need, "I need...," while declarative messages take a position, as in "I can, am, or will...."

Rowland and Rowland (1985) list eight strategies for effective communication. First, one should consider the objectives of the message in advance and then formulate a plan for communicating, which includes the answers to the who, what, when, why, etc. questions. One must formulate the message in a manner that is attuned to the receiver's self-interest as well as to the receiver's processing preferences. At the same time, one must be sensitive to differences in needs of others and their frame of references. Use of simple language that consists of the receiver's normal vocabulary is also important. Different channels should be utilized, and listening is especially important. Finally, one should follow up with a written form of the message.

An essential aspect of communication is listening. Listening means to pay attention, receive, or accurately perceive the message that is being sent. Rowland and Rowland (1985) described listening as being attentive, available, and accepting. There are two major barriers to listening. Our thought-speech processes, or the fact that our minds think faster than we either talk or process information, interfere with the ability to listen. The second major barrier to listening includes the receiver's preset attitudes, biases, and preconceptions. To overcome these barriers, it is necessary to be motivated to want to listen and then to listen with understanding (Rogers and Roethlisberger, 1983). When listening with understanding is the priority, there is not the impatience to make an evaluation, come to a conclusion, and begin talking. Rather, the priority involves concentrating on the message and the sender with no other immediate concern. Tramel and Reynolds (1981, p. 190) suggested lively listening as an active form of feedback. As a result of lively listening, one is able to let others know what is understood in regard to the message and to one's feelings. Leaders utilize listening as an effective communication skill in acquiring data, reinforcing the importance of the interpersonal relationship, and as a power tool.

Randsepp (1984) identified several listening skills that would enhance communication and decrease unnecessary conflict. Taking the time to listen seems like an impossibility in today's hectic society, but it will improve communication. The majority of people do not plan the purpose or content of their conversations, even when there is an important message to be communicated. As a result, it may take individuals a few statements before they are actually expressing the content they intended.

Interrupting is another barrier to effective listening. Individuals usually interrupt because they do not want to lose a point being made at that particular moment, or they have already reached a conclusion. Interrupting can also become a bad habit. By concentrating on the sender and the message, and by emphasizing the listening priority to be data gathering, the message may be completed by the time it occurs to the listener to interrupt.

By the listener considering it a responsibility to ensure good communication, reception of the message becomes a high priority. Included in receiving the message is listening to what is being said, as well as how it is being said. Not infrequently, the message can be obscured by an accent, speech impediment, or mannerism. Getting beyond these distractors is essential to effective listening. By concentrating on getting the message, a good listener does not jump to conclusions or make judgments. This listening skill is actually very difficult because the majority of people unconsciously tune out ideas that do not match theirs or that are perceived as threatening, and tune in to compatible ideas. This is illustrated by the fact that nurses may hear an infusion pump alarming halfway down the hall, but they may not hear the siren six blocks away that patients hear.

In addition to taking time to listen, listening between the lines can facilitate communication. People may initially converse about subjects that have created interest and kept the listener's attention on a previous occasion. Through the nonverbal communication technique of sitting down, the listener conveys to the message sender that he or she can talk about anything. By not responding with pat questions or answers and by concentrating on the message, accurate communication may truly begin. Finally, by listening with one's eyes, the messages being conveyed by the sender's nonverbal behavior can be received.

Types of Communication

There are a number of types of communication processes that can be useful skills for any nursing leader to possess. The ability to use confrontation can sometimes be a very effective way to resolve a conflict. Confrontation involves a direct approach between sender and receiver that focuses directly on the conflict issue. The confrontation message emphasizes "I" messages, not "you" messages or negative messages (Tappen, 1983).

The use of persuasion is another communication skill. In persuasion, there is discussion, not arguing. The other individuals are not labeled as wrong. Persuasion begins with agreement. The other concerned parties are encouraged to talk. These individuals are then credited for their contribution. A persuasive leader will use plenty of empathy and then dramatically present her idea in an enthusiastic manner, using a whole brain approach. The idea's ability to meet a specific need of those concerned is highlighted. The leader then uses questions to find out what is of interest or importance to others. The leader is willing to accept information and also disclose information about significant components of the idea. The persuasive leader is open, honest, and direct about her ultimate goal. Finally, she remains calm and repeatedly states her objective (Tramel and Reynolds, 1981).

Negotiation is the communication process that seeks a solution that is acceptable to all. Negotiation can occur concerning just about any matter that is not written in stone. This point is not always remembered by nurses who prefer to deal in absolutes. In reality, there are very few "absolutes" and therefore most things are negotiable.

The key elements that determine a successful outcome in a negotiation are power, time, and information. The amount of time is crucial. A negotiator should understand the time constraints of all involved parties and use this information to his advantage. Everyone has some form of deadline, either real or perceived.

The more information a negotiator has concerning the item of negotiation and the negotiators, the more effective a negotiator can be. More alternatives can be explored. The value associated with the item to the other parties is essential, whether the value be sentimental, economic, or time-invested. Ideally, all negotiations should end in some type of win-win solution. Unfortunately, "win-lose" is too real an outcome. Negotiation can usually occur when concerned parties are dealing from a perceived position of equal strength. The first step in the negotiation process is to identify the point of conflict. A leader will make the opening move by stating her position. This position should be extreme, well above the minimum, just short of ridiculous. Then follows a series of offers, counter offers, and elaboration that are frequently nothing more than smoke screens. When the bottom line is reached, the negotiation is complete (Tappen, 1983).

There are several strategies believed to be influential in the negotiation process. Emphasis should be on the similarities of those involved, as well as the importance and willingness for cooperation. Previous and current concessions should be pointed out. The sharing of information relevant to the negotiation is perceived as an act of good faith. Finally, the power to impose threats and rewards can be considered as an alternative. The question that then arises, however, is whether the parties are dealing from positions of equal strength and if it is true negotiation.

Levenstein (1984) emphasized several points to keep in mind during a negotiation. In addition to identifying the point of conflict, it is important to clarify the purpose or goal that the involved parties share. The negotiation must actually deal with the relevant issue, and not just a smoke screen. Terminology can be a problem during a negotiation because it is not unusual for individuals to use different words for the same thing, or use the same word for different things. Therefore, clarification of terms and actions is essential for a successful negotiation.

Negotiations occur in the reality of an environment composed of limited resources. Therefore, the emphasis on abstract principles or theories has little place in the actual negotiation. Listening is critical during negotiations because it enables the participants to identify potential trade-offs. Likewise, as a participant, you must clarify your own goals and consider both short term and long term consequences. Negotiations involve persuading the other party, not alienating them. As such, the use of logic communicates your perception of the other party's intelligence. Looking for integrated solutions communicates an attempt to satisfy the other person's real purpose. In order to satisfy the other person's real purpose, a negotiator needs to understand the other person's background, needs, goals, personal interests, feelings, and achievements.

Networking

Networking is considered a strategy for improving work performance, although the network phenomenon is not restricted to the work culture. The improved work performance results from the increased information exchange

and shared problem solving that occur via networks. Indicative of the
association with the work culture, networking was defined by Javonovich
and Tanguay (1980) as a process of building contracts to enhance job search
and success. Pancrazio and Gray (1982) defined networking as an exchange
based on favors, loyalties, and personal influences. A less restrictive definition of networks is the sharing of information and the creation of personal
linkages (Green, 1982). Networking involves a system of interrelated people
or groups, offices or work stations, linked together for information exchange
and mutual support (Harris, 1985).

The theory of networking is most closely identified with Granovetter's
Strength of weak ties article, published in 1973. The strength of an interpersonal
tie is a combination of the amount of time, emotional intensity, intimacy,
and reciprocal services that characterize the tie. Strong interpersonal ties
serve important personal and sociological functions. Weak ties also have
significance for individuals and society because they serve as bridges or the
only path between the majority of individuals. The results of several studies
support the proposition that more people can be reached through weak ties
than through strong ones. This is because strong ties result from a set of
dense relationships. When a few people know each other very well, they
tend to know the friends of each other very well. On the other hand, weak
ties are associated with a less dense network. Weak ties are more likely to
link members of different small groups than are strong ones, which tend to
concentrate within particular groups. Strong ties are perceived as increasing
local cohesion at the expense of isolation from other groups. Weak ties, on
the other hand, are essential to social integration.

As a result of this theory and additional work being done in network
analysis and sociometry, networks are receiving greater attention by individuals and groups from all aspects of society. Networking is regarded as a
growing phenomenon that provides a bridge among those with common
concerns. Lipnack and Stamps (1982) describe a network as a web of freestanding participants linked by one or more shared values. As a matrix of
exchange, networks help people to avoid or solve problems. Additionally,
networks provide a new form of social kinship that offers both social and
emotional support, advice, and intimacy. Some networks are now perceived
as having powerful social, political, or economic force to leverage on issues
relevant to their purpose for existence (Harris, 1985).

Networks have existed for some time, and many have evolved to formal
structures. The Million Dollar Roundtable in Illinois is a network of 23,000
insurance salespersons who qualify for this association through their sales
records. The Teachers' Centers Exchange (Devaney, 1982) has been operating
since 1975 and emphasizes five services. The Exchange provides information
and referrals to individuals and centers; publishes directories, essays, and
develops audiovisual material; recognizes participants through mini awards;
establishes work parties to cement the network ties; and serves as liaison
with organizations outside the network. These two formal networks are only
two examples of the types of networks that now exist. The Network Institute

(Box 66, West Newton, MA 02165) is a clearing house of people networks throughout the world.

Less formal, but nonetheless influential, are the "good ol' boy" networks that exist within most organizations. The strength of these weak ties, according to Henning and Jardim (1977), lies in the participants' knowledge that their individual success is ultimately tied to the success of the group. This network may be composed of individuals who would not be compatible for a close strong relationship. The network is effective because the weakness of the relationship enables the individuals to tolerate one another to accomplish individual or mutual goals. This "good ol' boy" network is usually difficult for women to understand because they have a tendency to emphasize interpersonal relationships, or strong ties. The strength of the relationships has always been important for women, which may help to explain their difficulty in promoting weak ties. Nevertheless, nursing leaders can benefit from helping to develop and participating in "good ol' girl" networks, as well as nonsexist networks and electronic networks.

Networks can be accomplished formally or informally, personally or electronically, locally or globally, externally or internally. Naisbett (1982) perceived informational networks as one of the forces shaping our future.

Personal networks are usually free-forming and adaptive. Harris (1985) provided several characteristics of these networks. In personal networks, relationships are both abstract and qualitative. The boundaries of the network are not clear, and participants function independently and autonomously. Power, responsibilities, and decision making duties are distributed among the network. Participants assume various roles in personal networks, depending on whether they are functioning as an entry point, end point, or link in the network. There is a shared value or concern that provides the glue for the network. There also appears to be a balance in terms of the integrity and importance of personal worth and collective purpose of the network.

Personal networks can be facilitated by individuals being willing to be open to differences in each other, promoting the sharing of unique opinions and insights, being understanding and encouraging, and being willing to share or be democratic. Networks are often formed as a result of membership in some type of professional, trade association, or special interest group. Initially, someone takes on the catalyst or "weaver role" to bring people of common concerns together, and thus a network is born (Harris, 1985).

The rapid developments in telecommunications have facilitated the formation of electronic information networks. These networks link offices and data bases together. Electronic bulletin boards can provide a way to establish networks of geographically diverse groups with common problems. Although the concept of electronic networking and telecommunications may sound futuristic for nursing, nursing leadership already possesses the expertise needed to achieve this form of communication. Similarly, nursing is accumulating data bases of significance to a variety of health care providers and related disciplines that could be shared via this form of network.

Networking is perceived as a powerful synergistic tool to be employed by leaders in order to remain well informed. It is a means for improving professional and organizational relations and for furthering career development. Networks can be formal or informal, but networks are essential methodologies of communication used by the successful nursing leaders.

Mentors

A mentor is a person who leads, guides, and advises a person more junior in experience (Darling, 1985). The topic of mentors and the associated mentoring that occurs have received a closer look by nursing leaders in the last few years as part of the search for ways to improve the quantity and quality of available nursing leadership.

Being a mentor or a mentee, the person receiving the attention of the mentor, involves being part of a significant relationship. There are three requirements of a relationship to be considered a mentoring relationship (Darling, 1984). First, the mentee must be attracted to the mentor. There must be admiration for the mentor, or a desire on the part of the mentee to emulate the mentor. Second, the individual serving as the mentor must be willing to invest time and energy in behalf of the mentee. Third, there need to be positive feelings toward the individuals involved in the relationship. These positive feelings are perceived as respect, encouragement, and support by the mentor and mentee.

As a result of the attraction, action, and affect involved in the mentoring relationship, a mentor assumes several roles (Darling, 1984). In the inspirer role, the mentor attracts the mentee by being either a model that the mentee values or admires; an envisioner who communicates a meaningful vision or goal to the mentee; or an energizer who stimulates the mentee through personal enthusiasm. Another major mentor role is that of investor. As an investor, the mentor expends resources to communicate knowledge, skills, and values to the mentee. In the supporter role, the mentor provides emotional encouragement and reassurance. As a result of this encouragement and reassurance, the mentee develops confidence and will consider risk-taking behaviors. A mentor may also assume a variety of subroles that are appropriate to the mentoring relationship. These roles include functioning as a standard setter, prodder pusher, teacher, coach, eye opener, door opener, idea bouncer, problem solver, career counselor, and challenger.

Mentors may be considered major mentors or minor mentors (Darling, 1984). Major mentors are classified as traditional mentors, step-ahead mentors, co-mentors, or spouse mentors. A traditional mentor is described as usually being older than the mentee and possessing sufficient experience in a career to give wise counsel. A traditional mentoring relationship is frequently experienced during the early part of the mentee's career. The step-ahead mentor is again usually older and wiser than the mentee. Unlike the traditional mentor who does not have to be in a direct superior position to the mentee or within the same organization, the step-ahead mentor is perceived as paving the way for the mentee to follow in his or her footsteps. A co-mentor relationship involves a peer in age and/or experience who engages in a reciprocal or mutual relationship. A spouse mentoring relationship may be unilateral or reciprocal. Mentor relationships of these various types are fairly extensive within the business world (Roche, 1979), but their prevalence in the nursing profession is just beginning to come to light.

Effective mentoring involves several elements (Moore, 1982). The accessibility of the mentor to the mentee, in terms of the amount of time together and the quality of the relationships, impacts on the effectiveness of the mentoring. The number of opportunities the mentee has to become visible or known within the chosen environment is another element. Feedback to the mentee also determines the effectiveness of the mentoring relationship. The degree of commitment to the mentoring relationship is highly critical to the effectiveness. The willingness to remain open and risk failure on the part of both parties also determines the effectiveness of the mentoring relationship.

Darling (1985) also described her Goldilocks theory of mentor matching, which determines the possibility for a mentoring relationship to occur, as well as the effectiveness of the relationship. The match or fit of mentoring is similar to the three variables of Goldilocks' too hot, too cold, or just right. The mentees' experience with authority figures could bias their perception and receptivity to a mentor relationship. The mentees' pattern of learning may not be congruent with the mentors' pattern of teaching. For example, the mentee may not need a highly structured environment, but the available and interested mentor may not have a compatible teaching approach. Finally, an individual may be at a stage of development at which a mentor is not needed, or the type of mentor such as a co-mentor may not be available. In these cases, minor mentor or self-mentoring strategies may be appropriate.

Minor mentors (Darling, 1985) are individuals who perform supportive functions. These supportive functions are more limited than those of a major mentor, but they may still ultimately contribute to career fulfillment. The supportive functions provided by minor mentors include intimacy, sharing, emphasizing the individual's self-worth, assistance, guiding, and directing.

Self-mentoring strategies are very similar to self-development techniques (Darling, 1984). These strategies are performed by the individual without the presence of the significant mentoring relationship. An individual may seek resources to assist in career development, such as writing to inquire about scholarships. Continuing education or other forms of self-learning are now available from journal and other sources. Increasing one's ability to listen, inquire, and observe are other strategies an individual may perform in mentoring of self.

Mentoring of nurse leaders is an effective strategy that will benefit nursing by preparing capable and talented individuals to assume highly visible positions within nursing. At the same time, it creates a legacy to mentor future nursing leaders and secure the position of nursing within society.

Communication Strategies

Gail Wolf (1986) pointed out that today's business, human relations, and nursing literature leave little doubt that effective communications are essential foundations to personal and organizational excellence and success. Under the prospective payment system, quality nursing care must be delivered at the lowest possible price. The cost of nursing care is directly related to productivity. Productivity is the result of several factors, two of which are job performance and job satisfaction. Communication directly affects how nurses perform their job in several ways. Recruitment affects the cost of nursing care and can be positively impacted by the communication atmosphere within the organization, as well as the communication atmosphere external to the organization. Retention also directly impacts on the cost of nursing care, and the communication atmosphere directly affects retention. Effective communication to consumers of nursing care is essential in order to demonstrate the efficiency and effectiveness of nursing services. Effective communication strategies consist of both internal and external strategies.

Internal strategies involve communication, the use of mentors, and the development of networks. Dr. J. D. Pincus (1986) identified three areas of communication that a nursing leader must address. Developing a positive communication atmosphere within the nursing organization can be accomplished through specific tactics. Promotion of an organizational structure to facilitate all forms of communication is one such tactic. Delegation of appropriate authority, accountability, and responsibility to the most appropriate level for that organization contributes to a positive communication atmosphere because it implies trust, acknowledges capabilities, and demands participation.

Head nurse and staff communication was the second area of internal communication Pincus (1986) found to impact on staff nurse performance. Facilitation of this relationship can be accomplished by the nursing service administrator's recognition of the importance of this relationship. Specific support includes providing mechanisms for the head nurse to acquire the necessary skills and knowledge to communicate with her staff. Additionally, acknowledgement of these role responsibilities as being significant includes allowing sufficient time and resources to meet these responsibilities.

Pincus' (1986) third area of internal communication involved nurses' need for frequent, constructive personal feedback. Regardless of their position, all nurses can benefit from regular performance appraisal, career counselling, praise, and recognition. Simple as this may sound, research has consistently demonstrated the lack of these elements within most nursing service organizations.

Another internal communication strategy involves the development of mentor relationships within the nursing organization. The lack of nursing leadership could be directly affected if nurses in administrative positions developed a commitment to serve as mentors to nurses aspiring to become nursing administrators.

The possibility of developing mentor relationships between nurses and non-nurses within the organization can also be pursued on a more formal basis. Mentorships with non-nurses increase communication across disciplines, increase the knowledge base of the individuals involved, and contribute to the recognition of shared values.

Networking strategies within a nursing department and health care organization also improve communication. As more and more bridges occur, knowledge is more effectively used. The development of networks of individuals across units or departments involved with the management of Diagnosis-Related Groups (DRGs) can increase productivity. Likewise, the encouragement of network development across levels of employees can result when such groups of employees are regularly given the opportunity to interact.

External strategies to enhance communication can be both formal and informal. The nursing service administrator must be knowledgeable about the use of the public relations department in promoting the image of the nursing service organization. The image of the nursing service organization is also affected during communication activities of nursing students and nursing recruitment activities. The nursing administrator's availability and ability to participate in media interviews constitute one strategy to increase communication proactively with the public (Sevel, 1986).

Mentorships external to the organization can be more difficult than internal ones, but these mentorships can facilitate developing the nurse leader in an area that is relevant to her career goals, or expansion in her current role. Networking external to the organization can be an effective personal and professional communication strategy. Networks of women executives or nursing leaders in similar positions can provide resources and referrals for problem solving and career advancement. Professional networks enable nurses to save time and resources, as effective and efficient methods of nursing care can be shared between health care institutions. Similarly, data can be compiled from many sources to substantiate research activities. Networks can also serve to encourage individuals to consider nursing as a career choice. Membership in community organizations, as well as appointment to public boards, creates a weak tie to many individuals who otherwise have no bridge to nursing.

The successful nursing leader striving to establish a standard of excellence for the areas of her responsibility will actively acquire communication skills and implement communication strategies in order to achieve this level of excellence. Communication is the essential link of one individual to the rest of the world. Thus, it becomes the single most important process for the nursing leaders to understand, utilize, and promote. As our society evolves and the health care priorities of our society mandate continuing changes, communication is the vehicle to keep abreast of and meet these times.

GROUPS AND ORGANIZATIONS

Introduction

This section discusses the concepts of groups and organizations. Understanding group dynamics and being able to function effectively within organizations are obviously essential capabilities of any nurse leader. The health care sector is changing dramatically and drastically. Organizations are diversifying and becoming more complex in an effort to adapt to these changes in the health care demands of society. The design of the successful health care organization of the future has not yet been identified because of the current rate of change. However, there are some reports (Gardner, Kyzr-Sheeley, and Sabatino, 1985) and some suggested structures (Coleman, Dayani, and Simms, 1984) to use as springboards. Like a volcano erupting, the shape of the mountain afterwards is not yet clear and the way is open to molding the future by those brave enough to take a risk.

Despite the rate of change within health organizations, nursing leaders can achieve their expertise within current groups and organizations. The previously successful centralized and decentralized organizational structures are giving way to elaborate matrix organizations. Understanding these organizations as the basic elements of a system helps to simplify how these newer organizations function. Applying the concepts of system theory and group dynamics will assist the nurse leader in designing a thinner and flatter organization to accomplish the department's objectives in the future. This section presents characteristics found within most groups and organizations. The development of groups, which follows a predictable pattern, will also be discussed. Any discussion of groups should also include a section on group roles, including the leader role. For a nurse leader, a group may be composed of either a group of individuals from the professional orientation or a group of interdisciplinary members. The latter presents a slightly more difficult situation than a homogeneous group. However, a more homogeneous group may be more prone to develop a "group think" mentality or a reluctance to think independently of the group.

Groups

Discussions of groups and organizations generally utilize systems theory as a basis for discussion. Systems theory basically defines a system as being composed of two or more elements in interaction that are differentiated by identifiable boundaries and distinct from their environment. An open system is characterized by input, throughput, and output energy cycles. The total energy consumed by any organization or system is utilized in either task accomplishment or system maintenance (McFarland et al, 1984). Most large systems or supersystems have contained within them smaller systems or subsystems.

Health care organizations are considered complex open systems that have several well known characteristics. Within these complex open systems are numerous subsystems that may be either organized departments or informal groups. Within these health care organizations, there are usually well established routine events and formal processes. The majority of the elements are interdependent on one another. Individuals are identified distinctly by their position, function, status, and power. Information from both within and without the organization is used to regulate the functions of the organization and make its decisions (McFarland et al, 1984).

There are several models of group development. These include linear, cyclical, pendular, and life cycle models. However, most of these models incorporate five basic stages within the model. For discussion purposes, the five stages identified by Tuckman and Jensen (1977) will be used in this text.

The first stage experienced by most groups, whether small or large, formal or informal, is the *forming* stage. There is a general feeling of uncertainty and insecurity during this time. This is due to the lack of definitive boundaries of the group, as well as to the lack of clearly defined roles of the individual members of the group.

The second stage is called the *storming* stage. The honeymoon is over, and individuals are not interested in being polite. As individual roles are tested and defined, there is an increase in the amount of tension and conflict. At the same time, because of the greater expression, common bonds can be identified. Following the storming stage, most groups go through a *normative* stage, which provides a sense of relief to the individual members. Because roles are now defined, goals can be set and individuals have a better understanding of what their contributions are to those goals. The group is calmer now and follows an established pattern to some degree. It is at this point that groups enter the *performing* stage, which is the truly productive stage of any group. The atmosphere, although comfortable, is goal oriented and positive. The individuals feel comfortable as members of the group.

The final stage of a group's development is called the *adjourning* stage. This stage is only recently receiving the same amount of attention as the other stages as its contribution to the individual member becomes more apparent. Previous group research emphasized the work and product of groups. More recently, the contribution of group membership for individual members' personal growth and satisfaction has become more apparent. The adjourning stage allows for attention to both elements of production and personal satisfaction. A period of time allocated for adjourning of a group permits closure to occur, a formal signal of the end. Depending on the situation, the end of a group's work can mean any number of things to an individual, whether pleasant, unpleasant, or mixed. Without a period to adjourn, individual members may be left with feelings of dissatisfaction and uncomfortableness. Adjournment also allows for feedback and evaluation of the group's work and product.

Groups as organizations are considered another form of an open system. Composed of at least three people, groups can be either formal or informal. Groups are characterized by a common bond, which is usually the purpose of their existence. There is close physical proximity in that the group physically meets together, which is not necessarily true of an organization. Within this physical proximity, group members interact with one another. Although all groups are composed of individuals, the characteristics of a group are different than the characteristics of the individuals (Tappen, 1983).

Group characteristics have a significant impact on how the group matures and performs. The group background contributes to the effectiveness of the group. Why was the group formed? Are the members coming from a common department, or do they represent a cross section of the entire organization or corporation? The background of the group sets the stage for the existence of the group, and these factors that contribute to the background of the group are important.

The group climate also impacts on the group. Consider whether the climate is one of crisis or calmness. A longstanding group can also suffer from a stagnating climate.

Group norms are those rules that are accepted by the members of the group as being legitimate. These norms may include such housekeeping rules as smoking or eating during a group meeting. A group norm can also include processing functions such as speaking during a group meeting or written communication by the group. In either case, it is necessary to know what the group norms are, in order not to violate them. Violation of group norms can render the individual group member impotent.

The effectiveness of a group is also determined by the amount of cohesiveness the group can develop. Group cohesiveness is largely dependent on the individual characteristics of the group membership. Cohesiveness may occur faster and better when members have known one another prior to the group's existence. A common background can assist cohesiveness. Motivation of the individuals can also influence the cohesiveness of a group. Likewise, group goals have an impact on group effectiveness. If the group goal is the allocation of limited resources, the strategies of the individual members may be quite different than when the goal is planning for a party.

The characterization of the group participation is determined largely by two elements: communication patterns and roles assumed by group members. Communication as a concept is covered in another section. Types of communication within a group are discussed in terms of patterns, forms, and agendas.

Communication patterns within groups are illustrated diagrammatically. LaMonica (1983) presented three classic communication networks that occur in groups (Fig. 5–3). The nurse leader should recognize the pattern used

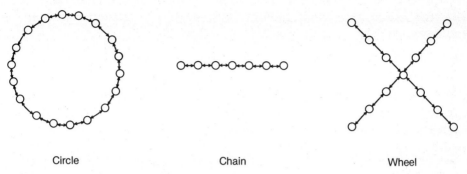

Circle   Chain   Wheel

FIGURE 5–3. Group communication network. (From LaMonica, E. L.: Nursing Leadership and Management: An Experiential Approach. Wadsworth Health Sciences, 1983, p. 145. Reprinted by permission of the present publisher, Jones & Bartlett Publishers, Inc.)

most frequently by a group. The importance of using different patterns at different times to achieve different purposes is also very relevant.

A circle network is not very efficient, nor accurate. It is difficult to identify the leader. Nevertheless, because of the involvement of each member, there can be a sense of satisfaction as well as an ability to adapt to a change. The chain network is more efficient than a circle network because no time is taken for extensive feedback. It is considered fairly accurate but low in member satisfaction and adaptability to change. Leadership may be more demonstrable in this communication pattern than in the circle network. The wheel communication pattern lends itself to leadership by the flow through a central person. Performance is usually efficient and effective. Individual satisfaction and adaptability to changes are considered low in this communication network pattern (Bavelas and Barrett, 1951; Leavitt, 1951). A nurse leader can employ these different communication network patterns, among others, depending on what she is attempting to control within the group.

Research about the different roles assumed by individuals within groups has been quite extensive. Transactional analysis (TA) is a method used to study behavior between individuals (Burne, 1964, 1972) and is frequently the basis for a discussion of group role. In TA, the three roles identified are parent, child, and adult. A group member can communicate in whatever person she chooses. Obviously, the communication that occurs between individuals behaving in adult roles is the preferred occurrence. Realistically, the nurse leader recognizes that group members communicate in different persons at different times, and it may be necessary for the leader to utilize different roles herself in order to be effective. The role of parent, child, or adult is not considered a particularly good or a particularly bad role within a group.

Another popular set of roles for nurses to assume is that of victim, rescuer, or persecutor. These roles, unlike parent, child, or adult, are rarely, if ever, desired roles within groups. They should be regarded as loser roles and avoided.

Tappen (1983) classified roles into three groups. Functional task roles are those roles that contribute to the completion of group tasks. Examples of these roles are initiator, contributor, information giver or seeker, opinion giver or seeker, disagreer, coordinator, elaborator, energizer, summarizer, procedural technician, and recorder. Individuals who assume these roles are considered as constructive members of the group because of their ultimate contribution to the evolution of the group through its stages. In specific instances, however, the disagreer or opinion giver may not be perceived so optimally.

Group building roles are the second group of roles classified by Tappen (1983). Individuals in group building roles encourage and support the group functioning as a whole, as well as encourage and support the individual members of the group. As such, these individuals are usually appreciated by the group members. These group building roles include the encourager, the standard setter, the gatekeeper, the consensus taker, the diagnoser, the expresser, the tension reliever, and the follower.

The third group of roles classified by Tappen (1983) are the individual roles. These roles do not contribute to the group in any way but rather detract and destroy group process and group goal achievement. As such, they are not appreciated by groups, and group members usually look to their leader to be effective in diffusing these individual roles. Most nurse leaders have experienced the aggressor, the recognition seeker, the monopolizer, the dominator, or the block player. These individuals can be very difficult to control. A nurse leader can learn effective strategies through the use of role playing.

The group leader has responsibility to the group. One such responsibility is to establish a clear understanding of the purpose and goals of the group as quickly as possible. This assists the group to move out of the forming stage and through the storming stage more quickly. A leader needs to have the ability to communicate effectively with the individuals of the group, understand the communication process, and interpret both communication content and process. Establishing the optimum balance of these skills in the group leader enhances group cohesiveness that is not at the expense of individual's freedom. A group leader maximizes the use of the different abilities of the individual group members. Finally, a group leader must know how to effect optimum decision making and secure the commitment of the members to those decisions (Lippett and Seashore, 1980).

The need for the development of effective group methods has resulted in professionals from a wide range of disciplines entering the field with approaches originating from various theories and practices. The Tavistock method (Grosling, 1967) refers to a diversified portfolio of approaches being developed and tested by members of the Tavistock Clinic and Institute in Britain. Utilizing psychodynamic principles derived from object relations theory as it applies to group functioning, and group dynamic principles, this approach is within the context of group psychotherapy.

There are several basic assumptions concerning the activities of a group and the roles assumed by the leader of the group underlying the Tavistock method. Small groups are engaged in two tasks simultaneously. The first task is the accomplishment of the stated purpose of the group. The second task of the group involves the satisfaction of emotional needs that are obscure and largely unacknowledged by the individual members.

Leadership of a group is dependent upon the needs of the group to accomplish these two diverse tasks. As a result, a successful leader acknowledges and works with the unstated task of the group in order to simultaneously achieve the stated purpose of the group. Therefore, a leader of a small group has five distinct functions or responsibilities. The leader functions as an expert, both in terms of how emotional needs can be manifested in group behavior, as well as in terms of goal achievement. The leader has a role in maintaining the boundary of the group. As a boundary keeper, the leader has to possess both an internal perspective of the group's two activities as well as an external perspective. As a teacher, the leader educates group members largely through the manner in which the leaders treat the group processes and the individual members. The leader also functions as the designator of the model or framework the group will use. As such, the leader does not impose his own order, but accepts and works with the order arising from the dynamics of the group. Finally, the leader has an important function as a listener (Grosling, 1967).

Stogdill and Coons (1957) formed four Ohio State leader styles that leaders may utilize to achieve group process. The correct style is dependent on the unique group and must be chosen appropriately. The styles are composed of two components: structure and consideration. Structure consists of organization, delegation, and decision making processes. Consideration refers to the interpersonal aspects of group process.

One of the four styles is the high structure, low consideration style. This style can be very effective in situations in which speed and efficiency are a priority. A high structure, high consideration style is very effective in situations in which a leader is dealing with a short term group that is composed of individuals inexperienced in group process. Another leadership group style is the high consideration and low structure style. This style is effective in a group consisting of a homogeneous group of individuals who are well experienced and skilled in group process. Another example may be a situation in which the goal is open ended or the process extended. The last style of leadership is the low structure and low consideration style. This is considered an effective style when little leadership is desired and group members can be free to evolve to their own decisions in their own time.

Within the leadership role of groups, research has identified the existence of sex role bias (Beauvais, 1977). This research has identified that group members, both male and female, perceive the task of leadership as a masculine role. Maintenance roles, such as those identified as group building roles, are perceived as female roles by group members. Whenever a female assumes a leadership role, it creates some tension among group members. Obviously, this research is not applicable to groups within a nursing service department, which is usually over 90% female. But it is noteworthy for the nurse leader who finds herself frequently involved in groups outside of nursing. In this situation, the group may be composed of members from a variety of disciplines.

There are four factors that the nurse leader must also take into consideration about the group in this situation. First, there is a difference in the vocabularies used by individuals of the group. Second, there is a difference in uniqueness of the professional concepts. Third, there are different levels of knowledge among the individuals in the group. The fourth factor deals with the ethno-cultural differences that are present among the individuals in the group. These four factors can significantly affect communication within the group and thus must be considered by the group leader and group member (Epstein, 1982; Castillo, 1981).

Organizational Theory

Formal organizational theory is founded in Max Weber's bureaucratic theory. Weber believed that a monocratic bureaucracy was capable of attaining the highest degree of efficiency and was superior to all other forms in stability and discipline. This ideal perception of bureaucracy by Weber arose out of contrast to feudalism, the only other organizational form known at the time, the early 1900's. Clark (1985) ascribed the popularity of Weber's bureaucratic theory to its fit with the problem-solving model of the administrators, its emphasis on rational-legal authority, and Weber's theory linkage of capitalism and Protestantism. Weber's theory was based on rational grounds that included (1) an organization bound by rules, (2) a systematic division of labor, (3) necessary authority to carry out functions, (4) a hierarchy of offices, (5) competency, and (6) knowledgeability. This bureaucratic theory lent itself well to both organizational research and practical implementation.

The Getzel-Guba model is a popular organizational model with roots in Weber's theory, which proposed that an organization consisted of two dimensions. The first dimension consisted of the institution with its roles and role expectations. The second dimension consisted of the individual with his personality and needs. Social behavior in an organization, according to the Getzel-Guba model, is derived from the interaction of these two dimensions.

There followed a decade of research and writing on human relations within organizations defined by Weber's bureaucracy. The resulting work in management theory has been classified into several historical phases. The first of these phases is called the classical management phase, which is estimated to have begun around 1910 and is closely identified with the work of Frederick Taylor. Principles resulting from Taylor's work included the development of the ideal or best way to accomplish a task. The best way was the result of an in-depth analysis that included time and motion studies. A second major principle was the selection of the right person for a job, and the training of that person in the best way. Combining the right worker with the right way, and using incentives to overcome worker resistance to the change, resulted in both increased production and increased earnings for the worker. Another important principle was cooperation between managers and workers, with the managers being responsible for the planning and preparation of work.

Other major contributors to management theory during this period were H.L. Gantt (1916), Harrington Emerson (1912), and Frank and Lillian Gilbreth. It was through F. Gilbreth's efforts that bricklayers' movements were reduced from 18 to 5 movements, and thus output was improved from 120 to 250 bricks per hour. Within this classical management phase, these contributors were frequently regarded as being concerned with rational or scientific techniques (Filley, House, and Kerr, 1976).

While the contributors noted above focused upon production, Henri Fayol was studying organizations in France. Fayol, a French industrialist, concentrated on explaining the workings of the administrative levels of the organization. There were 14 principles of management that Fayol felt could be universally applied to any type of organization. Although Fayol wrote his work in 1916, it was not available in America until 1930 (Filley, House, and Kerr, 1976).

The human relations theory phase occurred with a wave of enthusiasm for personnel management that occurred after World War I, and the labor relations movement that developed in the 1930's. The focus of the human relations theory was on the worker's feelings, beliefs, perceptions, and ideas. Considered by many to be the landmark occurrence of this phase, studies conducted at the Hawthorne Plant of the Western Electric Company resulted in the classic *Management and the Worker*, by Roethlisberger and Dickson in 1939. The findings from the Hawthorne studies suggested that a management approach that balanced efficiency and morale would probably be the most effective approach (Filley, House, and Kerr, 1976).

Behavioral science research came into popular use in the 1950's, although major contributions were published in the 1940's. The three levels of behavioral science focused on the individual, the group, and total organization behavior. Chester Barnard's work served as a landmark contribution to the organization theory. *The Functions of the Executive*, published in 1938, is considered a classic. Barnard tied the needs of the organization to the needs of the individual, and stressed cooperation as the main way to achieve both individual and organization success. Many of Barnard's ideas concerning organizational structure and the use of sociological concepts to management were expanded upon by Herbert Simon, author of *Administrative Behavior* (1947). These theorists perceived the organization as a system of deliberately coordinated activities of two or more people. Efficiency and effectiveness were of equal importance in determining the survival of an organization.

Informal organizations are a necessary component of any formal organization, and contribute to communication and cohesiveness within the organization (Filley, House, and Kerr, 1976).

Mary Parker Follett stressed the group principle in her works, because she believed that the group took precedence over the individual. Participation, communication, cooperation, and shared authority were characteristic of the concepts found in her writing (Hodge and Anthony, 1982).

Another major contributor to the behavioral school was Douglas McGregor and his Theory X and Theory Y of human motivation. Other behaviorists discussed in more detail in the section on motivation include Abraham Maslow and Frederick Herzberg.

The operations research or systems research phase in organizational theory occurred during World War II. The focus in this phase is on the use of quantitative analysis. Theories from mathematics, statistics, and economics were frequently adapted for use in studies during this period. The human element was de-emphasized and concentration was on the properties of the operation, which would not change even if the human variable changed (Filley, House, and Kerr, 1976).

The concept of heterarchy has been an important force within the development of organization theory. Schwartz and Ogilvy (1979) described heterarchical order in terms of a net of mutual constraints and influences. This concept has provided an antagonistic and challenging view of the hierarchial concept present in Weber's bureaucratic theory. As a result, heterarchial order has served as a stimulus for further research into these two concepts.

Clark (1985) has summarized the evolution of organizational theory with the following conclusions:

1. Traditional or classic organization theory, which Clark attributes as originating in Max Weber's bureaucratic theory, has fit the belief system of Western society so completely that it has stood the test of time.

2. Diverse organization perspectives, such as expectancy, need, and contingency theories, remain only modifications of the classical Weberian theory.

3. Contemporary theorists, aided by contributions from the social and behavioral sciences, are beginning to provide alternative views of the organization.

A contingency theory has also been proposed. Contingency theory proposes that there is no one best way or fixed framework because goals, technical tasks, accessibility to clients, and the organization itself vary in complexity. Organization theory development has benefited from emphasis in several key areas within the make-up of an organization. The importance of goals to organizations has received significant attention. Different internal organizational structures are caused by the degree of complexity in the environment. Organic and dynamic systems are in response to a fast-changing environment, whereas stable organizations result from stable environments. According to contingency theory, organizations can change their form, and managers have some control over their destiny. Contingency theory specifies what to look for inside the organization, identifies the complexity of specializations and the amount of uncertainty in the decision process, and then designs information systems to fit this environment.

Galbraith (1973) also proposed a theory that included the same cause and effect concept embodied in the contingency viewpoint. According to his theory, all organizations must develop internal jobs and communication systems to fit the complexity of the environment. This theory includes concepts of organizational stage of maturation. An organization matures into an increasingly complex organization, and this maturity is usually the result of a crisis that occurs at the end of each stage. Contingency theory has been considered to be more concerned with the current state of the environment, whereas the Galbraith model accounts for longer periods of organizational growth (Hampton, Summer, and Weber, 1982).

Aldrich (1979) and McKelvey (1982) are credited with contemporary population ecology models in organizational theory. These theories are derived from Darwin's *Origin of Species* and from Herbert Spencer's application of Darwin's concepts to the evolution of social organizations. A classification based on organizational differences is proposed for different organizational populations. A process of variation has caused these species to be different. Given these variations, and given the fact that there are not enough resources in society to support any and all organizations, society engages in a natural selection process. Society selects the organizations that best fit society's needs and retains them. According to the population ecology view, managers do not have direct control of whatever causes organizational success. Rather, it is the environment that determines the survival of the fittest. Managers can create structural variations that can result in a superior fit of goals and activity systems to the environment. This view is in sharp contrast to the strategic view of organizational evolution (Hampton, Summer, and Weber, 1982).

The concept of organizations, environment, and strategic choice is central to strategic theory. The strategic view of organizational evolution holds that managers have unlimited choice to select what kind of environment the firm will operate in, and have choice to shape the organization form to match present and future environments. Internal resources of the organization and external outputs are of equal importance in strategic theory. The concept of environment is multidimensional, which differs from the contingency emphasis on the environment's complexity. Time span, within the strategic viewpoint, deals with the very long term life cycle of organizations.

Strategic choice consists of two kinds of decision behavior, policy formation and strategy formulation. These behaviors are performed simultaneously and relate to each other through the processes of elaboration, reformulation, institutionalization, and interdependence. Elaboration occurs when strategies are developed into more specific detailed actions. Reformulation is the focusing on a particular portion of a strategy that is causing problems. Institutionalization is the slow assimilation by clients, suppliers, and organizational members of a new culture. Interdependence occurs when strategists connect bits and pieces during policy formulation in a logical, progressive way to enact their strategic choice. As a result, strategists conceptualize holistic, comprehensive visions of all elements of organization form (i.e., products, markets, and internal competencies) and formulate pieces of strategy to align with the ever-changing environment (Hampton, Summer, and Weber, 1982).

Most recently, McFarland (1986) proposed the development of macromanagement theory as a paradigm for organizational theory. Today's organizations are increasingly managed with reference to their roles as social institutions. Macromanagement theory suggests that greater attention to interorganizational relationships can help manage the organization, as well as the enormous complexities of the world.

Organizations

Organizations, like groups, can be discussed from an open systems perspective. Nadler and Tushman's (1980) model for diagnosing organizations provides a useful way to think about health care organizations (Fig. 5–4). The major input variables include the environment, resources, and history of the organization. The environment places constraints, makes demands, and provides opportunities for the organization. The amount, type, and quality of resources available to an organization have significant impact on the product of the organization. Recognition of the impact of the organization's history, including critical events, previous decisions, and evolving values, is an especially attractive feature of this particular model. Strategies concerning the goods and services of the organization are developed within the context of these inputs.

The key elements of the organization are the task, the individuals, the formal organization arrangements, and the informal organization. The outputs of this organizational system are goods and services that are produced at the individual, group, or organizational level. The emphasis of this model is on the fit or congruence among all of the different variables. The majority of all organizational structures can be analyzed using this model. When viewed in this context, it is easier to identify the function of any one group or individual and how they contribute to the goods and services produced by the organization. This model, then, has a potential to help reduce conflict among individuals or groups within an organization because it enables them to visualize their interdependence within the system.

There is a perspective, not illustrated by this model, that can contribute to conflict or incongruence between individuals and subunits within the organization. This perspective involves the orientation to the task by the individual or group performing the task. Even though the task may ultimately contribute to the outcome of the organization, because the emphasis, out-

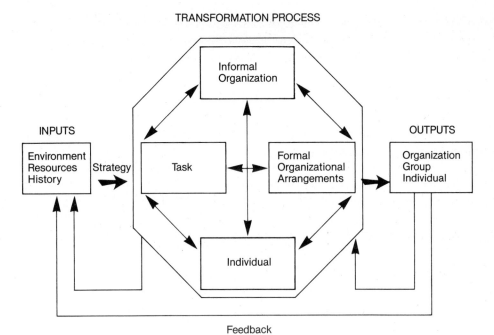

TRANSFORMATION PROCESS

FIGURE 5–4. A congruence model for organizational analysis. (Nadler, D. A., and Tushman, M. L.: A Model for Diagnosing Organizations. Reprinted, by permission of the publisher, from ORGANIZATIONAL DYNAMICS, Autumn, 1980. © 1980, American Management Association, New York, All rights reserved.)

come, and standard of evaluation differ, there remains potential conflict among the individuals or groups within the organization.

There are six orientations to the task that can be held by groups or individuals within the organization. The *professional* orientation is frequently ascribed to the medical or nursing staff. The target of these groups is the needs of the client, and efforts are directed at the reduction or elimination of the client's problem. Success is determined by the individual characteristics of the problem. A successful outcome can range from an uncomplicated newborn delivery to a pain-free death. Groups or individuals with a *bureaucratic* orientation perform their tasks with an emphasis on maintaining the integrity of the institution. As a result, success is determined by the proximity to maintenance of policies and procedures. A *craft* orientation concentrates strictly on the task for which individuals are responsible. The appearance of the product determines the success of the endeavor. Individuals or groups with *technical* orientation are preoccupied with the purpose of their task. Task completion or efficiency is valued by these people. For example, biomedical technicians or engineering department personnel have a much narrower perspective or emphasis on their role within a healthcare system than do nurses. *Service* oriented personnel are concerned with keeping clients satisfied and complying to meet the clients' demands. As a result, these people can often be at odds with individuals of technical or bureaucratic orientation. Finally, those individuals with an *entrepreneurial* orientation are primarily concerned with the profit maximization resulting from the task. These individuals may find themselves at odds with the professional and service individuals, among others (Georgopoulos, 1972).

This orientation perspective of the various individuals and groups found within organizations is offered so that the nurse leader or manager can use it in communication efforts. The tasks that are important to these individuals do vary, as do the targets of the tasks, the outcome resulting from the tasks, and the criteria whereby the tasks as well as the individual performing the tasks are evaluated. Armed with this knowledge, the nurse leader can communicate, emphasizing those aspects that are the most important and meaningful to the respective group. If these orientations are not taken into consideration, unnecessary conflict occurs because individuals or groups don't see eye to eye or appear to be working toward the same goal.

ORGANIZATIONAL STRUCTURE

Organizational structure divides tasks within systems and then promotes the coordination of the people involved in those tasks. Initially, there were functional organizations that were highly centralized. These organizations are still appropriate and are effective in limited application. As the size of an organization and complexity increased, decentralization of the organization was found to be very effective. Although decentralization was begun as early as 1921 by DuPont, it did not reach its height of popularity until the 1970's. Decentralization was perceived as being able to move responsibility and authority downward within the organization. A disadvantage of decentralization was a decrease in standardization. This disadvantage has become more pronounced in the 1980's, when increases in regulation and technology have required more standardization (Waterman, Peters, and Phillips, 1980).

As organizations have become even more complex and external forces have mandated better control, the matrix organization structure has developed. A matrix organization is a multiple command system. As such, it does not emphasize the division of tasks, which was the emphasis of the other models, but rather it emphasizes coordination and flexibility. The difficulty with a matrix structure is that individuals attempt to comprehend all the various dimensions and layers. The key to understanding matrix structures is the ability to zero in on those aspects of the organization that are the most critical at any given point in time. In other words, a matrix structure provides an even greater degree of flexibility for an organization to be responsive to a changing environment.

Matrix organizations have resulted in product line management. In other words, there is an organization around a given output. These types of structures encourage better information processing among individuals and groups involved in tasks contributing to a particular product. A matrix structure is believed to be more efficient in the use of resources because there is the potential for less waste. Another advantage promoted by this type of structure is that it leaves existing groups of employees intact yet encourages an interdisciplinary experience. Difficulties associated with this type of structure include its complexities, which can lead to dual authority, conflict, and confusion. It has also been successfully used to fragment nursing and regulate nursing to no higher than middle management authority. Figure 5–5 is an example of a segment of a current organizational structure that utilizes matrix concepts and demonstrates product line organization. The highest level of identified nursing authority is found in the middle, at the third level of the organization. Obviously, this is a step backward for nursing. As Stuart (1986) emphasized, nursing must be involved in high level decision making in order to enact power. This is difficult to accomplish at the third level of administration. It also denies the application of the concept of centrality and discourages interdependence, which are other sources of organizational power.

Fortunately, many organizations moving toward product line management utilize existing administrative personnel to initially enact this structure. As a result, vice presidents for nursing practice are assuming associate executive directorship positions. In reality, this is not changing their level within the organization. It does, however, alter their span of control. Although nurses functioning in associate executive director positions may no longer organizationally be responsible for all nurses within the organization, they do become accountable for other services. Functionally, these nurse associate executive directors may be responsible for all nurses, thereby retaining group identity to some extent. The institution is also able to meet JCAH requirements and can also attempt to retain the authority to standardize wherever desirable. The concern remains, however, that nurses may not recognize the need to seek these positions within their career alternatives. Poor preparation by nurses in these roles will quickly result in their replacement by health service administrators, of which there are many eager new graduates. Nurse leaders and managers have to be very careful about these organizational changes. But, more critical is understanding where and how nursing can make its major contribution to the organizational goals. The nurse leader must be clearly able to delineate why and how he or she is the most qualified to control patient services.

TOMORROW'S STRATEGIES

The problem that health care institutions face today is how to organize in order to effectively deal with a future that is both unstable and uncertain. Because the future is so ambiguous, the transition or movement in the direction of the future is inevitably also ambiguous. Because the end state is uncertain, the process of achieving it is also uncertain and therefore usually will take longer than a known process would take. As a result of this

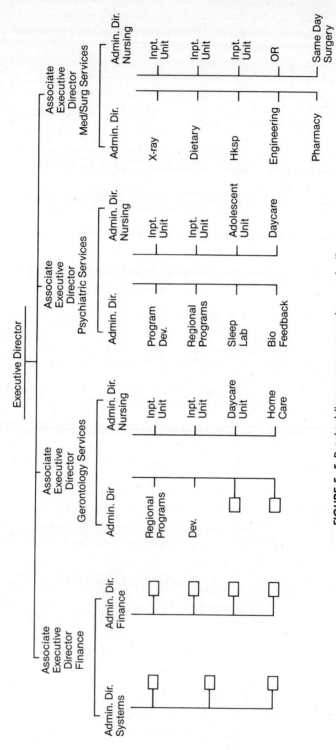

FIGURE 5–5. Product line management organization.

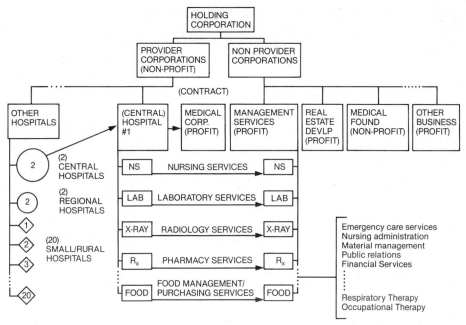

FIGURE 5–6. Super System—year 2000. (Reprinted with permission from Coleman, J. R., Dayani, E. C., and Simms, E.: Nursing Careers in the Emerging Systems. Nursing Management, *15*(1):19–29, 1984.)

uncertainty, the level of anxiety among all involved parties is greater and political activity increases. The increasing political activity, combined with the lack of defined direction, makes control immensely more difficult. All of these factors create a turbulent and very threatening environment that consumes an inordinate amount of valuable resources and time. Maintenance functions for the organization can fall by the wayside as a result of the emphasis on the future crisis. Yet, organizations cannot stand still (Nadler, 1982).

Organizational structures of the future will continue to evolve from the matrix model. As the size of various multi-hospital and multi-institutional systems grow, "super systems" will evolve, utilizing major matrix concepts (Fig. 5–6). At the same time, matrix concepts will formulate into temporary ad hoc models in an effort for organizations to increase flexibility and decrease response time. Successful organizations will be able to focus a temporary system for a limited time on a single priority or goal. This system will be able to effectively mobilize the best resources of the organization. When this system or temporary structure has achieved its purpose, it will be dismantled. At the same time, strategies to deal with the uncertain future states will also be required of organizations. These strategies include deliberate efforts to maintain a stable culture for employees (Waterman, Peters, and Phillips, 1980). In order to achieve this stability, the organization will need to instigate methods to shape and direct the political activity that occurs. Emphasis on constructive behavior in moving forward is another strategy. Moving forward in small steps, rather than in quantum leaps, can also be an effective strategy (Nadler, 1982). Finally, attention to the maintenance functions of the organization will help to promote a stable culture for the employees.

References

Leadership

American Academy of Nursing Task Force on Nursing Practice (1983). *Magnet hospitals: attraction and retention of professional nurses.* Kansas City, MO: ANA.

Baird, Jr., J.E. (1982). *Quality circles leader's manual.* Prospect Heights, IL: Waveland Press, Inc.

Calkin, J.D. (1980). Using management literature to enhance new leadership roles. *The Journal of Nursing Administration, 10*(4), 24–30.

Claus, K.E., and Baird, J.T. (1977). *Power and influence in health care: A new approach to leadership.* St. Louis: C.V. Mosby.

Collins, E.G. (ed.) (1983). *Executive success: Making it in management.* New York: John Wiley and Sons.

Diers, D. (1979). Lessons on leadership. *Image II* (3), 67–71.

Douglass, L.M., and Bevis, E.O. (1983). *Nursing management and leadership in action.* St. Louis: C.V. Mosby.

Epstein, C. (1982). *The nurse leader: Philosophy and practice.* Reston, VA: Reston Publishing Co.

Fiedler, F.E. (1967). *A theory of leadership effectiveness.* New York: McGraw-Hill.

Goble, F. (1972). *Excellence in leadership.* American Management Association.

Hersey, P., and Blanchard, K.H. (1977). *Management of organizational behavior: Utilizing human resources* (3rd ed.). Englewood Cliffs, NJ: Prentice-Hall.

Herzberg, F. (1966). *Work and the nature of man.* Ohio: World Publishing.

Hollander, E.P. (1978). *Leadership dynamics: A practical guide to effective relationships.* New York: Free Press.

Kotter, J.P., and Lawrence, P.R. (1979). *Mayors in action: Five approaches to urban governance.* New York. John Wiley and Sons.

LaMonica, E.L. (1983). *Nursing leadership and management: An experimental approach.* Belmont, CA:Wadsworth Health Sciences Division.

Leadership for improving instruction: 1960 Yearbook. Washington, D.C., Association for Supervision and Curriculum Development, 1960, p. 182.

McFarland, G.K., Leonard, H.S., and Morris, M.M. (1984). *Nursing leadership and management: Contemporary strategies.* New York: John Wiley and Sons.

Mintzberg, H. (1977). Folklore and fact: The manager's job. *Review,* January, 32–35, 66, 69.

Ouchi, W.G. (1981). *Theory 2: How American business can meet the Japanese challenge.* Reading, MA: Addison-Wesley.

Prentice, W.C.H. (1983). Understanding leadership. In Collins, E.G.C. (ed.). *Executive success: Making it in management.* New York: John Wiley and Sons, pp. 140–150.

Schein, E.H. (1970). *Organizational psychology* (2nd ed.). Englewood Cliffs, NJ: Prentice-Hall.

Schreisheim, C.A., Mowday, R.T., and Stodgill, R.M.: Crucial dimensions of leader-group interaction. In Hunt, J.G., and Larson, L.L. (eds.). *Crosscurrents in leadership.* Illinois: South Illinois University Press.

Stevens, B.J. (1981). The role of the nurse executive. *The Journal of Nursing Administration, 11*(2), 19–23.

Tannenbaum, R., and Schmidt, W.H. (1983). Effective leadership. In Collins, E.G.C. (ed.) *Executive success: Making it in management.* New York: John Wiley and Sons.

Tappen, R.M. (1983). *Nursing leadership: Concepts and practice.* Philadelphia: F.A. Davis.

Tramel, M.E., and Reynolds, H. (1981). *Executive leadership: How to get it and make it work.* 'Englewood Cliffs, NJ: Prentice-Hall.

Yura, H. (1984). Nursing leadership evaluation. *The Health Care Supervisor, 12*(3), 16–28.

Yura, H., Ozimek, D., and Walsh, M.B. (1981). *Nursing leadership: Theory and process.* (2nd ed.). New York: Appleton-Century-Crofts.

Zaleznik, A. (1977). Managers and leaders: Are they different? *Harvard Business Review*, May–June.

Power

Benziger, J.P. (1982). The powerful woman. *Hospital Forum*, May–June, 15–20.
Brown, J.C., and Kanter, R.M. (1982). Empowerment: key to effectiveness. *Hospital Forum*, May–June, 6–12.
Claus, K.E., and Bailey, J.T. (1977). *Power and influence in health care: A new approach to leadership*. St. Louis: C.V. Mosby.
Kalisch, B.J., and Kalisch, P.A. (1982). *Politics of nursing*. Philadelphia: J.B. Lippincott.
Kanter, R.M. (1983). Power failure in management circuits. *In* Collins, E.G.C. (ed.). *Executive success: Making it in management*. New York: John Wiley and Sons, pp. 249–266.
Kotter, J.P. (1983). Power, dependence and effective management. *In* Collins, E. G. C. (ed.). *Executive success: Making it in management*. New York: John Wiley and Sons, pp. 306–323.
Leininger, M. (1977). Territoriality, power and creative leadership. *Power—use it or lose it*. NLN Pub. 52–1675.
McClelland, D.C., and Burnham, D.H. (1983). Power is the great motivator. *In* Collins, E.G.C. (ed.). *Executive success: Making it in management*. New York: John Wiley and Sons, pp. 289–305.
Peterson, G.G. (1979). Power: A perspective for the nurse administrator. *Journal of Nursing Administration*, July, 7–10.
Sheflett, N., and McFarland, D.E. (1978). Power and the nursing administrator, *Journal of Nursing Administration*, March, 19–23.
Silber, M.B. (1981). Nurse power: Projecting self and ideas. *Supervisor Nurse*, July, 65–68.
Stevens, K.R. (1983). *Power and influence: A source book for nurses*. New York: John Wiley and Sons.
Stuart, G.W. (1986). An organizational strategy for empowering nursing. *Nursing Economics*, 4(2), 69–73.
Zaleznik, A. (1983). Power and politics in organizational life. *In* Collins, E.G.C. (ed.). *Executive success: Making it in management*. New York: John Wiley and Sons, pp. 267–288.

Decision Making

Dalkey, N. (1969). *The Delphi technique: An experimental study of group opinion*. Delphi, CA: Rand Corporation.
Delbecq, A., and Van de Ven, A. (1971). A group process model for problem identification and program planning. *Journal of Applied Behavioral Sciences*, July–August.
Douglass, L.M., and Bevis, E.O. (1983). *Nursing management and leadership in action*. St. Louis: C.V. Mosby.
Drucker, P.F. (1983). The effective decision. *In* Collins, E.G.C. (ed.). *Executive success: Making it in management*. New York: John Wiley and Sons, pp. 464–475.
Etzioni, A. (1967). Mixed scanning: A third approach to decision making. *Public Administration Review*, 27, 385–393.
Fishburn, P.C. (1979). *Utility theory for decision making*. Huntington, NY: Robert E. Krieger.
Greenwood, W.T. (1969). *Decision theory and information systems: An introduction to management decision making*. Cincinnati, OH: South-Western.
Hough, L. (1970). *Modern research for administrative decision*. Englewood Cliffs, NJ: Prentice-Hall.
Janis, I., and Mann, L. (1977). *Decision making: A psychological analysis of conflict, choice and commitment*. New York: Free Press.
Jedamus, P., and Frame, R. (1969). *Business decision theory*. New York: McGraw-Hill.
Kassouf, S. (1970). *Normative decision making*. (Prentice-Hall Foundations of Administration Series, H.A. Simon, ed.) Englewood Cliffs, NJ: Prentice-Hall.
Koberg, D., and Bagnall, J. (1974). *The universal traveler*. Los Altos, CA: William Kaufman.
Lancaster, W., and Lancaster, J. (1981). The leader as decision maker. *Nursing Leadership*, 4(4), 7–12.
McFarland, G.K., Leonard, H.S., and Morris, M.M. (1984). *Nursing leadership and management: Contemporary strategies*. New York: John Wiley and Sons.
Menges, G. (1974). *Economic decision making: Basic concepts and models*. London: Longman.
Osborn, A. (1979). *Applied imagination*. New York: Scribners.
Tappen, R.M. (1983). *Nursing leadership: Concepts and practice*. Philadelphia: F.A. Davis.

Motivation

Alderfer, C.P. (1972). *Existence, relatedness, and growth: Human needs in organizational settings*. New York: Free Press.

Aronson, E., and Carlsmith, J. (1962). Performance expectance as a determinant of actual performance. *Journal of Abnormal and Social Psychology*, 65, 178–182.

Atkinson, J.W., and Feather, N. (1966). *A theory of achievement motivation*. New York: John Wiley and Sons.

Becker, G., and McClintock, C. (1967). Value: Behavioral decision theory. *Annual Review of Psychology*, 18, 239–286.

Dawis, R., Lofquist, L., and Weiss, D. (1968). A theory of work adjustment (a revision). *Minnesota Studies in Vocational Rehabilitation*, 24, 1–263.

Deci, E.L. (1975). *Intrinsic motivation*. London: Plenum.

Edwards, M., and Powers, R. (1982). Turning staff frustration to satisfaction. *Nursing Management*, 13, 51–52.

Eysenck, M.W. (1982). *Attention and arousal, cognition and performance*. New York: Springer-Verlag.

Festinger, L.A. (1962). *A theory of cognitive dissonance*. Stanford, CA: Stanford University Press.

Freud, S. (1942). *The ego and the id*. London: Hogarth Press.

Futrell, C.M., and Parasuraman, A. (1981). Impact of clarity of goals and role perceptions on job satisfaction. *Perceptual and Motor Skills*, 52, 27–32.

Harvey, O.J., and Schroder, H.M. (1963). Cognitive aspects of self and motivation. *In* Harvey, O.J. (ed.). *Motivation and social interaction: Cognitive determinants*. New York: Ronald Press.

Heider, F. (1958). *The psychology of interpersonal relations*. New York: John Wiley.

Herzberg, F., Mausner, B., and Snyderman, B. (1959). *The motivation to work*. New York: John Wiley.

Hollon, S., and Garber, J. (1980). A cognitive-expectance theory of therapy for helplessness and depression. *In* Garber, J., and Seligman, M. (eds.). *Human helplessness: Theory and applications*. New York: Academic Press.

Hull, C. (1943). *Principles of behavior*. New York: Appleton-Century-Crafts.

Jones, E.E., and Davis, K. (1965). From acts to dispositions: The attribution process in person perception. *In* Berkowitz, L. (ed.). *Advances in experimental social psychology* (Vol. 2). New York: Academic Press.

Kelley, H.H. (1967). Attribution theory in social psychology. *In* Levin, D. (ed.). *Nebraska symposium on motivation* (Vol. 15). Lincoln: University of Nebraska Press.

Lewin, K. (1951). *Field theory in social science*. New York: Harper.

Maslow, A.H. (1954). *Motivation and personality*. New York: Harper and Row.

Maslow, A.H. (1968). *Toward a psychology of being* (2nd ed.). New York: D. Van Nostrand.

McFarland, G.K., Leonard, H.S., and Morris, M.M. (1984). *Nursing leadership and management: Contemporary strategies*. New York: John Wiley and Sons.

Monte, C.F. (1977). *Beneath the mask*. New York: Praeger.

Rotter, J.B. (1954). *Social learning and clinical psychology*. New York: Prentice-Hall.

Rowland, H.S., and Rowland, B.L. (1985). *Nursing administration handbook*. Rockville, MD: Aspen Systems Corp.

Scanlon, B.K. (1976). Determinants of job satisfaction and productivity. *Personnel Journal*, January.

Storms, M.D., and Nisbett, R.E. (1970). Insomnia and the attribution process. *Journal of Personality and Social Psychology*, 16, 319–328.

Timmreck, T.C., and Randall, G.J. (1981). Motivation, management and the supervisory nurse. *Supervisor Nurse*, March, 28–31.

Vroom, V.H. (1982). *Work and motivation*. Malabar, FL: Robert E. Krieger Publishing Co.

Weiner, B. (ed.) (1974). *Achievement motivation and attribution theory*. Morristown, NJ: General Learning Press.

Communication

Baird, J., and Baird, L. (1985). Key attitudes differ among nursing personnel. *Aspen's Advisor for Nurse Executives*, 1(3), 7–8.

Berlo, D. (1960). *The process of communication: An introduction to theory and practice*. New York: Holt, Rinehart and Winston, p. 72.

Burk, B., Gillman, D., and Ose, P. (1984). Brain research for educators. *The Journal of Continuing Education in Nursing*, 15(6), 195–199.

Burk, B., Gillman, D., and Ose, P. (1984). Nursing orientation: A whole brain approach. *The Journal of Continuing Education in Nursing*, 15(6), 199–204.

Claus, K.E., and Bailey, J.T. (1977). *Power and influence in health care*. St. Louis: C.V. Mosby.

Cringle, R.K. (1984). *Communication in nursing: From concept to practice.* Bowie, MD: Robert J. Brady Co.

Goble, F. (1972). *Excellence in leadership.* New York: American Management Association.

Kelly, L.S. (1985). The making of a nurse influential. *Nursing Outlook, 33*(6), 275.

Lamar, E.K. (1985). Communicating personal power through nonverbal behavior. *The Journal of Nursing Administration, 15*(1), 14–44.

LaMonica, E.L. (1983). *Nursing leadership and management: An experimental approach.* Belmont, CA: Wadsworth Health Sciences Division.

Levenstein, A. (1984). Negotiation vs confrontation. *Nursing Management, 15*(1), 52–53.

McFarland, G.K., Leonard, H.S., and Morris, M.M. (1984). *Nursing leadership and management: Contemporary strategies.* New York: John Wiley and Sons.

Pincus, J.D. (1986). Communication: The key contributor to effectiveness—The Research. *The Journal of Nursing Administration, 16*(9), 19–25.

Raudsepp, E. (1984). Seven ways to cure communication breakdowns. *Nursing Life, 4*(1), 50–53.

Rogers, C. (1965). Dealing with psychological tensions. *Journal of Applied Behavioral Science, 1*(1), 6–25.

Rogers, C.R., and Roethlisberger, F.J. (1952). Barriers and gateways to communication. *Harvard Business Review, 30*(4), 28–32.

Rogers, C.R., and Roethlisberger, F.J. (1983). Barriers and gateways to communication. In Collins, E.G.C. (ed.). *Executive success: Making it in management.* New York: John Wiley and Sons.

Rowland, H.S., and Rowland, B.L. (1985). *Nursing administration handbook.* 2nd ed. Rockville, MD: Aspen Systems Corp.

Selber, M.B. (1981). Nurse power: Projecting self and ideas. *Supervisor Nurse,* July, 65–68.

Sevel, F. (1986). Are you prepared to meet the media. *The Journal of Nursing Administration, 16*(3), 21–24.

Sheridan, D.R., Bronstein, J.E., and Walker, D.D. (1984). *The new nurse manager.* Rockville, MD: Aspen Systems Corp.

Springer, S.P., and Deutsch, G. (1981). *Left brain, right brain.* CA: W.H. Freedman and Co.

Tappen, R.M. (1983). *Nursing leadership: Concepts and practice.* Philadelphia: F.A. Davis.

Thiry, R.A. (1977). Relationship of communication satisfaction to need fulfillment among Kansas nurses. Unpublished doctor dissertation, University of Kansas.

Tramel, M.E., and Reynolds, H. (1981). *Executive leadership: How to get it and make it work.* Englewood Cliffs, NJ: Prentice-Hall.

Wolfe, G.A. (1986). Communication: Key contributor to effectiveness—A nurse executive response. *The Journal of Nursing Administration, 16*(9), 26–28.

Networks

Backwell, J.E. (1983). *Networking and mentoring: A study of cross-generational experiences of blacks in graduate and professional schools.* Atlanta: Southern Educational Foundation.

Devaney, K. (1982). *Networking on purpose.* San Francisco: Far West Laboratory.

Granovettes, M.S. (1973). The strength of weak ties. *American Journal of Sociology, 18*(6), 1360–1381.

Green, M.F. (1982). A Washington perspective on women and networking: The power and pitfalls. *Journal of NAWDAC,* (Fall), 17–21.

Harris, P.R. (1985). *Management in transition.* San Francisco: Jossey-Bass.

Hennig, M., and Jardim, A. (1977). Women executives in the old-boy network. *Psychology Today, 10*(8), 76–81.

Javonovich, J., and Tanquay, S.L. (1980). Networking. *Journal of Placement,* (Fall), 30–34.

Lipnack, J., and Stamps, J. (1982). *Networking: The first report and directory.* New York: Doubleday.

Pancrazio, S.B., and Gray, R.G. (1982). Networking for professional women: A collegial model. *Journal of NAWDAC,* (Spring), 17–21.

Mentors

Campbell-Heider, N. (1986). Do nurses need mentors? *Image, 18*(3), 110–113.

Darling, L.A. (1984). What do nurses want in a mentor? *The Journal of Nursing Administration, 14*(10), 42–44.

Darling, L.A. (1984). Mentor types and life cycles. *The Journal of Nursing Administration, 14*(11), 43–44.

Darling, L.A. (1984). So you've never had a mentor . . . not to worry. *The Journal of Nursing Administration, 14*(12), 38–39.

Darling, L.A. (1985). Mentor matching. *The Journal of Nursing Administration*, 15(1), 45–46.

Darling, L.A. (1985). *The Journal of Nursing Administration*, 15(3), 42.

Darling, L.A. (1985). *The Journal of Nursing Administration*, 15(4), 42–43.

Darling, L.A. (1985). *The Journal of Nursing Administration*, 15(9), 41–42.

Felton, G. (1978). On women, networks, patronage and sponsorship. *Image*, 10(3), 58–59.

Moore, K. (1982). The role of mentors in developing leaders for academe. *The Educational Leader*, (Winter), 23–28.

Roche, G. (1979). Much ado about mentors. *Harvard Business Review*, 57(1), 14–16, 20, 24–28.

Groups and Organizations

Aldrich, H. (1979). *Organizations and environments*. Englewood Cliffs, NJ: Prentice-Hall.

Bavelas, A., and Barrett, D. (1951). An experimental approach to organizational communication. *Personnel*, 27, 366–371.

Beauvais, C. (1977). Dilemmas for women in authority. Paper presented at the U.S. Commission on Civil Rights, Washington, D.C., September.

Bradford, L.D. (ed.) (1978). *Group Development* (2nd ed.). San Diego, CA: University Associates.

Christman, L. (1979). The practitioner-teacher. *Nurse Educator*, 4, 8–11.

Clark, D.L. (1985). Emerging paradigms in organization theory and research. *In* Lincoln, Y.S. (ed.). *Organizational theory and inquiry: The paradigm revolution*. Beverly Hills: Sage.

Coleman, J.R., Dayani, E.C., and Simms, E. (1984). Nursing careers in the emerging systems. *Nursing Management*, 15(1), 19–29.

Filley, A.C., House, R.J., and Kerr, S. (1976). *Managerial process and organizational behavior*. Glenview, IL: Scott, Foresman and Co.

Galbraith, J. (1973). *Designing complex organizations*. Reading, MA: Addison-Wesley.

Gardner, S.F., Kyzr-Sheeley, B.J., and Sabatino, F. (1985). Big business embraces alternate delivery. *Hospitals*, March 16, pp. 81–84.

Georgopoulos, B.S. (1972). *Organizational research on health institutions*. Institute for Social Research. Ann Arbor, MI: The University of Michigan.

Grosling, R. (1967). *The use of small groups in training*. New York: Grune and Stratton.

Hampton, D.R., Summer, C.E., and Webber, R.A. (1982). *Organizational behavior and the practice of management* (4th ed.). Glenview, IL: Scott, Foresman and Co.

Hodge, B.J., and Anthony, W.P. (1982). Early contributors. *In* Magula, M. (ed.). *Understanding organizations: A guide for the nurse executive*. Wakefield, MA: Nursing Resources.

LaMonica, E.L. (1983). *Nursing leadership and management: An experimental approach*. Belmont, CA: Wadsworth Health Sciences Division.

Leavitt, H. (1951). Some effects of certain communication patterns on group performances. *The Journal of Abnormal and Social Psychology*, 46, 38–50.

Lippett, G., and Seashore, E. (1980). *Group effectiveness: A looking-into-leadership monograph*. VA: Leadership Resources.

March, J.G., and Simon, H.A. (1958). *Organizations*. New York: John Wiley and Sons.

McClure, M.L. (1984). Managing the professional nurse. Part I. The organizational theories. *The Journal of Nursing Administration*, 14(2), 15–21.

McKelvy, W. (1982). *Organizational systematics: Taxonomy, evolution, classification*. Berkeley: University of California Press.

Nadler, D.A. (1982). Managing transitions to uncertain future states. *Organizational Dynamics*, 11(1), 37–45.

Nadler, D.A., and Tushman, M.L. (1980). A model for diagnosing organizations. *Organizational Dynamics*, Autumn, 1980.

Schwartz, P., and Ogilvy, J. (1979). *The emergent paradigm: Changing patterns of thought and belief*. Menlo Park, CA: SRI International.

Stogdill, R., and Coons, A. (eds.) (1957). *Leader behavior: Its description and measurement*. Research Monograph No. 88. Columbus, Bureau of Business Research, Ohio State University.

Tappen, R.M. (1983). *Nursing leadership: Concepts and practice*. Philadelphia: F. A. Davis.

Tuckerman, B.W., and Jensen, M.A. (1977). Stages of small group development revisited. *Group and Organization Studies*, 2(4), 419.

Waterman, Jr., R.H., Peters, T.J., and Phillips, S.R. (1980). Structure is not organization. *Business Horizons*, 23(1–3), 14–29.

NURSING LEADERSHIP THEORY

INTRODUCTION

This chapter presents a conceptual framework based on the work of Yura, Ozimek, and Walsh (1981), and of Epstein (1982), for discussing nursing leadership at the executive, middle, and first line levels within an organization. Nursing hierarchies vary from organization to organization and may consist of many or few layers of supervision. Three levels are discussed with the assumption that conceptualization, synthesis, and interpretation can be accomplished for individual and specific needs.

A presentation of leadership theories and leadership behaviors for nursing is based on the assumption that this knowledge and these behaviors are valued and expected by the nurse and the organization within which he is functioning. By this point in nursing's history, it would be expected that a leadership role is an accepted role within a health care institution. Unfortunately, there remain vestiges of the Dark Ages, in which administrators' and medical staffs' expectations continue to revolve around the "nurse" capabilities of the individual at various levels of the nursing organization. The emphasis on the leadership role as opposed to the nurse role depends to some extent on the level of organizational functioning. However, nursing leadership functions at all levels of an organization. Those organizations that

6

do not value leadership usually do not value leadership throughout the entire system, not just in nursing. Nevertheless, within these restrictive systems, leadership can be all but impossible. As a result, individuals with leadership capabilities will usually move on to more conducive environments.

THEORETICAL BASIS

Yura (1984) defined nursing leadership "as a process whereby a person who is a nurse affects the actions of others in goal determination and achievement." This process consists of "the behaviors of deciding, relating, influencing and facilitating." This definition encompasses the perspective of nursing leadership from both above and below the organizational level. A perspective of nursing leadership from staff nurses is presented in the American Academy of Nursing Task Force's *Magnet Hospitals* report (1983). Effective nursing leadership behaviors identified in that report included being knowledgeable, strong, qualified, supportive, accessible, and communicative. Claus and Bailey (1977) promoted a conceptual model of nursing leadership that was composed of power, authority and influence. These authors perceived nursing leadership as essentially a relationship. Within this relationship, actions occurred that influenced members within the relationship to move toward goal setting and goal attainment. Additionally, leadership included managerial and human relations behaviors, the use of influence strategies, and the wise use of power (p. 5). Douglass and Bevis (1983) explain this concept of leadership further:

> The leadership role is interactional in nature and cannot be learned or enacted out of the social context of complementary roles. In other words, every leader, to be a leader, must have someone, some group to lead. The role of being led is the role that complements the role of leader. A leader must learn not only the leadership behaviors that enable the assumption of the leadership role, but also the role of the led (p. 7).

Here again, one sees the concepts presented earlier. There is the identification of the concepts of goals, participant involvement, and the leader's behavior. These authors also subscribe to the understanding and use of authority, power, and influence by successful nursing leaders. Additionally, the effects of leader's and follower's personality, behavior, and situational factors are viewed as primary influences on the leadership style that will be effective. This is similar to the factors identified by Tannenbaum and Schmidt (1983) and the evolution of leadership theory to encompass the interaction of all of the variables involved in this phenomenon.

Epstein (1982) preferred to define leadership operationally in terms of a philosophy of life. To this end, she espoused a theoretical framework that utilized Maslow's concept of need hierarchy and self-actualization along with the concepts promoted through humanism. Leadership is a process in which individuals are encouraged and enabled to become the best they can be as the result of three groups of leadership behavior. These behaviors include rational thinking, education, and interdisciplinary communication. Although labeled somewhat differently, these groups of leadership behaviors contain the majority of the same behaviors identified through leadership research. Epstein emphasized the active, conscious, autonomous follower as carrying equal weight or emphasis with the leader in the leadership phenomenon. Additionally, Epstein incorporated most of the variables previously identified. These variables include the effect of the situation and organization, time of occurrence, importance of goal, and the potential for other group members to function as leaders. The main difference in Epstein's proposal appears to center around the argument against the use of power and authority. Although an interesting proposition, it is unique to this literature.

After reviewing this significant material on leadership and nursing leadership, it becomes apparent that except for consistent variables involved in the phenomenon, leadership theory continues to mature. There remains sufficient latitude to define leadership for each unique occurrence. How, then, can nursing, within a changing organizational setting, learn, apply, and grow, based on this knowledge base? There are several ways. First, nurses who aspire to be leaders should become familiar with the literature on leadership theory. Despite the lack of concreteness, leadership theory is widely read and utilized within formal organizations. Knowledge of specific concepts such as power and authority enables the nurse leader to evaluate the actions of those around him as well as himself. His leadership will undoubtedly be evaluated on the basis of these concepts. Before one can acquire skill and expertise, an individual must have a firm knowledge base.

Leadership theory may be evolving as a result of changes in our societies and cultures. Leadership theory attempts to describe, explain, and predict the phenomenon of leadership of human beings. Since humans and their societies are not static, neither will leadership be static. Therefore, nursing must be somewhat cautious about rigidly applying leadership theory to future situations. What adequately explained effective leadership in the twentieth century may not be valid for the twenty-first century. For this reason, nursing leadership should be well versed in what *is* valid, in order to assertively seek out and experiment with new approaches. This, then, is a second reason for nursing leaders to be knowledgeable about leadership theory. In many respects, nursing is in a unique situation and is therefore in a position to conduct research on leadership theory in nursing. Not only would this make a valuable contribution to the body of knowledge that is nursing, but it would also add to the general body of leadership knowledge.

Yet another way for nursing leaders to utilize this knowledge base is in the development of new nursing leaders. Novice nurse leaders can learn skills and expertise based on the knowledge that is available through formal and informal education. Nursing, like many professions, suffers from an insufficient number of leaders. Time after time, nursing authorities lament this and encourage the education and development of new nurse leaders.

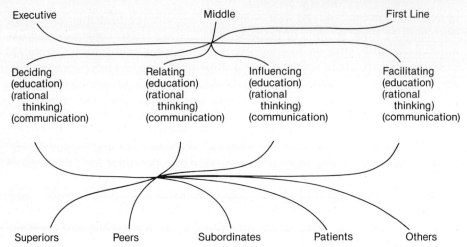

FIGURE 6–1. Conceptual framework for nursing leadership behaviors at different organizational levels. (Based on Yura, H., Ozimek, D., and Walsh, M. D.: Nursing Leadership: Theory and Process, 2nd ed. New York, Appleton-Century-Crofts.)

In order to achieve this, there must be an available curriculum, learning experiences, and mentors.

Finally, as nurses become more knowledgeable about leadership, nurses can incorporate this theory into their relationship with the patient. This would assist the staff nurse in being a more effective patient advocate. Also, patients could learn leadership behaviors that would enable them to have more control over their own lives.

Nursing leaders need to have a firm foundation in leadership theory in order to develop skills and expertise utilizing a variety of behaviors that enable them to adapt to any situation. This, in turn, will enable them to be flexible in meeting changes within the American culture and society that are constantly occurring.

A FRAMEWORK OF NURSING LEADERSHIP BEHAVIOR

This section utilizes a conceptual framework based on Yura's (1984) and Epstein's (1982) leadership process framework to examine nursing leadership behavior at the executive, middle and first line level (Fig. 6–1). The four behaviors within the leadership process include deciding, relating, influencing, and facilitating. Inherent within each of these behaviors are the components of education, rational thinking, and communication. Each level of nursing—executive, middle, and first line—exhibits leadership in this manner to supervisors, peers, subordinates, patients, and others.

Deciding Behaviors

The behavior of deciding encompasses a number of activities. Of these activities, goal setting and planning constitute two significant processes. Since organizational and department goals are usually fairly broad, the nurse executive needs to possess the ability to think conceptually as well as rationally. The decisions the nurse executive makes need to be based on a sound knowledge base. Rational thinking utilizes the best available information; self-awareness; and objective and honest analysis of the inputs, throughputs, and outputs in a logical manner. In that regard, rational thinking parallels scientific thought and the nursing process. Incorporated within the rational thinking process used in the deciding behavior is the process of evaluation. Data from the knowledge base are evaluated for their relevancy. Ultimately, the decision itself is evaluated.

Conceptual thinking is not constrained by facts and figures, as is the process of rational thinking. Rather, conceptual thinking is a skill whereby ideas are generated as the result of a synthesis of a broad, rich, and varied base. Decisions made by the nurse executive include the philosophy of nursing that guides the nurse executive's practice, as well as the practice of the individuals who work in the nursing department. This decision relates to the nurse executive's superiors because this philosophy needs to be compatible with the institution's philosophy.

The acquiring of the knowledge base used in both rational and conceptual thinking carried out by the nurse executive is accomplished through formal and informal education. Advanced degrees in either nursing administration or business are now essential. Continuing education enables nurse executives to recharge their knowledge base and contributes significantly to their perspective. Informal education occurs primarily in the form of mentorships. In addition to another nursing service administrator, the chief executive officer, as well as a board member, can function in this capacity. The nurse executive utilizes educational principles with subordinates to increase their understanding of how and why the nurse executive reached a particular decision.

Communication skill and techniques are essential for nurse executives in the decision making process. They utilize communications for acquiring data to add to their knowledge base. Through the process of inquiry, probing, and validating, the nurse executive is more clearly able to analyze the situation. In providing feedback to both a superior and subordinates, the nurse executive indicates the process that has been completed, the value ascribed to various pieces of data, and the impact of a decision on them.

Decisions made by the nurse executive, even though frequently general in nature, do impact on patients and their families. That is why communication, feedback, and evaluation that include one of the primary consumers of nursing, the patients, must be included. The other primary consumer of nursing services, the physician, is also a key variable considered by the nurse executive in decision making. Likewise, communication prior to decision making, feedback, and evaluation that includes physician input is required. Public relations and image have recently become a more significant concern. For these reasons, the nurse executive also takes into consideration information or data from other individuals or groups that may be affected by the decision, even if only remotely. Education and communication with these others, whether they are consumers or providers of related interests, can ultimately determine the success or failure of a particular goal or decision.

Frequently, decisions at the nurse executive level are not highly specific and can be actualized in a variety of ways. As health care changes, however, the decision making process for the nurse executive will become even more critical. The nurse executive should be in a position to become involved in corporate decisions at an early stage. This means involvement with the board of directors/trustees and any strategic or long term planning activities that occur. Changes sometimes occur very rapidly, so the nurse executive must stand ready to make a decision quickly or change a decision rather than continuing on a doomed course. Many decisions made by nurse executives are in response to or in reaction to circumstances perceived to be beyond their control. When nurse executives are able to articulate the impact they have on any given decision, their participation will be more solicited. Action rather than reaction sounds like a nice idea, and it is, despite its difficulty. Reaction can never be eliminated because of the role and responsibilities of nurses and departments of nursing. However, the ability to better control the activity of a nursing service department can be better achieved through rational thinking, education, and communication. Rational thinking helps take a lot of the "risk" out of the risk taking decisions made by the nurse executive.

To what extent decisions are the middle nurse manager's responsibility varies depending on the institution. The middle manager assumes different roles in decision making. The nurse executive may delegate certain decisions to the middle management level, either individually or as a group. Likewise, the middle manager may decide to delegate certain decisions to subordinates. The middle manager may be, as can be all nurse leaders, involved in formulating decisions and goals, planning their implementation, and predicting the outcome of the decision or goal attainments. The middle manager can use experience and education in a specialty area of nursing or management to educate the nurse executive. Likewise, the middle manager utilizes principles of adult education in communicating decisions to subordinates. A large part of the middle manager's job is dealing with interpersonal issues and communicating upwardly and downwardly within the nursing department the data used in decision making, as well as the decisions themselves. Although removed from frequent and regular direct patient contact, the middle managers may find themselves in a decision making position for crisis situations. Again, the principles of learning as much as possible about the situation, rationally thinking through the problem to reach a decision, communicating the decision to relevant participants, and educating those involved to prevent similar crises serve the middle manager well.

First line nurse managers have numerous opportunities to demonstrate leadership behaviors, including those involved in decision making. Although head nurses are frequently perceived as being dominated by the overwhelming bureaucracy of the organization and system, in truth head nurses are in the best position to lead and experience goal achievement for themselves, their staff, and their patients. Many of the decisions head nurses have to make are more technical and short term compared with the conceptual and broad decisions made by the nurse executive. Nevertheless, the head nurse also uses rational thinking, education, and communication in reaching those decisions.

Relating Behaviors

"Relating to others requires an ample degree of charity (love), feeling and value for one's fellow man. Trust and respect for another, be he client or co-worker, are essential elements in establishing a relationship that is productive of good effects" (Yura, Ozimek, and Walsh, 1981). Self-awareness, self-confidence, personal energy levels, and certainly communication skills are also essential components of relating behaviors.

Relating behaviors for the nurse executive include socializing, interacting, conversing, cooperating, and attending to peers and superiors. Considered by some to be a form of networking and by others to be demoralizing, relating behaviors remain for the nurse executive a critical set of behaviors in determining an effective leader. Nurse executives educate themselves about the personal and professional lives of the individuals who are their superiors and peers. This information enables them to initiate phatic conversation. Phatic conversation is establishing an atmosphere of sociability and revealing or sharing feelings. The use of phatic conversation demonstrates a genuine interest and value of the other person as an individual and establishes areas of commonality. Relating behaviors have to do with the socialization of males and females. Males are socialized to relate to one another through team sports, whereas historically females are not. This is not to imply that the female nurse executive strives to relate to peers and supervisors as "one of the boys." You don't have to take up racquet ball, tennis, running, or golf to be an effective nursing leader. However, any mutual areas that enhance relating to a peer or supervisor should be identified and utilized in that relationship. For example, *Newsweek* (1985) magazine reported that golf has become an effective vehicle for establishing business connections and relationships because of its social attributes.

The use of rational thinking by nurse executives in relating behaviors enables them to discriminate among their alternatives, identify what kind of bargaining needs to occur, and critically project the phases of interacting that need to occur. Rational thinking also serves to override any temptation to relate to peers or superiors in an emotional manner. Self-awareness in combination with rational thinking enables the nurse executive to remain in better control of self and act logically rather than react.

How the nurse executive relates to subordinates has a great deal of impact on his or her effectiveness and success as a leader. Self-awareness provides nurse executives with a realistic understanding of their own strengths and weaknesses. This lessens any feelings of being threatened by a subordinate who has a particular expertise. A sensitivity toward others, combined with a knowledge of human behavior, is the basis for determining the relating behavior. Nurse executives who feels they are better than their middle or first line managers are not likely to utilize a philosophy of educating subordinates to help them achieve their maximum potential. This superiority attitude will also be apparent in the communication that occurs. The nurse executive will project this superior attitude by being critical, withholding or concealing essential information, gossiping, or cutting off or ignoring the needs and contributions of the subordinates. Successful nurse executives, on the other hand, use rational thinking to determine the best way to relate to subordinates. They objectively evaluate their relationship and through communication provide definitive cues to clarify the executive's and subordinate's role.

Nurse executives, unless they are in a small institution, do not do a great deal of relating directly to individual patients. Visibility is not relating. Regular sampling of patients by the nurse executive accomplished during rounds is also not true relating. One mechanism to enable a meaningful relationship between patients and the nurse executive would be to place a consumer on some of the nursing committees, such as patient education, or seek patient input about policies and procedures that directly affect patients. The same could be said for the nurse executive's relationship with staff nurses. There must be a conscious effort on the executive's part, owing to a sincere concern and value of the staff nurse, to establish a relationship. As with the patient, the creation of situations that promote a relationship has to be initiated by the nurse executive.

The nurse executive is in a position to relate to a variety of other groups that contribute to success and effectiveness. Obviously, a main group is physicians. Education, rational thinking, and communication are essential ingredients of this relationship. Other groups include the crossing of interdisciplinary lines to express concern and interest in their issues. This can also occur outside the hospital setting and can include the business community, the education and political arena, or environmental concerns.

Middle managers' ability to relate with their superior, the nurse executive, as well as with other superiors can significantly impact on their present and future success as nursing leaders. The peer relationships of a nurse middle manager are also of significance because they too contribute to the department's smooth and coordinated functioning. Fragmentation, one-upsmanship, and competition at the middle manager level can be destructive behaviors that affect all levels of nursing. Likewise, the middle manager's ability to achieve cooperation from subordinates is second only to the ability to communicate and listen effectively. The middle nursing manager is in a somewhat better position than the nurse executive to relate to a select group of patients. This provides a different perspective from that of the first line manager as well as feedback for the first line manager. The use of rational thinking by middle managers enables them to filter, synthesize, and interpret data to those above and below.

The first line nurse manager's relating behavior to superiors enables the manager to effectively educate and communicate the needs and contributions of the nurse manager's department unit to the overall effectiveness of the department. Relating to peers effectively accomplishes collaboration and the more efficient use of resources. The first line manager has to be effective in relating behaviors with staff in order to elicit cooperation from them as well as from support personnel and interdisciplinary health care team members. An integral part of relating behaviors is the ability to listen effectively and simultaneously remove barriers to communication. Education of first line nurse managers provides them with a knowledge of human behavior, which they use extensively in relating to staff and others. Likewise, education of her staff and others communicates the value of these individuals to the first line nurse manager.

Rational thinking by the first line manager determines which relating behaviors are the most appropriate for staff, physicians, patients, and others. Because of the first line manager's daily and regular relationship with the two main consumers of nursing, patients and physicians, the manager can evaluate the mechanisms and directions for needed changes as well as the reactions of these two groups.

Influencing Behaviors

Influence is defined as the act or power of producing an effect without apparent exertion of force or direct exercise of command (Mish, 1983, p. 620). Claus and Bailey (1977) stated that influence is the result of power and is largely determined by the relationship the leader has with the followers. In other words, the leader will only have as much influence on the followers as they, the followers, want to give the leader. The emphasis in this discussion is on positive influence, not negative influence, although illustrations of negative influence are occasionally provided.

In order to perform influencing behaviors, the nurse executive utilizes education to acquire and demonstrate a high level of expertise. Acquiring education also enables the nurse executive to understand and deal with manipulative behavior. Also as a result of education, the nurse executive can utilize motivational theories to create a positive climate within the department. Education of counseling and coaching techniques assists the nurse leader to develop the leaders within the department and assist the nurse executive to serve as a model and mentor. The influence of mentors on leaders from multiple disciplines is consistently reported and should not be under-emphasized. Knowledge of the power structure and holders of power within the department and organization impacts on the nurse executive's ability to influence others.

Rational thinking impacts on the nurse executive's influencing behaviors in several ways. It allows better control over the work situation, as well as provides the basis for challenging conflict and utilizing legitimate authority in many ways. At the same time, rational thinking provides the process for identifying a range of strategies for goal achievement, enables the nurse executive to deal concretely with the real present, and frees the nurse executive to conceptualize and anticipate the future.

Communication is an essential component of influencing behaviors by the nurse executive, whether dealing with superiors, peers, or subordinates. The obtaining and sharing of information occur largely through communication and provide a significant source of influence. The ability to establish and maintain contacts with supervisors and peers occurs as the result of communication. The nurse executive influences subordinates significantly through the communication of approval or disapproval.

The middle nurse manager exhibits influencing behaviors primarily to peers and subordinates. The middle nurse manager can, however, influence the nurse executive through the controlling and interpretation of upward information and by advocating a particular course of action. Through competition, challenge, or role model, the middle manager can influence peers. Through the process of communication, the middle manager can convey ideas, opinions, expectations, and goals to first line nurse leaders. The middle nurse manager is also in a position to provide reinforcement for the first line nurse manager.

The first line nurse manager performs significant influencing behaviors, primarily to staff. The first line nurse manager is responsible for interpreting, promoting, persuading, inspiring, directing, and advancing specific actions that will result in goal achievement. Through the use of personal education, this manager possesses the knowledge base to identify the what, how, when, and why of a specific decision or goal. Education of staff influences not only their motivation to perform, but also their ability to perform as well. Rational thinking provides the first line nurse leader with the total perspective of the influencing behaviors. Communication is the agent of actualization of influence in many cases. The first line nurse manager is in a position second only to that of the staff nurse in the ability to influence patients and physicians. This nurse manager possesses knowledge that is critical to patients' and physicians' successful outcome. The nurse manager's influence on staff creates the climate and the goal setting that support or deny successful patient outcomes. The head nurse or first line manager reinforces this influence through discipline or corrective action that enhances productivity and goal-oriented behavior. Yet at the same time, the amount of influence the first line manager has is dependent on knowledge and responsiveness to the individual needs and differences of the staff.

Facilitating Behaviors

Facilitating behaviors are those behaviors that make goal attainment easier. Facilitating is a more active and frequently more direct process than influencing. These behaviors may include the actual allocating or providing of resources needed to reach a goal. Facilitating is helping to make things happen. Facilitation occurs when all other conditions and requirements have been met or accounted for to the fullest extent possible. By this, it is meant that decisions have been made, relationships have been established, and influences have been accomplished (Yura et al, 1981, p. 105).

The nurse executive is in a position to facilitate goal achievement for superiors and peers because of the knowledge of a very complex system, because of control of the majority of the resources within the institution, and because of the significant relationship between the nursing department and the consumers of the institution's goods and services, the patient and physician.

Rational thinking provides the nurse executive with the problem solving abilities required to identify various strategies that enable goals to be achieved. This type of thinking also identifies the proper time and sequence to activate the chosen plan. Included in this is the nurse executive's development of an effective nursing service organizational structure that can be responsive to changing trends and patterns. The nurse executive must be knowledgeable and be able to apply change theory and implement the change process. Without these skills, the nurse executive will not facilitate anything successfully.

Communication is obviously essential when a goal is facilitated unless it is strictly a physical or mechanical process of facilitating. However, the nurse executive should not lose sight of the value of communicating involvement in the ultimately successful and desired outcome. In other words, nurse executives should not be afraid to blow their own horns.

The middle line nurse manager does a lot of facilitating for the nurse executive, and for the first line nurse manager, because so much of the middle nurse manager's role is composed of coordinating, directing, and communicating activities. This manager, too, must be knowledgeable and comfortable with change theory and change process.

The first line nurse manager ultimately facilitates goal achievement for higher level nurse managers. This manager uses management and clinical knowledge along with rational thinking to plan, direct, control, and evaluate the staff's performance. The head nurse uses education to maximize the efficiency and effectiveness of staff and other resources. Through communication skills, this manager establishes the work climate and motivates staff. The first line nurse manager facilitates staff satisfaction and growth through stimulation, education, stress reduction, feedback, and reinforcement. As a result, the first line nurse manager facilitates patient and physician goal achievement.

TOMORROW'S STRATEGIES

The effective use of deciding, relating, influencing, and facilitating behaviors by the nurse executive is the key to successful leadership. Each level of nursing leader in varying ways may impact on the goal achievement or outcome within his department and within the institution. Another key behavior for the nurse leader is communication. Closely tied to each behavior just described, communication is essential to establish good relationships, resolve problems, and develop plans for the future. The strategy for the nurse leader at any level, then, revolves around the ability of the leader to communicate effectively and utilize the described behaviors to accomplish goals and objectives that place nursing in the forefront of health care.

References

American Academy of Nursing Task Force on Nursing Practice (1983). *Magnet hospitals: Attraction and retention of professional nurses.* Kansas City, Missouri: ANA.

Claus, K.E., and Bailey, J.T. (1977). *Power and influence in health care: A new approach to leadership.* St. Louis: C.V. Mosby.

Diers, D. (1979). Lessons on leadership. *Image*, 11(3), 67–71.

Douglass, L.M., and Bevis, E.O. (1983). *Nursing management and leadership in action.* St. Louis: C.V. Mosby.

Epstein, C. (1982). *The nurse leader: Philosophy and practices.* Reston, VA: Reston Publishing Co.

Lamonica, E.L. (1983). *Nursing leadership and management: An experimental approach.* Belmont, CA: Wadsworth Health Sciences Division.

McFarland, G.K., Leonard, H.S., and Morris, M.M. (1984). *Nursing leadership and management: Contemporary strategies.* New York: John Wiley and Sons.

Mish, F.C. (1983). *Webster's ninth new collegiate dictionary.* Springfield, MA: Merriam-Webster, Inc.

Rowland, H.S. and Rowland, B.L. (1985). *Nursing administration handbook* (2nd ed.). Rockville, MD: Aspen Systems.

Tannenbaum, R., and Schmidt, W.H. (1983). Effective leadership. In Collins, E.G. (ed.). *Executive success: Making it in management.* New York: John Wiley and Sons.

Tappen, R.M. (1983). *Nursing leadership: Concepts and practice.* Philadelphia: F.A. Davis.

Yura, H. (1984). Nursing leadership evaluation. *The health care supervisor*, 12(3), 16–28.

Yura, H., Ozimek, D., and Walsh, M.B. (1981). *Nursing leadership: Theory and process* (2nd ed.). New York: Appleton-Century-Crofts.

FOUNDATIONS OF MANAGEMENT

A continuously changing health care environment with emphasis on reduction of costs and improvements in productivity has directed those at executive levels toward a renewed interest in and a need for improved management skills. The nursing administrator, no longer the senior nurse or best clinician, must now be prepared to manage her departments as any business manager would. Management of patients and personnel, while important, is no longer sufficient for the successful nursing administrator. Instead, emphasis is placed on business concepts, strategic management, financial management, productivity, and marketing. In each of these areas, principles exist that may be applied to the thinking and activity of the nursing administrator to guide her toward success.

Management is that process through which actions are coordinated to achieve goals. The process of management includes functions of planning, directing, organizing, coordinating and controlling. The function of planning involves predicting the future and making decisions in relation to that prediction. Directing refers to directing of actions toward the desired goal. Organizing is the process of bringing together the various resources necessary to achieve the goal. Coordinating is ensuring that the resources remain balanced and function together during the process. Finally, controlling refers to monitoring and regulating performance. In each of these activities, the manager must deal with information and people, and must make decisions based on data obtained.

The five chapters in this section address the topics just listed and describe the application of management functions as appropriate. The effect of these variables on current practice and their impact on the future direction of nursing practice are discussed. Through the use of basic concepts and principles applied to health care and nursing administration, Section III provides an overview of management foundation and strategies for tomorrow.

BUSINESS CONCEPTS

INTRODUCTION

The consideration of health care institutions, such as hospitals, as businesses has been a somewhat controversial issue. Until recently, health care institutions were thought to be service organizations, most of which were categorized as non-profit. Non-profit in this context refers to tax status rather than whether a "profit" was generated. While the major function of health care organizations is the provision of health care to the public, it is, in fact, this type of service that necessitates the functioning of these organizations as businesses. Health care institutions, much like other busi-

7

nesses, "deal in a commodity—the commodity of life" (Holyfield, 1983, p. 2).

Health care cost the American economy roughly $425 billion in 1985. Approximately 7% of the nation's work force is employed in health care. All these numbers mean big business. The economic viability of health care institutions relies heavily on the utilization of business principles. The importance of business operations in health care institutions is reflected in the trend toward business degrees by health care management level employees.

Business concepts may be divided into principles that are basic to all businesses and principles that are especially applicable to health care institutions. Principles that are basic to all businesses are discussed in the first section of this chapter. These principles are found to some degree in the various types of businesses, including health care. Structured organizations, human resource programs, productivity programs, quality control, management systems, strategic planning, and some mechanism for obtaining capital are principles essential to businesses. Businesses also have common characteristics, which may include positive operating margins, customers, competition, marketing, regulations by government, bad debts, technology, and especially a product orientation. Characteristics of a business, as they apply to health care businesses, are discussed in the second section of the chapter. The role of entrepreneurialism in health care is covered in a third section.

BASIC PRINCIPLES

The business environment can be quite complex, but there are several fundamental areas that are common to all business organizations. The maturity of the health care organizations as businesses may be measured by the amount of growth the organizations have attained in each of the areas described. All businesses, health related or not, will have reached some degree of activity in each fundamental property, although one area may be at a very basic level whereas others are extremely well developed and quite mature.

Structured Organizations

A structured organization is one aspect of the business environment that applies to all businesses. The head of the corporation or business may have one of several titles, but essentially has ultimate responsibility for the operation of the organization. Within the structure may be found a board of directors or trustees in whom is placed the final decision making power related to the organization. Organizational structures define the lines of authority and communication within the organization.

The structure may be quite simple, with a minimum number of management personnel reporting to the head of the organization; or there may be quite a complex framework, as noted in the corporate structure, with several organizations under the corporate umbrella with separate boards, separate organizational structures, and multiple levels of management personnel between the corporate head and the worker who produces the final product or service. Matrix organizational structures are even more complex, with individuals reporting to multiple supervisors in which responsibilities are numerous or in which departments are complex. For example, the Oncology Unit Head Nurse or Manager may report to a Nursing Director responsible for management of nursing staff and to the Director of Oncology Services responsible for the overall oncology program.

Hospitals and other health care institutions easily fit the model applied to other businesses. From simple to complex structures, the health care organization may conform to any one of the wide variety of industries or multiple other organizations that must have some form of structured organization in order to function effectively. Because of the diversity in services provided within one health care organization, the structure of a particular institution may be quite complicated, but the fundamental structure must be present to some extent.

Human Resources Program

Human resources are essential in every business, including health care. The sheer numbers of people in health care emphasize the need for appropriate management of those human resources. The development of programs to manage personnel is another area common to businesses of all types and sizes. The level of sophistication of the program varies significantly with the type of business and its size.

Human resource management covers the spectrum from the simple programs with hourly wages and associated Social Security and income tax deductions to the more complex programs, which may have multiple benefit packages, complicated personnel policies, and employee development plans. Even in health care organizations, which are extremely labor intensive, the range of programs for managing human resources is a broad one. More than half the revenue of an average hospital is spent on employee wages and benefits. Much emphasis in human resource programs is based on obtaining and retaining a wide variety of professional and non-professional employees. Unlike many other industries in which jobs may be eliminated by technology, health care technology tends to produce a requirement for higher skill levels in the trained personnel working with the newer technology (Holyfield, 1983).

Human resource programs are necessary in businesses to control the multitude of problems related to employees. Such programs may include simply hiring, payment, and termination, but more often will also encompass activities related to wage and hour regulations, Equal Employment Opportunity Commission (EEOC), unemployment compensation, workmen's compensation, employee grievance, and all disciplinary measures. The extent to which the program operates will depend to a large extent on the complexity of the business. The importance to a business of a good human resources program is identified in excellent companies that have a respect for the individual employee, train him, and set reasonable expectations for him to perform his job (Peters and Waterman, 1982).

Productivity Program

Productivity measurement is one key to a business' knowledge of itself. Productivity programs for many businesses have been in operation for many years. These programs typically determine the level of productivity and help to determine how productivity may be improved. While many factors may influence the success of a business, the most significant one may well be productivity performance (Miller, 1984). A business such as a health care institution may improve efficiency and cut expenses through consolidating departments or positions. For example, one secretary/receptionist may handle calls and other secretarial duties for two small departments to eliminate one staff member and improve the productivity in each department. In a nursing department, a unit secretary or transporter may be shared between departments to improve productivity.

Productivity may be defined as the work or product produced from a specified amount of resources or the amount of resources required to produce a certain amount of work. Improvements in productivity may mean more product for less overall cost. Measurement of productivity becomes necessary to improve efficiency of the operation of a business.

Since health care has been faced with major changes in reimbursements, the emphasis on measuring and improving productivity has increased (Harji and Sabatino, 1984). As large portions of operating budgets continue to be committed to wages and salaries, the areas targeted most for productivity gains are those of staff-to-patient ratios. Programs aimed at measuring and improving productivity are fundamental in current and future business environments. See Chapter 10 for a more detailed review of productivity, including methods for productivity measurement and management.

Quality Control

Paralleling the necessity for productivity programs are quality control programs. Sacrificing quality for productivity serves no purpose in maintaining survival of a business. Particularly in health care, in which concern has been raised that quality will suffer as health care institutions attempt to cut costs, the importance of quality control programs is evidenced. All businesses, whether service or product oriented, need some program for controlling quality at the same time that productivity is being measured and improved. Development of standards as measures of quality and tools in quality control is an important consideration for the business.

As customers evaluate products and services, one major criterion in selection of the product or service is the quality of that product or service. The cost of the product or service is certainly tied to the quality, but customers will seek the product or service that is the "best" (quality wise) for the money. In the business of health care, quality often carries considerably more weight than cost. Customers of health care frequently demand "only the best." Controlling the quality of the service and products of health care, then, has a high priority in the health care business.

Quality assurance programs in health care have also received more emphasis than perhaps in other business because of regulatory and accrediting agencies that serve to protect the public interest. The development of quality assurance programs is discussed in Chapters 15 and 17.

Management Systems

In today's business environment, businesses need yet another system in place to operate management systems effectively. From simple accounting and reporting of day to day operations to sophisticated forecasting for multiple complex theoretical situations, management systems can develop as the organization develops. As computerization becomes more common, even in very small businesses, the greater is the role of management systems (such as computerized information systems, productivity reporting systems, etc.) in the success of businesses.

Health care organizations, because of the complex technology associated with medicine and related disciplines, already utilize data management systems in varying degrees. Computerized reporting of laboratory data, order entry, productivity management reporting, staff utilization reporting, and various studies to identify problems related to productivity or efficiency may all be included in management systems programs. Management systems are yet another control mechanism to ensure success in the business environment.

Strategic Planning

Strategic planning is essential to any business. One major difference between success and failure in business is the ability to control the business environment (Taylor, 1982). This can be done at least partially through strategic planning. Strategic planning for many businesses, including health care, may not realistically be necessary or possible for a long range period.

TABLE 7–1
Characteristics of a Business

Positive operating margins
Customers
Competition
Marketing
Government regulations
Bad debts
Technology
Product orientation

In the presence of rapid change, for example, long range planning becomes difficult, whereas strategic planning is a key to success.

Strategic information obtained from a variety of sources allows the business to make a strategic assessment of both the external environment and the situations in which the business finds itself. From the assessment, strategies and objectives may be established to guide the organization toward its goals. Adequate planning provides resolutions for problems before they occur, keeps the organization headed in the right direction, and improves productivity by preventing wasted time spent on the wrong track.

Capital

Capital formation or obtaining capital is necessary for the function of any business. Revenue may be obtained through charges for a product or service or in a variety of other ways, including investments and interest earnings. Health care institutions, like many other businesses, may have hidden resources (such as foundations) for funding that can improve the overall capital picture. Maintaining a good mix of financial resources will maximize the leverage a business has in its financial affairs (Petty, 1982). Management of capital is another fundamental for businesses. Identification of resources, obtaining funds, and maximization of investments are a few ways in which good financial management contributes to the success of the business.

CHARACTERISTICS OF A BUSINESS (Table 7–1)

Positive Operating Margins

All businesses must have a positive operating margin. Even those not-for-profit health care institutions (those that are considered non-profit for tax purposes and that do not have shareholders to whom dividends are paid) cannot survive if they do not make money. A break-even operating margin only delays the organization's demise. As with other businesses, health care institutions need money to put back into their facilities in order to offer other services, to replace or buy equipment, and to meet increases in operating costs. For-profit institutions additionally must disperse profits to their owners or investors. If money is unavailable for new programs or services, for new equipment or technology, or for increases in operating expenses, the ability to compete with other similar organizations may be significantly reduced.

The operating profit margin at which the organization functions reflects the operating effectiveness of the organization (Petty, 1982). Several factors may influence this margin, but evaluation of the margin in comparison with other like industries or organizations is necessary to determine if improvements can be made.

Customers

Businesses that provide services or products have another common characteristic. Every business, including health care institutions, has customers. While some industries have a specific audience to whom they provide services or for whom they produce, health care institutions have several customers (Holyfield, 1983). The customers of health care institutions fall into several primary categories. One customer is the physician who, especially in the past, has made the decision about where the patient was admitted for his health care. Even today, physicians exercise much control over the type and quantity of services the patient receives. It is also the physician who controls the course of treatment and the amount of time the patient is hospitalized.

The major consumer of health care services is the patient. Unlike customers of other businesses, the patient would usually prefer not to return to the health care institution. Patients who require hospitalization are generally utilizing the services of this business when they least feel like evaluating that service. This group of customers desires a health care "business" that can provide services that literally may be life-saving or at least will certainly enhance their lives.

Another group of consumers of health care services are employers. The popularity of health maintenance organizations and preferred provider organizations demonstrates the interest by employers in health care. These employers, who offer health care services as an employee benefit, desire quality at the lowest possible costs.

Yet another set of customers are those insurance companies and government programs that are the third party payers for patients. This group continually seeks to obtain for the patients services at lower costs. The insurance companies especially and the government programs such as Medicare desire that health care institutions reduce the amount of time the major consumer is served, as well as the number of services provided.

Many of the demands of the customers of health care businesses are contrary to the basic premise of other businesses (Holyfield, 1983). The major consumer, the patient, does not usually wish to be a patient—does not wish to be a customer of the health care business. The customer who can leave the setting of the major health care institutions (hospitals) sooner is best satisfied.

As with other businesses, the major customer of health care institutions (the patient) seeks high quality service and the lowest possible costs. Physicians, other customers of this business, seek the same quality/cost ratio but additionally have demands for control in decision making. Employers, insurance companies, government entitlement programs (Medicare, Medicaid), and special interest groups often seek to control other factors related to health care services, such as costs, access, quality, decision making, and even length of stay or actual admission.

Competition

Competition among health care organizations does not differ substantially from the competition among other businesses. Under TEFRA (Tax Equity and Fiscal Responsibility Act) cost-plus reimbursement, because there was not an incentive to reduce costs for health care, competition was not as obvious or as necessary as it is under current third party payment systems. The 7000 hospitals in the United States are now set in a very competitive market place, yet are different economically from many other businesses because of the third party reimbursement system (Holyfield, 1983).

Other businesses have regular sales of products or services, and competition for purchases of those services or products is evident as money paid for the product or service appears. The third party payment for products and services that characterizes health care in America masks to some extent the payment for services in such a way that competition is often less obvious than in many other types of business. For example, many physicians and boards of trustees do not support any type of "advertising" of services in a forthright manner but prefer to use "good public relations" to make the public aware of services. The competition is often subtle and is certainly often directed beyond the consumer of the service (the patient) to the physician, the employers, and the third party payers.

There has been concern that a new competition for patients being introduced into health care will affect the quality of that health care (Relman, 1980). Although competition among medical practitioners for admission to medical schools and for various positions in health care institutions has existed for some time, the different type of competition—a competition for patients by both physicians and health care institutions—has created a shift in American culture away from the protected and subsidized health care market ruled by the medical profession (Light, 1983).

The purpose of competition is to prevent unrestrained excesses among competitors and to balance the interests of those competing with one another.

The concern about quality raised primarily by the medical profession and health care organizations does require consideration. There is general consensus that the *clinical quality* of American health care is good. *Social quality*, or the quality of care as it relates to societal health needs, may not be viewed as favorably, since the focus has been on specialized, highly technical and acute episodic care as compared with primary, preventive, and long-term care needs (Starr, 1982). However, it has only been in the last decade that primary preventive and long-term care needs have assumed an increased value by our society. The *relative quality*, or how quality is related to price, is another area in which America has rated low (Starr, 1982). The emphasis on specialized and highly technical care has been quite costly, and the lack of effective competition has made our society tend to assume that resources were unlimited.

Competition impacts on all three types of quality just identified. Although studies that compare clinical quality in proprietary versus non-profit hospitals are lacking, clinically inferior care could be a potential result of cost containment efforts related to competition. This certainly is an area that needs safeguards, and the education of consumers is one such safeguard.

Quality is one of those vague terms that means different things to different people. Quality is measured by an individual's or group's standard, and may vary from group to group or individual to individual. Consumer satisfaction is one measure of quality that, while frustrating to providers of health care, may be utilized in the competition for the consumer. Consumers often judge quality not by the nursing care, lack of complications, or healing process, but by how quickly their call light is answered or their request for pain medication is fulfilled. This is further complicated by perceptions of the individual consumer. Even the personality of the provider may play a significant role in how that consumer rates the quality of his care. Therefore, clinical quality is related, at least in part, to consumer satisfaction, and consumer satisfaction is a major goal of competition.

Competition in health care affects both social quality and relative quality. Reduction in length of stay, preventive health care, and a level of care suited to the diagnosis are more likely to occur with competition. Under the current prospective payment system, payment for Medicare patients is directly related to the diagnosis and the incentive to reduce costs is related to the reduction in length of stay. Problems that are associated with this particular system and the reduced length of stay include the fact that the patient may be sent home too soon and may therefore develop complications or have a relapse, resulting in another hospitalization and higher costs for health care. Because immunizations and health care for the poor are unprofitable health care services, these services may not, on the other hand, receive consideration in the competition among providers. Ethical dilemmas related to this type of issue are unlikely to be resolved by competition. A number of factors may influence the conditions in which competition exists. For this reason, competition may or may not significantly improve the amount of these particular services provided for the dollar.

A major factor in the health care competition is the customer who seeks good care for the most reasonable cost. This does not always mean the best care regardless of cost, but, just as consumers of restaurant food may be willing to pay a bit more for a filet mignon instead of a sirloin, the consumer of health care will consider what he is receiving for the amount paid. The cheapest care may be unacceptable because of poor quality. For this reason, as competition increases, health care providers must consider the quality of the care as well as the costs. The key to competition, then, is efficient use of resources to provide high quality care at competitive prices.

Marketing

Businesses of all kinds must be concerned with their market. The market is defined as the number of people and their total potential for spending in relation to the service or product of a particular company within the geographic area capable of being served by that company (Riccardi and Dayani, 1982). Because marketing has in the past been considered an evil, wasteful practice used to take advantage of innocent customers, the importance of marketing within health care has been given minimal consideration until relatively recently (Cunningham and Cunningham, 1981). Now with the changes occurring in reimbursement and the necessity for competition, marketing has become a key factor in the success of these health care institutions.

Marketing performs several vital functions for society (Cunningham and Cunningham, 1981). It serves to provide an information network that links the customers with those who provide the service or produce the product. The information flow between consumer and provider is essential for a business to operate cost effectively. To operate efficiently, the health care institution needs to know the costs of supplies, labor, and other overhead in providing the service as well as the amount the customer is willing to pay for that service.

Marketing may also serve to equalize the demand for a particular service with the service that is available (supply). An understanding of demands for new or old services by the consumer of the services or the market is essential to the health care institution. In such a labor intensive business, providing services is dependent on the effective utilization of the human resources of the organization. The availability of those human resources in the right numbers at the time the demand for service is there is extremely important. This is made even more difficult by the variety of personnel required for specific services. Identifying the services desired and selling those services at a time when the institution can provide them, as well as determining the time the services are most desired, are functions of marketing that assist in equalizing supply and demand.

Centralization is another function of marketing. Marketing can provide a centralized mechanism for bringing the customer to the various products or services available in one location, rather than that customer seeking out those products and services in separate locations.

The role of marketing within health care institutions, as within other businesses, relies heavily on the state of the demand for the services provided by the institution. The demand may vary from no demand to too much demand. The role of marketing is to change the demand state to one that is more desirable. Marketing is an essential part of a business, necessary for the effective performance of the business. Chapter 11 discusses marketing in more depth as it applies to health care and to nursing administration.

Government Regulations

Increased government regulations have had significant effects on all businesses. Most recently, health care institutions have been targeted more strongly because of rising health care costs. Now among the most heavily regulated of all industries, hospitals are regulated by over 100 federal, state, local, and quasi-governmental agencies (Holyfield, 1983). Since the federal government purchases a large percentage of health care, it requires strict regulations to control reimbursement received for Medicare patients. The result of the regulations is more rising costs in order to satisfy the regulations rather than a reduction in costs.

Current regulations related to reimbursement are called the prospective payment system, or PPS. Under this system, the government has offered a set fee based on medical diagnosis. If the health care institution can care for the patient for less cost than the amount assigned to the specific diagnosis related group (DRG), the institution will make a profit from the admission. If, however, the institution's costs exceed the amount paid, the institution must absorb the loss. Rarely is consideration given to a specific patient (outliers). Institutions whose costs are high for whatever reason or that have high percentages of charity or Medicare patients may have difficulty competing successfully with other institutions because of inability to control revenues more successfully. It is this specific legislation—PPS—which had targeted cost control, which now also contributes significantly to the continuing rise in health care costs. This is related to the additional personnel needed to certify admissions, monitor DRGs, monitor length of stay, etc. The potential danger to patients from reduced length of stay or delayed admissions is another negative impact of the system. Another potential problem is related to a two-tiered health care system in which patients with Medicare might receive one level of care while the insurance or "private pay" patients receive another. These negatives are products of the system.

Beyond the regulations controlling payment or reimbursement, the standards or rules of numerous other agencies contribute to costs for delivery of health care services. The Occupational Safety and Health Administration (OSHA) tightly controls all kinds of safety practices, including whether or not plastic garbage can liners are used. The Food and Drug Administration regulates syringes and major technological devices, as well as pharmaceuticals. The Internal Revenue Service, Social Security Administration, and Environmental Protection Agency are involved in health care regulation. The Department of Labor oversees employee relations. Even the Federal Trade Commission and Federal Aviation Administration (air transport of patients) can become involved.

State agencies involved in regulations related to health institutions are nearly as diverse as the federal agencies. They range from health planning agencies to fire and health departments, insurance commissions, and employment/unemployment agencies.

Professional organizations and the quasi-public agencies are added to the list of regulatory agencies. Joint Commission on Accreditation of Hospitals, and laboratory and radiology certification organizations are examples of these types of agencies that regulate health care institutions. Voluntary compliance with regulations and certification requirements may result in benefits to the institution, such as fewer survey visits or association with residency programs. However, the fact remains that health care institutions must spend huge amounts of dollars and time to satisfy these many regulations.

Bad Debts

Besides the cost of doing business and of satisfying the numerous regulations, health care institutions have yet another characteristic of businesses. That characteristic is bad debts. Many consumers feel that health care is a right, not requiring payment. Health care is often the last bill paid by the consumer. Most businesses average 1 to 3% in bad debts, whereas hospitals may lose 12 to 15% of their billed revenue. These losses have in the past been either subsidized by insurers or handled through cost shifting (Holyfield, 1983).

Much of the problems related to bad debts can be associated with third party payers. Often the patient never sees the entire bill. The insurance carrier pays, and the consumer does not realize how ultimately the entire bill is being paid by all consumers. Additionally, consumers can go to health care institutions without advance payment. This practice has become increasingly more difficult, and the trend toward advance payment, a common business practice, is becoming more accepted by the consumer. The practice of admission without payment is uncommon in other businesses. Hotels, for instance, require a credit card or a deposit. Lay-away, or payment for purchases over time, is still common in many businesses, but the product is not released until payment is completed. Credit is common in many businesses, but additional charges occur through service charges or interest payments. Bad debts in other businesses are frequently handled through collection agencies or legal pathways with which many health care institutions are hesitant to openly be associated for fear of bad public relations.

Technology

Increasing technology or improvements in equipment/procedures are common to most industry or business. Because consumers of health care have demanded state-of-the-art equipment and procedures, and because of cost-plus reimbursement that funded unlimited capital expansion, technology in health care has grown at a more rapid pace. Research in medicine has also encouraged change in technology, and the new breed of physicians relies heavily on fast and accurate diagnostic tools.

Technology has been identified in many industries or businesses as a mechanism to reduce the number of jobs, therefore improving productivity. Technology in health care frequently means advanced skills for personnel and, if anything, may increase the number of jobs (Holyfield, 1983). Additionally, health care facilities such as hospitals typically replace a large portion of their equipment every five to seven years to keep up with advances in technology.

Technology may result in costs savings or may increase costs significantly. Businesses, including health care institutions, must evaluate technology for maximal utilization and cost effectiveness (Echevesti, 1982). If new technology improves services but is so costly that it is not affordable by a good portion of the market, it is not reasonable to purchase the technology. Adapting to changing practices through changes in technology, however, is essential to any business.

Product Orientation

"Building a better mousetrap" has resulted in many innovative ideas for changes in the major product of a business. Successful businesses, whether providing a service or another commodity, continually strive to create an improved product. This product orientation or desire to identify what it is the customer wants most and to develop that product (or service) is found in the health care business as well as in others.

For decades, health care organizations were thought of only as providing the service of caring for the ill. However, to operate efficiently as a business, it has become quite clear that health care institutions, like other businesses, must focus on the product demanded by the consumer. That product (including programs, procedures, etc.) must be produced in a quality manner, marketed to the customer, and regularly evaluated for its appeal and sales. Failure to focus on the product may result in failure of the organization to provide desired services or products to the customer. The customer, then, may look elsewhere for the desired product. In the competitive health care market, such losses would eventually lead to the failure of that health care organization.

ENTREPRENEURIALISM

Health care institutions, faced with financial difficulty in the era of prospective payment, are diversifying in multiple ways. New ventures range from clinics to emergency care centers to exercise centers to health maintenance organizations and preferred provider organizations. Beyond these health-related activities, organizations are forming other corporations to purchase real estate, operate retirement centers, and run hotels and restaurants.

There are many advocates for these joint or single ventures who argue that these activities support the health care institution's resources so that the ill and injured may receive better care. Others raise concerns that the risk to the security and effectiveness of institutions on which the public depends is too great (Cunningham, R., 1983). Whether risky or not, entrepreneurialism in health care is increasing at a rapid pace. The goals of such activity may vary from institution to institution, but several goals emerge as significant. These include additional funding, marketing, and improved relationships with physicians or others.

Provision of a secondary source of funding for the institution or corporation is one goal of entrepreneurial activity. Whether funneled through for-profit, separate corporation, or obtained through health-related, not-for-profit ventures, the source of income may be increased when other programs are added. This income may be the result of foundations created specifically for the purpose of channeling gifts to the institution or may be incidental to the creation of a program desired by the consumer.

A second goal of entrepreneurial activity may be marketing of the institution itself. Identifying programs desired by the consumer and providing them is just one way in which the institution may be successfully marketed. The use of preferred provider or health maintenance organizations to tie into other businesses is frequently a successful mechanism to improve or maintain the market share of a particular institution. For instance, although health maintenance organizations may discourage hospitalization, when the hospitalization becomes necessary, the institution would prefer that the hospitalization not occur at a competitive institution. Even programs that do not "make money" for the institution may improve the image and visibility of the institution and, therefore, be worth the cost.

Improving the relationship of an institution's management with physicians or other groups might be considered a third goal for entrepreneurialism. Joint ventures with the physician(s) or with other groups may serve two purposes. They may indirectly bind the group or individual to the institution, hopefully binding the loyalty simultaneously, and they may enhance the number and/or types of admissions to the institution. If the physician or group has a vested interest in a part of the institution, he (it) hopefully would appreciate the necessity for the success of the institution.

Considering that these goals are achievable through entrepreneurial activities, it may be that any concerns related to such activities are overshadowed by the benefits to be gained. In the business environment, in which good cash flow, assets or net worth, and return on investment are keys to success, creative development and implementation of entrepreneurial activities may result in more business-like health care.

Entrepreneurialism expands beyond health care to nursing to meet the same types of goals described. Providing funding or revenue and marketing are achievable in much the same manner. Groups of nurses or individuals with or without support from the health care institution may find ways to become entrepreneurs. Examples are numerous: consultation, education, clinical private practice, health care facilities, and wellness programs. Nurses provide consultation in a variety of ways, including planning, program development, patient classification, and clinical problem-solving. Consultation with the nursing staff may be offered by a nursing administrator to other facilities, or an individual may provide consultation independently. Education has grown tremendously in its outreach, or its ability to reach out to groups beyond the traditional educational institution's walls. Seminars and workshops of all types are offered in a variety of locations by multiple sources such as private consultants, health care institutions, associations representing specialty health care groups, or educational institutions. Seminars may be available through an institution or developed solely by the entrepreneur nurse.

Entrepreneurial activity within nursing departments can be a part of strategic thinking and management which is discussed in the next chapter. Assessment of needs or requirements does not always need to be addressed in a traditional manner. New approaches to old problems require creative thinking and risk-taking—both of which are characteristic of the entrepreneur. The nursing administrator is in a position to be that entrepreneur—to develop a durable equipment business to expand the scope of home health services or initiate a rehabilitation program for cardiac patients. These are important strategies for the nursing administrator's future.

NURSING AND BUSINESS

A nursing department must operate as any other department in the health care institution. Whether nursing care is specifically charged or included in "room and board" charges, the department is definitely revenue producing and has expenses that offset that revenue. Although finances are discussed in depth in Chapter 9, the financial management of a nursing department is a part of its business operation.

Nursing departments fit well into an organizational structure with lines of authority and communication able to be clearly defined. Nurse managers at the department level are common, and the responsibilities of these managers have evolved significantly over the years. Today, the unit manager generally has fiscal responsibility as well as human resource management responsibility. These responsibilities include management of productivity and quality. Planning responsibilities may to various extents include involvement in strategic planning, marketing, and competition.

The nursing administrator's role extends far beyond that of the nurse (unit) manager to include involvement not only in the business end of department management, but also to involvement in institutional ventures. Organizational planning, marketing, competitive program development, and compliance with governmental regulation are aspects of the nursing administrator's expanded role. Entrepreneurial activities provide additional methods by which the nurse executive may develop business strategies to ensure future successes.

SUMMARY

Successful businesses of various kinds have in common the principles and characteristics described in the above paragraphs, as well as a few characteristics not always found in the businesses that are unsuccessful. Peters and Waterman, in their book *In Search of Excellence* (1982), identify eight characteristics of successful businesses. It is interesting to note that many of these eight characteristics evolved from a basic principle for business.

"Staying close to the customer" certainly is one of those characteristics. Learning what the customer desires and providing those services or products is good marketing strategy. Tied closely to this strategy is the "bias for action" characteristic, which provides for many of those products or services without excessive delays in committees, evaluation, or study (Peters and Waterman, 1982).

Peters and Waterman also identify several characteristics that address the structure and mission of the business. Preserving a simple form with few management or administrative layers addresses the issue of structure. An insistence that the executive of a business maintain the firm's essential business is another key point, and "sticking to the knitting" or staying with the business best known by the company is tied to this. Over-diversification has resulted in many losses to many companies.

Some characteristics of successful companies are related to the people working with the business. "Productivity through people" is another phrase used by Peters and Waterman in describing the motivation of employees of a particular business to perform exceptionally well in order to share the benefits of success. Having identified central values in the business yet encouraging autonomy in production or in the delivery of the service(s) is yet another characteristic of success in businesses (Peters and Waterman, 1982).

The goal of business is to improve net worth while quickly providing the customer with desired products or services at acceptable standards and for reasonable prices. The difficulty for health care institutions may be in achieving the business environment in which this may be accomplished successfully.

To survive in the economic climate today, health care organizations must operate in much the same way as any other business. Financially sound business practices certainly are a portion of that operation (see Chapter 9, Financial Management). However, a number of other principles apply as well to the health care business.

Some structure or form is needed for every business to define responsibility and the framework for the organization. Employee programs that help to train the employees who produce the product or provide the service is another key principle. Employees are often the first impression the consumer has of the company. If the multiple problems associated with employees are not controlled, the customer/business relationship may not be well established (Mescon and Mescon, 1985).

Some measure of productivity and quality control are necessary to the organization's well being. Management systems, capital formation, and strategic planning are also necessary for functional businesses.

Businesses must also characteristically maintain positive operating margins, have customers, and compete with like businesses. Marketing of the services or products is necessary to ensure the sale of the product or service. Like other businesses, health care is regulated by the government and other agencies. Bad debts may plague health care as well as the other businesses.

The increasing technology in business is common in health care and has produced multiple problems and multiple changes in practice, but it has been advantageous in many ways to health care. The product orientation of businesses has become the focus for health care institutions as well. These characteristics are as necessary as the others for functional businesses, including health care. Maintaining success as a business is dependent on the successful combination or mixture of the identified principles and the amount of emphasis on each of them.

References

Bromberg, M. (1983). Entrepreneurialism in medicine. *New England Journal of Medicine*, *309*(21), 1313.

Cunningham, W., and Cunningham, I. (1981). *Marketing: A managerial approach*. Cincinnati: South-Western Publishing Co., pp. 4–7.

Echevesti, D. (1982). Marketing and business. In *The nurse entrepreneur* (Richard, B., and Dayani, E.). Reston, VA: Reston Publishing Co.

Harji, M., and Sabatino, F. (1984). Productivity efforts on the rise. *Hospitals*, *58*(22), 89–90.

Holyfield, D. (1983). The cost of doing business. *Horizons* (Fall), 2–8.

Light, D. (1983). Is competition bad? *New England Journal of Medicine*, *309*(21), 1315–1318.

Mescon, M. and Mescon, T. (1985). To foster the best, begin at the bottom. *SKY*, 116–120.

Miller, D. (1984). Profitability = productivity + price recovery. *Harvard Business Review* (May–June), Number 3, 145–153.

Peters, T., and Waterman, R. (1982). *In search of excellence*. New York: Warner Books.

Petty, J. (1982). *Basic financial management*, 2nd ed. Englewood Cliffs, NJ: Prentice-Hall.

Relman, A.S. (1980). The new medical-industrial complex. *New England Journal of Medicine, 303,* 963–970.

Riccardi, B., and Dayani, E. (1982). *The nurse entrepreneur.* Reston, VA: Reston Publishing Co.

Starr, P. (1982). *The social transformation of American medicine.* New York: Basic Books.

Taylor, C. (1982). The business ownership game. In *The nurse entrepreneur* (Richard, B., and Dayani, E.). Reston, VA: Reston Publishing Co.

STRATEGIC MANAGEMENT

INTRODUCTION

Strategic management is a term used to encompass both strategic thinking and strategic planning. It deals with review of mission, organizational growth, strategy development, and change processes needed to implement strategic plans (Ansoff, Declerk, and Hayes, 1976). This approach is particularly suited to health care institutions that are facing frequent and significant changes. As a problem solving process, strategic management is directed at identifying new and better relationships between the institution or agency and its environment (Bopp and Hicks, 1984). As Waterman (1982) pointed out, such links between organizations and the environment may require changes in the elements of the organization—the strategy, skills, style, systems, staff, shared values, and structure. It is precisely because of these changes and their necessity that strategic management is important.

8

As a major component of the foundations of management, strategic management provides the theoretical approach to thinking and planning for the nursing administrator. In the practice of nursing administration, strategic planning and thinking are necessary in the management of patient care, of personnel, and of risks. This problem solving process is critical to the nursing administrator, who must react to change and must be proactive in creating an environment conducive to success. With this foundation, the nurse administrator may determine direction, identify goals, and implement strategies for that success.

The concept of strategic planning began in the battlefield of war and has developed in businesses over the years because of its success there. Previously, long range planning for five, ten, or more years was a more common practice in business, but this was found to fall short of the needs of business. Although long range planning was not necessarily intended to specify a particular number of years, there was an implication that the planning covered a "long" period of time. The period might vary from one business to another, and the frequency with which such plans were reviewed might also differ with the organization. To further complicate matters, decisions from "long range planning" became more necessary for the present and immediate future than for a period several years away. Finally, a rapidly changing economy, technology, and direction in a business resulted in a need to reconsider and/or change long range plans so frequently that planning for a long period became less feasible.

Planning has conventionally been oriented toward the past, the present, the future, or combinations of these. Although some crossover occurs or variations may be noted in these types of planning, the planners within organizations generally have had an orientation toward one of these planning modes.

Reactive planning occurs when planners are dissatisfied with the current situation and wish to change it by returning to a previous, more comfortable state (Ackoff, 1982). Reactive planners frequently consider technology as the cause of problems. Each problem is dealt with separately without integration with the whole organization. Reactive planning has several attractions: an appreciation of history; an avoidance of abrupt, disruptive, and poorly understood changes; and security through preservation of traditions.

A second type of conventional planning is called inactivism. Inactivists consider the status quo as the stable environment, and they avoid change (Ackoff, 1982). Planners who prefer the present state of affairs expend much energy preventing change and maintaining conformity, but do the least that is necessary to return to equilibrium. This group would prefer palliation to cure for problems.

A dominant style of planning in the United States is one referred to by Ackoff (1982) as preactivism. Preactive planners seek accelerated change. They prefer technology as a principal cause of change. Unsatisfied with the past or present, preactivists believe the future is always preferable. Preactivists do not value experience but rely on prediction of and preparation for the future. Even inaccurate predictions fail to deter this type of planner because of their proneness to contingency planning.

The fourth type of planning is called interactive or proactive. Planners who fall in this category consider the past, present, and future and attempt to plan the future of their organization rather than react to it. Adaptation is considered one of the key requirements because of the rapid environmental changes.

Although Ackoff (1982) believes that strategic planning falls into the preactive planning category, it may actually be considered proactive when it is examined more carefully. Strategic planning offers an alternative to traditional types of planning, including "long range planning." All planning is directed at accomplishing goals, but strategic planning is a systematic approach to decision making. Strategic planning may also include, as Drucker (1974, p. 125) suggests, "organizing efforts necessary to carry out these decisions" and evaluation of outcomes. Formalized strategic planning, then, determines outcomes, specifies action needed, and evaluates the success of the action (Fox and Fox, 1983). Strategic planning, however, cannot be rigid or static in its approach to the future, but must continually be reviewed and revised as situations and the environment change (Steiner, 1979). Strategic planning implies no time frame but rather a type of approach.

Differentiation of strategic thinking and strategic planning is important in understanding the role of strategic planning in businesses, including health care. Strategic planning, by its nature, may hinder strategic thinking. Because strategic thinking helps determine the direction in which the organization moves, it must be responsive to changes in the environment. Planning tends to focus on goal development and achievement, and, while strategic planning considers the environment and situations, strategic thinking precedes strategic planning in its focus on problem solving.

This chapter will describe the benefits of strategic management and, more specifically, of strategic thinking and planning. The basic principles of and factors influencing strategic management will be identified and discussed. The actual process of strategic management will be described as well. Application of the process of strategic management to MBO (management by objectives), forecasting, and program development will also be addressed.

BENEFITS OF STRATEGIC MANAGEMENT

Strategic management has many benefits for the health care organization. The sense of direction that results from strategic management is especially beneficial. Strategic management accomplishes this task through specific processes that examine the factors that can influence the direction taken and the alternatives available. Strategic management determines the limits and monitors the variance from the intended pathway that the organization has chosen. When it functions appropriately, strategic management will consistently address complex or complicated projects in an organized fashion (Fox and Fox, 1983).

Cost reduction may also be a benefit of strategic management. Crisis management and short term problem solving too frequently result in use of costly resources. Planning activities for departments using well defined objectives reduces the waste of both human and material resources by giving departments direction. Strategic management matches the strengths of departments, programs, and the organization as a whole to the opportunities in the environment.

The control mechanisms that are provided through the strategic planning process will indicate the degree to which the organization as a whole or its individual departments may be deviating from the selected direction as well as the appropriateness of the deviation. Strategic management is primarily flexible. It permits adaptation with relative ease and encourages changes in direction when appropriate. The rewards in strategic management occur in problem resolution and adaptation rather than in sticking to the original plan.

Development of projects in stages is well suited to strategic management. The examination of the various factors that influence the outcome of decisions is an important step in the process and is particularly valuable with complex projects. Interrelated tasks necessary to accomplish the objectives in this type of project can be addressed successfully in the strategic planning process at each stage.

Strategic planning may be beneficial in the method by which it is accomplished. Involvement of key individuals in the planning process provides satisfaction at both personal and professional levels. Such involvement of individuals enhances motivation and may stimulate the process as well as providing results (Fox and Fox, 1983). Once the planners are involved in the strategic thinking process, they feel a sense of importance to the organization, which will result in that needed motivation to identify alternative directions and to choose the appropriate direction in view of the environment.

Strategic management provides these benefits, which serve the purpose of strengthening the competitive position of an organization, increasing the effectiveness of the organization's management, and improving the overall performance. Controlling the direction of the organization; cost effective management; involvement of suitable persons; and evaluation of the interrelationships of groups, departments, or projects are key components of strategic management.

BASIC PRINCIPLES IN STRATEGIC MANAGEMENT

Fox and Fox (1983) have identified several principles that are considered basic to strategic planning and strategic management. Others consider the basic purpose of strategic management to be its focus on the environment (Hofer and Schendel, 1978). Each principle identified here will be discussed in more detail as the strategic management process is explained.

One major principle of strategic management is environmental analysis. As changes in the health care environment continue to occur at an ever rapid pace, internal and external environmental factors must rank high among those factors requiring consideration in health care planning. This environmental assessment or analysis would identify, monitor, and forecast trends or could affect the implementation of organizational strategies (Bopp and Hicks, 1984).

Internal environmental factors may include organizational characteristics, technical assets, financial picture of the organization, ability of the organization to market itself, and human resources. Strengths or deficiencies of the organization in these key areas would be analyzed. The political climate, the role of government agencies, and the legal climate would be external environmental factors requiring consideration during the environmental analysis.

Another principle basic to strategic management would be adaptation or flexibility. Strategic management would require an adaptability to environmental changes. Important to this principle is the ability to adapt when appropriate without excessive delays or extensive research. Adaptation after a crisis rather than in such a way as to avoid the crisis is reactive. Strategic management requires proactive thinking and planning. Changes in health care occur so rapidly at times that the flexibility to adapt rapidly may be necessary to the survival of the organization.

An important principle in strategy formulation that is a key feature of strategic management is consideration of the past, present, and projections for the future. Drucker (1974) asks the questions related to where the organization has been, where it currently is, and where it wishes to be. Although these questions seem relatively simple, it is surprising how many organizations look only to where they wish to be without considering where they have been and where they are now. The process of strategic management involves examination of the organizational strengths and weaknesses, which requires a look to the past and present. An understanding of what the organization has faced, what it has achieved, and where and why it has failed is important to the process of strategic management because it guides the organization away from previous mistakes, considers the situations in which that organization developed and grew, and can help the organization build on its strengths. Evaluation of organizational opportunities continues to an examination that includes the future. This evaluation of opportunities for the future is based on the strengths and weaknesses that resulted from the past and present experiences of the organization. From this, the future of the organization may be directed.

As early as 1975, the importance of listening to the consumer and to the employee was being stressed (Ryan, 1975). The needs and desires of the organization, its employees, and especially of its customers are basic considerations of strategic management. There is a sense of importance felt by those groups who are consulted in the planning process. The internal assessment can provide planners with information related to the needs of the employees. Evaluation of trends and examination of issues will identify the needs or desires of the customers of the organization.

The process of strategic management would be incomplete without one other major principle. Measurement of outcomes to help accurately determine the effectiveness or success of implemented changes is a key feature in the strategic plan. The data gained may then become an important part of the environmental analysis as the process continues.

STRATEGIC MANAGEMENT PROCESS

The process of strategic management is not a complicated process, but rather a framework within which decision making can readily occur. The problem solving approach—identify, plan, implement, evaluate—can easily be fitted into the strategic management process. However, strategic management is certainly more complex and hopefully more beneficial than this simple approach. The framework around which organizations build and grow is obviously extremely important in the current health care climate. Health care organizations, of necessity, cannot be limited to planning for the future. Gluck, Kaufman, and Walleck (1982) have determined that effective strategy formulation based on key issues facing businesses is the framework necessary for successful planning.

The process of strategic management has been considered by Ansoff, Declerk, and Hayes (1976) as dealing with four major areas: organizational growth and renewal, development of appropriate strategies to achieve growth, determination of mission, and organizational changes necessary to effectively implement strategies. Each of these areas can be subdivided into parts, which include the basic principles of problem solving. A general systems conceptual framework simplifies the otherwise complex interactions that occur in health care organizations. Figure 8–1 illustrates the process used in strategic management.

Review of Organization

Before any successful plan can be developed, the position of the organization must be reviewed. Health care organizations are closely related to society. Society originally initiated health care institutions as service organizations whose major purpose was to meet the health care needs of society. The mission of a health care organization is its guiding philosophy, derived from beliefs or values that the organization has deemed to be of primary importance. It should identify the publics for which services are to

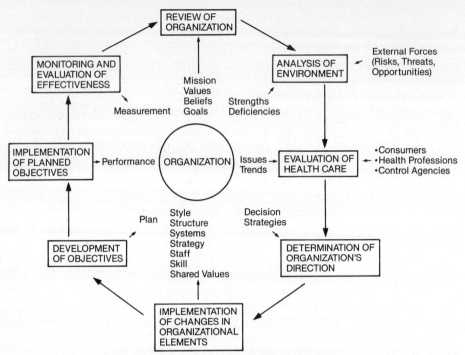

FIGURE 8–1. Model for strategic management.

be performed and the type of service (such as "health care"). In some health care organizations, a general mission statement and a more specific philosophy statement may exist, which may detail the expectations of those delivering a service and the expectation in terms of quality or productivity.

As long as the needs of society are being met through health care organizations, such organizations may survive. However, if society fails to recognize that its needs are met, such health care organizations may fail. It is of great importance to realize that, as with everything, change occurs in the needs of society. What may have stimulated the need for a particular type of health care program at one time may be irrelevant and unnecessary at another time. Another important factor that must be considered is that what society needs must be determined by society. While "experts" may feel a type of program is not needed or justified because of small numbers of individuals affected or because of the small impact on society, society may perceive that the program not only has value but is needed. Response to the perceived needs of society, then, may be one very important part of the organizational mission.

The values that an organization has will most certainly influence the direction the organization may take. Values are the basic beliefs or ideas that an individual or group of individuals hold dear. These values or beliefs may be very simple and straightforward or may be very complex and interwoven.

Key individuals within an organization develop the institutional philosophy from a composite of individual values, so that the philosophies of two otherwise similar organizations may vary significantly from each other.

Before any real strategic planning or strategic management may occur, an understanding of the organization's values and its mission must occur. The progressive relationship of values and beliefs to philosophy and mission must continue toward the institutional goals and objectives found at the departmental or even lower hierarchical levels of the organizational structure. The relevance of each objective and goal to the mission and values requires consideration in the strategic management process. This may seem an extremely time consuming task but can be accomplished in a variety of ways and at multiple levels. Goals, for example, require review at the top management level. Although goals describe the desired outcome, they generally are non-specific and not easily measurable. Many specific objectives can address a single goal, which may be reached "if the target of the objective is met." Progress toward a goal can be measured by how well objectives are achieved.

Review of the organization must include a review of its values or beliefs, its mission or philosophy, and its goals and objectives. The potential for a change in any or all of these is an important consideration in view of the role health care plays in society and the need for health care organizations to be able to respond to societal pressure (Bopp and Hicks, 1984).

Analysis of Environment

Freeman (1984) describes an approach to environmental analysis that considers that individuals or groups may have an interest in the direction an organization may take. The interest may be related to the problems of the organization or to the outcome of the planning process. A preparatory step in the environmental analysis, Freeman's approach involves identifying and analyzing what he refers to as stakeholders. Those individuals or groups who have opinions on the major issues affecting the organization and those who might be able in any way to influence any part of the planning process would be considered stakeholders. Any group or individual who should be interested in the direction the organization takes should also be included.

Analysis of the stakeholders in several categories provides for the planners two important pieces of information. The analysis will provide the focus for further study of issues that might prove to be essential or critical to the organization's future. Analyzing the stakeholders may also provide information to the planners about the relationship the stakeholders have with the organization.

How important the stakeholder is to the organization can be determined only after a thorough analysis. The areas of interest the stakeholder has with the organization may be identified. The concerns of the organization and stakeholders in relation to one another must also be reviewed. Any trend or

TABLE 8–1
Considerations in Stakeholder Analysis

Areas of interest in relation to organization
Concerns/questions of organization about
  stakeholders
Concerns/questions of stakeholder in relation to
  organization
Issues or trends that impact on interaction
  between organization and stakeholder
Departments and/or individuals who would deal
  with stakeholders
Relative importance of stakeholder to
  organization
Factors influencing ability of organization to
  effectively manage the stakeholder

issue that would impact on the interaction between a stakeholder and the organization should be analyzed. Once this analysis has been completed and the individuals or departments within the organization that may deal with the various stakeholders have been identified, the relative importance of the stakeholder to the organization may be determined. Dependent on the factors that might be an influence, the ability of the organization to effectively manage the stakeholder may then be decided. Table 8–1 lists the areas to be considered in stakeholder analysis.

The information gleaned from the stakeholder analysis is essential in the more in-depth environmental analysis. Analysis of the environment has two major foci: internal and external. Assessment of the internal environment is difficult because very often the planners lack objectivity. It is therefore helpful if the planners are directed by specific guidelines in examining the organization's internal environment.

INTERNAL ASSESSMENT

The purpose of the internal assessment is the identification of the organization's deficiencies or weaknesses and its strengths. The analysis of the organization should consider especially the seven variables identified by Waterman (1982) as those elements that compose the unique culture of the organization. The culture of an organization refers to the manner in which it has developed or matured. It includes the physical surroundings of the organization, but, more importantly, that culture has been shaped by historical forces, societal forces, and patterns of interaction between the organization and others. Since the demands upon an organization by its customers or publics and the expectations of multiple groups interacting with an organization differ significantly from one organization to another, each organization's culture is unique.

The *structure* of the organization and the protocols that determine who reports to whom and how departments are interrelated represent one of the variables that needs analysis. The relationship of the structure to the other elements is an important aspect of the analysis. Consideration must include the formal and informal structure of the organization, since the informal organizational structure may hold power not recognized formally but that could significantly affect the strategies of the organization.

Because of its effect on the direction of the organization, management *style* plays an important role in the organization. The style of the key figures within the organization determines the level and depth of communication to the staff. Verbal and non-verbal communication may differ greatly, depending on the style of management. The analysis of style should include such factors as how expectations are communicated, public statements, reports reviewed, treatment of staff, and how time is spent by the leader (Bopp and Hicks, 1984). The style of management may also affect communication horizontally and upwardly.

The *staff* of the organization is a third element in the culture of the organization. The group of individuals who compose the staff of the organization are human resources. The efficient use of these resources requires evaluation. An examination of the development of the staff to include the appropriate education/training to promote the professional growth is another important aspect of the analysis. The skill level of the staff as a whole may play a role in the development of strategies and must therefore be contemplated.

The *systems* that determine how smoothly the organization functions are often a key element in the internal environment of the organization. Those procedures or processes that specify the way the institution operates may include protocols for operations, performance management systems, quality control or quality assurance systems, accounting and budget systems, and information systems. Understanding the role of the various systems in the organization is important to the overall evaluation of the internal environment.

The attributes or capabilities of the organization contribute continually to its success or failure in the business of which it is a part, just as personal attributes determine the success of an individual within a certain position. These *skills* must be identified in the internal environmental analysis so that decisions made at a later point in the strategic management process may include decisions related to new skills or replacement of skills if necessitated by beneficial changes.

The *shared values* previously discussed, which compose the philosophy of the institution, serve several functions (Waterman, 1982). The values of the organization will determine the appropriateness of relationships among organizations or among individuals and the organization. They will also denote legitimate controls for behavior within the organization. Description of acceptable characteristics and behavior for members of the organization may also be a function of the shared organizational values. Finally, the manner in which the organization should deal with the external environment is derived from the shared values of the organization. An analysis of the organization's values begun in the first step of the strategic management process must continue as the elements of the organization's culture are reviewed in light of its efficiency and effectiveness.

Strategy is the last element to be reviewed in the culture of an organization. How organizational strategy aligns with the other elements is important in the assessment of an organization's ability to operate successfully. Although strategy can and should be adjusted, this adjustment can be accomplished only in relation to the other six elements.

Internal assessment may begin with an evaluation of each of the seven elements described in the previous paragraphs as they relate to one another. Assessment of the current and projected assets and liabilities of the organization is yet another part of the internal assessment. Much of the information obtained from the evaluation of the elements can be used in identifying the organizational assets or liabilities. Consideration should be given to the resources available to the institution.

Technical resources such as equipment and facilities and human resources including the number and qualifications of the staff may head the list of assets and liabilities. The systems available for managing these resources efficiently may be added to the list. The structure and management of the organization receive consideration as well. The financial situation of the organization is yet another characteristic that must be assessed, and the market capacity of the organization is equally important. (Refer to Chapter 9, Financial Management, and Chapter 11, Marketing for Health Care.)

As the analysis of the internal environment occurs, it will be important for the nursing administrator to relate each step to the department of nursing. While no department can be separate from the whole institution, the role of the nursing department of any health care institution cannot be overemphasized. The needs of the consumers for nursing care, for example, are part of the analysis of the market capacity for the organization. How well nursing works within the predetermined framework of the organization is important to the analysts who are identifying the assets and liabilities of the organization. Implications for nursing practice of all identified liabilities or assets must be carefully evaluated by the nursing administrator in the process of strategic management.

EXTERNAL ASSESSMENT

External environmental assessment requires somewhat more work by the managers and planners, since research of sorts may be necessary. Many external forces or phenomena impact on health care organizations in a direct or indirect manner, producing risks, threats, or opportunities. It is better, then, for an organization to err by overanalyzing the external environment than to incorrectly assume that some aspect of the environment is unimportant. Analysis should therefore begin with the very broad social and economic factors and with the governmental policies that may impact on health care.

The economic climate in which health care finds itself is generally felt by all businesses and the general public. However, the impact of this economic climate on health care may vary significantly from the impact on any other business. It is the impact on health care and even more specifically on nursing that must be analyzed. The financial market is part of the economic climate and would include potential funding sources, interest rates, or other investment opportunities for the health care institution.

Government regulation has certainly been an external force that has seriously impacted on health care. The changes in the role of the government in relation to health care have been so dramatic since the 1930's that the variance between costs and available revenues has produced drastic change in reimbursement and will continue to produce changes in health care delivery (Kolderie, 1983). The role of the government in health care should be assessed by considering several factors: the role as provider of services, the policy-maker role, and the fund-provider role. In each of these roles, government regulation or action may impact positively or negatively on the future of a health care institution.

Social factors that may affect the health care institution cover a range from the characteristics of the population to consumer expectations. Age of the population and shifts toward a different age group are a portion of the demographics that could alter the types of programs and type of nursing care needed. Consumer attitudes related to health care and to wellness/illness are seriously affecting the health care industry and would necessarily need to be evaluated during the external environmental assessment. General and broad or slow trends in the demographic appearance of the population should also be included.

Technology has been a major issue in health care changes over the years. The wide expansion of technology in health care and the conflicting cries for better technology but lower costs must be analyzed. This will even involve evaluation of research related to improvements in technology and the related costs of such technology.

The labor market is another focus of the assessment of the external environment. How much and how well trained labor can be expected to be will be a necessary component of the evaluation. Even the attitudes of the labor market toward the health care organization could be important and should be considered.

The political and the legal climate need consideration by the analysts in relation to any impact they may have on the health care organization. If, for example, the laws of a particular state require each physician to carry a minimum amount of malpractice insurance, the effect on the institution may be significant should a number of physicians decide to move from the area because of the climate—political or legal.

Finally, and often most importantly, the competition with which a health care institution must deal is a major portion of the external assessment. Competition may include not only other health care institutions with similar full services, but any of the single service organizations (urgent care, surgicenters), entrepreneurs (free standing centers, private practitioners), suppliers, or contractors for services. Even professional groups, creditors, and volunteer agencies must be considered as competitors in the evaluation of the external environment, since in planning comprehensive programs, there may be overlapping of services that the organization desires to offer.

Health care institutions may be able to perform the environmental analysis or may require the services of a consultant. Large corporations in health care generally have planners whose expertise is in assessment and planning. Consultants can fill this role when the health care institution is unable to. Consultants should not be asked to make the decision, but rather they should assist with analysis and evaluation. Whether or not a consultant is used in the internal and external assessment, it is very important that a data base be established and maintained for the information that is gathered. Such a data base can be crucial when the organization is ready to forecast for future programs or services. Use of computerized data base systems is one way in which this may be accomplished. At a later point in the process, the consultant may be able to assist in identifying alternatives.

Identification of Issues and Trends

The trends and issues that may be impacting on health care institutions are an important part of the strategic management process. These trends or issues may be occurring within health care or may be only peripheral. In either case, a careful examination of them will be helpful in identifying the risks, opportunities, or threats that are associated with the trends and issues. There is a close relationship between the external forces that impact on health care and the issues or trends outside health care that may influence it.

Naisbitt (1982) has identified numerous trends that may impact on health care. These trends include a move toward wellness and holistic care, home health care, and movement toward healthy activities including diet/exercise programs and programs for prevention of illness. While these are only examples of trends, they demonstrate the effect a trend might have on the health care industry.

Ethical issues are surfacing at a tremendous rate, as concerns for quality of life or the effect of cutting costs arise. These issues, too, will impact on health care and should be carefully evaluated. Legal issues may be tied to many of the ethical issues, and these relationships require careful analysis.

Issues and trends may find their source in consumers, health professions, or controlling agencies. In each of these groups, there will be information that can assist health care institutions in the decision making process involved with strategic management. Steiner (1979) stresses that, in order to accurately gauge the impact of changes, a systematic assessment of environmental factors and key trends or issues is of great importance. Each issue or trend will need to be prioritized and addressed according to its influence in the formulation of strategies for the organization. For example, issues relating to nursing practice may be minimal in one particular state but nursing may be in jeopardy in another state. Prioritization of the issue in view of the effect or impact it could have must guide the process (Lukacs, 1984).

Determination of Organization's Direction

Much of the work necessary to the strategic management process will have been completed at this point. That work has provided the foundation from which strategies may be developed (Bopp and Hicks, 1984). An objective analysis that began with a review of the organization itself, continued to an assessment of the internal and external environment, and finally involved an evaluation of health care from an issues and trends perspective, would most certainly have provided additionally a learning process for the organization.

The knowledge gained through this analysis, when integrated with the knowledge already found within the institution, will result in the formulation of strategy. Andrews (1980) refers to strategy as the "pattern of decisions" that an organization would develop to produce its goals, policies, or plans. The extent to which an organization may expand or the changes it may initiate to meet its goals are of significance in view of the major changes continually facing health care.

Health care institutions, as with any other business, must determine and define their business during this strategic management process. Based on the findings of the strategic assessments, health care organizations may choose not to change, or may determine that a new direction is needed. An attitude of tolerance to previously considered radical direction may be in order. Health care institutions may need a direction that opens doors to diversification of activities, from traditional inpatient acute care to ambulatory services, or horizontal integration to form multi-hospital systems, for example. As health care institutions reach this stage of the process, they may need to reconceptualize the mission and values to determine the direction for survival.

Changes in Organization's Elements

The seven elements of an organization's culture described by Waterman (1982), which were discussed in the section on environmental analysis, are interconnected. How well an organization can implement a *strategy* it has determined to be appropriate will depend on how well these variables can be realigned with one another. Changes in the culture of an organization may be very necessary to achieve specific strategies and outcomes desired. For a particular strategy, one or more of the other six variables may require some change. For example, if specific skills are needed for a type of service to be offered, the type of staff in the organization may require change to offer the service. Inability or unwillingness to change the other variables may result in failure in implementation or reduced effectiveness of a strategy (Bopp and Hicks, 1984).

The *structure* of the organization may inhibit or support a particular strategy. Once a strategy has been determined reasonable, necessary, and appropriate, the organizational structure should be evaluated to decide whether it can support or will inhibit implementation of the strategy. If it cannot support the strategy, a reorganization may be necessary. The extent of reorganization will vary, depending upon the support required for the success of the strategy. A good example of how this may be accomplished is seen in a strategy to provide modern and non-traditional maternity services. These services could be provided through the use of LDRP (labor, delivery, recovery, post-partum) rooms to enhance family involvement and bonding. In order to accomplish this, the obstetrical department might need to be structured differently. This same concept could apply to an organization-wide strategy.

Another variable that will need to be evaluated before success can occur in relation to a particular strategy is *systems*. Information and financial reporting systems as well as specific policies and procedures may need to be revised or changed to effect successful strategies. Many of these systems address the smooth operation of the organization, so consideration must be given to how systems changes will affect the proposed strategy as well as the continuing strategies or other operations within the organization.

The *shared values* of the organization may be contrary to a defined strategy determined to be necessary for organizational success. Values are often the most difficult to change of the variables attributed to an organization's culture. However, the manner in which behavior is controlled or guided and in which the relationships between groups or individuals are prescribed or defined can certainly affect the success of a strategy. Even the long term goals of the organization that are part of the shared values may change to support survival strategies.

Skills of the staff and of the organization, evaluated earlier in the process of identifying strengths and weaknesses of the organization, may need revision or strengthening based on the newly determined strategies. New skills, both in technological and people capabilities, may be necessary to support new strategies.

The demographic make-up of the *staff* of an organization may influence the strategies that have been determined as necessary to move the organization in a specific direction. The staff mix that is necessary to effect the desired changes within the organization may or may not be present. Willingness to evaluate those needs and to develop, allocate, or recruit the desired mix may be a key component in the success of the organization as it moves in new directions.

Finally, the *style* or the behavior of management as perceived by the organization can impact significantly on the success of the strategies of the organization. The actions of management can communicate their priorities

TABLE 8–2
Elements of the Organizational Culture

Structure
Style
Staff
Skill
Systems
Shared values
Strategy

and expectations to other members of the organization (Bopp and Hicks, 1984). Changes in organizational direction can signify a need to change the style of management as well.

Each of the variables (Table 8–2) associated with an organization's culture should be evaluated in relation to strategy to ensure that the connection between the variables is balanced well. An imbalance between variables or the lack of consideration of one or more variables as it affects the strategy can result in failure or reduced effectiveness. An example of the changes that might be important with a particular strategy is illustrated in the following examples.

Assume that a hospital has determined through a strategic management process that a hotel services program is necessary to the success of the hospital in the highly competitive marketplace of health care. The *strategy* is implementation of a hotel services department. The *structure* change required means combining under one manager departments that previously have operated quite independently of one another. Furthermore, the size of this new department is such that administration may need to create another assistant administrator position. Certainly, at the very least several assistant administrators will be affected, and reporting lines will be altered. *Systems* changes necessary to support this strategy will include policy and procedure changes. Productivity measurement tools will require alteration, and information systems reports format will need to be changed as well.

The change in the organization's *shared values* will have already occurred for this strategy to have been reached, but additional value changes will need consideration. The long term goals of the organization and the pre-scribed relationships among individuals and groups may need change. Such a program as hotel services necessitates a more cooperative inter-departmental relationship specifically related to meeting the objectives of the program.

The organization's capabilities or *skills* may need change, too, to support the strategy. Technological advances such as computerization, knowledge acquisition, new equipment, or guest relations programs for the staff are examples of changes that may be necessary. The *staff* may require supplementation in numbers or in demographics to achieve the identified objectives. For example, a more assertive and outgoing supervisory staff in the house-keeping department or a higher educational level among the security force may be important to the success of the strategy.

The change in the *style* of management that is needed to successfully implement this strategy may be even more important. Management may need to take a more active role in observation and supervision. Visibility of management and positive reinforcement for positive behavior would be an essential element in this type of program.

Each of the variables, then, required some type of change to support the strategy described. The amount of change required might be minimal or quite extensive, depending on the state of the organization at the time the strategy was implemented. The important point to be made is that any one of the variables may need to be changed to support specific strategies of an organization.

Development of Objectives

There is a progressive linkage in the strategic management process from mission to current goals to objectives. Actualization of the organization's mission occurs through this process (Fox and Fox, 1983). Management by objectives, which has been emphasized by many business organizations as important to successful operation, can certainly be applied to health care organizations. Management by objectives (MBO) has advantages and disadvantages. The development of objectives is undeniably a component of the strategic management process. The place of the MBO philosophy within this process may, however, be questioned.

Management by objectives follows two basic principles: (1) results orientation and (2) basis in human behavior (Cain and Luchsinger, 1978). The concept of MBO is based on behavioral theories that address motivation of individuals to achieve desired goals. Mutual goal setting by the individual and his or her supervisor is a major aspect of MBO and as such has significant advantages in motivation of the individual to achieve. An assumption must be made that managers want to satisfy employees' needs for self-esteem and self-actualization and that the employees are achievement oriented. Only through the achievement of results will the needs for self-esteem and self-actualization be met. MBO, then, offers the opportunity to systematically meet the high level needs described. MBO also offers the objective criteria by which job performance can be measured, i.e., achievement of expected results.

The problems or concerns related to MBO should be considered, then, before it becomes a part of the strategic management process (Levinson and LaMonica, 1980). MBO can, for instance, stifle creativity by forcing the focus of reward to be on the agreed upon objectives. While creativity may occur at the time of development of objectives, there may be little acceptance of new ideas later. If rewards are given for achievement of expected results of objectives, innovation and spontaneity of service at other times may go unrewarded. Psychologically, the MBO philosophy can be extremely stress producing because of limitations in the choice of objectives. The MBO process itself may be utilized at least in part in the strategic management process. However, consideration of disadvantages or problems should occur before major emphasis is placed on such a process. Although creativity, rapid response, risk taking, and entrepreneuralism are the buzz words of the 1980's, they do not totally preclude sound business practices such as MBO. In large organizations, such as hospitals, both extremes of sound business practice and risk taking have a valuable contribution to make in moving health care into the 1990's.

The steps in the MBO process parallel the remainder of the steps in the process of strategic management. These steps will be discussed separately, and their place in strategic management will be reviewed. The development of goals may be a "top down," "bottom up," or combination process. The first phase in MBO is development of goals. Objectives are then developed, which define the manner in which the goal is to be achieved. Regardless of the approach used, several basic principles apply to objectives.

Objectives should be clearly written and able to be reached. They should also be measurable. Realistic is a term often applied to objectives and essentially means that they can be attained as described. Quantification of objectives is preferred to ensure that measurability. A completion date for objectives is essential with MBO, since success is dependent upon achievement. Objectives may be developed at several levels from subordinate to supervisor, but they should involve the individuals whose performance appraisal includes the results of their achievement.

Objectives in strategy management must follow the strategies identified and the direction determined to be best for the organization. Depending upon the management philosophy, the organizational culture, and the flexibility resulting from the process, objectives may initially be developed at the top management level and filtered down to the individual employees or may be developed at the level of individuals or units and progressively built to the top. Essential to the process is keeping always in sight the overall strategies for the organization and continually monitoring and updating as necessary the plans that have been developed.

Several other steps that are included in MBO are covered in the next sections of this chapter, since they apply to much broader aspects of strategic management than MBO. They include action planning, evaluation, and performance appraisal. Each of these, with the exception of performance appraisal, fits into the model for strategic management. Performance appraisal is more appropriately covered in Chapter Sixteen, Human Relations Management.

Implementation of Objectives

Once objectives have been established, an action plan for implementation is needed. The plan for action is sometimes considered to be the sub-objectives or the steps necessary to achieve the objectives. Planning for implementation can be very simple or very complicated, depending on the objective. Some objectives may require a series of steps before they can be accomplished.

Actual implementation of planned objectives may be stalled because of limited staff, lack of commitment, or errors in judgment (Lukacs, 1984). Because cooperation between departments can determine the success or failure of the strategy, planning must address the interdepartmental relationships. The implementation of planned objectives is the area of the process in which many personnel are actively involved—work performance. As such, it requires much of a manager's energy and must fit well with other management functions.

Evaluation of Effectiveness

Implicit in the continuous process of strategic management is the evaluation of effectiveness. Effectiveness is defined for this discussion as "producing the desired effect." Rather than a final step, evaluation is reviewed as a preceding step to organizational review. Continual monitoring throughout the implementation phase permits identification of change in environmental trends or conditions that might demand adjustment of an alternative or objective. This continual monitoring is often referred to as the formative evaluation. This type of evaluation is beneficial because it provides continual control by management.

A summative evaluation may be performed at the conclusion of a project to determine whether the objective was met or how effectively the objective was accomplished. Analysis of resource utilization, productivity, and impact on the department or institution is generally included in a summative evaluation. Quantitative comparisons may also be included in this type of evaluation. The measurement of the final outcome of the program or project against objectives identified for that program or project is the purpose of the summative evaluation (Fox and Fox, 1983).

Several key components should be considered in the evaluation for effectiveness. Resources—personnel and supplies or equipment—are one component necessary for the successful completion of an objective. Lack of adequate resources would certainly influence the objective. Stability of the environment in relation to the objective is another component requiring consideration. Changes in either the internal or the external environment may, in fact, impact significantly on the completion of an objective. Changes in the organization culture through changes in one or more of the variables of the culture could produce important effects on the entire organizational direction. For example, a change in the structure of an organization to provide for better product line management could have significant negative effects on the nursing care provided by the organization. To meet the objectives for the product line manager of one area, team nursing might be used, while in another area primary care might continue. The inconsistency between areas could over time be noted and criticized by the customers of the organization (patients, physicians, employees). Also, because of the different types of nursing, there could be reduced flexibility in staffing, which could adversely affect the organization's expenses.

Model for Strategic Management

Strategic management, although it involves strategic planning, goes beyond the simple process for planning to include thinking and action. Figure 8–1 illustrates a model for strategic management. Each step involved in the strategic management process has been explained and fits into the sequence identified in the model.

Much of the process involves the organization producing, identifying, or determining what is happening with the organization and what is desired to happen. The review of the organization, environmental analysis, and evaluation of health care issues and trends exemplify the identification of what does exist. External sources of data contribute to the pool of information in these steps. External forces may also produce risks, threats, or opportunities for health care organizations. Consumers; health professionals such as physicians, nurses, or therapists; and control agencies such as JCAH, and federal and state agencies may identify additional trends and issues that impact on health care. Once the organization has taken an analytical look at itself, it also must make the decisions about its direction. The decision about organizational direction is an important one for future success.

After the decision regarding direction is made, the impact of the decision is felt by the organization. Elements of the organization's culture may be changed to accomplish the goals developed to carry the organization in the direction in which it is moving. Those changes are fed back to the organization as part of the continual strategic management process. Objectives that are developed and implemented become another component of the system that impacts on the organization. Evaluation of the achievement of objectives is the final step before the organization once again must step back and deeply analyze itself.

The organization gives much of itself during a part of the process, but it gains much as it develops, learns, and grows through the changes that affect it and through the development, implementation, and evaluation of its objectives. The process of strategic management is continual and is sequential to an extent only. Evaluation, for instance, occurs throughout the process. Change, based on these evaluations, can also occur continually. It is of importance to stress that while the process of strategic management is continual, an organized approach to the process is necessary to ensure that no steps are overlooked and that consideration is given to each step. Failure to consider all factors throughout this process could result in failure for the organization.

A nursing department may utilize the strategic management model, for itself. In using the model, the nursing department may initially review the values, beliefs, and goals of nursing. A careful analysis of the internal and external environment follows. Strengths and weaknesses of the nursing department are identified internally. Externally, the risks, threats, and opportunities facing nursing are considered. The nursing department may have as a strength an all RN staff, but, externally, a shortage of RN's may produce a threat to the department, for example.

The issues and trends in nursing will need evaluation. Although ethical issues that continue to face nursing may head the list, any of the issues that are unresolved and the trends for the future will require consideration. Nursing administration may then decide on a direction for the department. That direction might, for example, be elimination of head nurses in the change to true primary nursing. Such a direction would certainly require changes in the variables of the organization's culture, specifically in the style, skills, systems, structure, staff, shared values, and strategy.

Objectives would need to be developed to support the new direction chosen for nursing. Each objective would be implemented and continually evaluated. As problems were identified, adjustments might be needed. The final evaluation might indicate success or failure in achievement of objectives, but certainly it would reflect on the values and beliefs of the organization as the strategic management process continued.

FORECASTING

Forecasting is the practice of predicting the future. In health care, forecasting is commonly done in the process of strategic management. This technique is most frequently utilized in planning for the budget but can be utilized in program planning as well. It is important for the manager to recognize that forecasting is only a tool and does not ensure accuracy. Successful forecasting can be beneficial for the manager but does not alleviate the need for flexibility.

There are at least 20 methods of forecasting currently in use, which vary in complexity, sophistication, and accuracy of results. Each method has specific limitations and advantages in terms of costs, time requirements, data needs, and outcome. Before a decision is made about a specific method, the manager should examine the dimension of each to identify the method best suited to particular needs.

The first dimension to be considered is time—the time the forecast is to cover as well as when it might be needed or need to be updated. Any limitations of a particular method should also be evaluated. These might include finances necessary to achieve the prediction (surveys, for example) or computer capabilities required. How easily environmental variables, shifts in trends, and management decisions could be fed into a specific method would need additional examination. Finally, before a decision on a method for forecasting is made, the manager would want to know the expected level of accuracy, detail, and turning points reflected. Generating a forecast for any lengthy period is difficult for health care institutions. Techniques may be combined to improve accuracy, and the use of judgment in any prediction is essential. Many techniques are very costly, so that an analysis of costs to benefit may be helpful. Table 9–14, Forecasting Methods, may be helpful in the selection process of a technique for forecasting (Georgoff and Murdick, 1986).

Forecasting is a very common practice in health care institutions. Several steps are necessary in the process of forecasting. Collection of historical data related to the department is the first step. If forecasting is to project the number of procedures or patients, the historical data for several years is preferred. Although historical data have questionable value in these rapidly changing times, use of these data will give a more accurate picture of the trend for the department. The next step is to collect other pertinent data that might influence the number of procedures or patients. This might include the opening or closing of another department (in this institution or a competing one), the change in patient mix related to other programs or units, a change in the number or mix of physicians, and the addition or loss of equipment. Any factor that could influence the numbers could be important.

Once the historical and the influencing data are collected, careful analysis of the information will be necessary. Analysis of the data must consider the rate of growth or decline in activity related to the department, the effect of other departmental activity on the department under analysis, and other factors that might influence the number of procedures or patients. Use of a graph such as that illustrated in Figure 8–2 is useful in the analysis.

The graph in the illustration indicates that an annual growth rate of approximately 10% occurred from 1980 to 1983, but a decline of approximately 10% per year occurred from that point. Assuming no other factors would influence the activity, one could forecast a continued decline of 10% for the following year. Unfortunately, one must also consider the previously mentioned factors. The closing of a similar department at a competitive hospital might result in an additional 4,000 patients per year, which would mean a forecast of 12,100 patients for 1987 instead of a decline of approximately 800.

Forecasting involves a careful look at the historical trend of the department to which additional patient days, procedures, and other data may be added or deleted to reach the "best guess" for the future. Such a determination must serve as a guide only, and must consider all available data. Forecasting is simply a prediction, and flexibility in its use is essential to successful management.

PROGRAM DEVELOPMENT

Development of new programs is a task assigned ever more frequently to nurse administrators. Such responsibility requires considerable study and

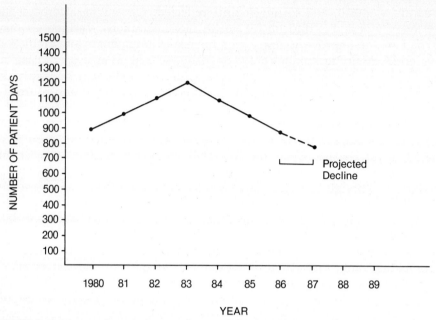

FIGURE 8–2. Forecasting growth potential. This example projects patient days based on trend from previous years.

planning to achieve success. Initially, the administrator responsible for the program must determine the feasibility and desirability of the program. Additional planning must also occur prior to any program. The steps that should be followed in program development are outlined as follows:

1. Identification of need for program
2. Determination of feasibility of program
3. Planning for program
4. Implementation of program
5. Evaluation of success of program

Identification of a need for a program can occur through several mechanisms. The consumers of health care may demand that the program be developed. Physicians may see the need and request that the program be developed. Competition may indicate the need for a program to ensure successful competition or to provide a competitive edge. A program may naturally "fall out" as a result of other activities. Once a program need is identified, an analysis is needed to determine the feasibility of the program.

Financial feasibility is certainly an important aspect of the feasibility analysis, but there are other factors that also require consideration. The impact of the program on other departments and on public relations, and the long term impact should be considered. For instance, a specific program may always lose money but a side effect of the program may be an increase in patient admissions that would not otherwise have occurred. The program

---

TABLE 8–3
Feasibility Worksheet

I. Start-up costs: A. Planning: _____ hrs. @ $__ $ _____
/hr.

B. Contract $ _____
development _____ hrs. @
$_____/hr.

C. Legal fees $ _____
D. Subtotal (A + B + C) $ _____
E. Expected number of procedures $ _____
F. Cost per procedure (D ÷ E) $ _____ I.

(Spread over one
year)

II. Equipment costs: A. Cost of equipment $ _____
B. Useful life of equipment—years   _____
C. Subtotal (A ÷ B) $ _____

D. Annual maintenance contract $ _____
E. Yearly equipment costs (C + $ _____
D)
F. Expected number of procedures   _____
G. Costs per procedure (E ÷ F) $ _____ II.

III. Labor Costs: Total hours required per procedure
(_____)
Multiplied by hourly rate ($ ____) $ _____ III.
(NOTE: Several employees may be required for a
procedure—each salary must be considered and each
individual's time computed per procedure)

IV. Supply costs: Per procedure $ _____ IV.
V. Total direct costs: (I + II + III + IV) $ _____ V.
Per procedure   A. Add profit margin (% profit $ _____
multiplied by V)

VI. Charge per   Total charge required (V + A) $ _____ VI.
procedure:

---

may be desired because of the effect it has on another area (i.e., patient days). Another program that may never pay for itself monetarily may be worth the investment because of the positive public relations it produces.

In considering financial feasibility of a program, several factors are important. The cost of initiating such a program (start-up costs) would include human resources to plan and implement the program, equipment and supplies, and construction or renovation. Equipment could be depreciated over its expected life, and the start-up human resource time would generally be spread over the treatments or procedures of one year. The other costs would include personnel costs per procedure and supplies per procedure. After all costs were assessed, the profit margin required or desired would be added to determine the charge needed to support the program (see Table 8–3 for a sample worksheet).

Besides these actual cost figures, consideration should be given to several other factors that would influence the financial feasibility. Reimbursement by third party payors, bad debt ratios, and the financial picture of other programs in the institution should be a part of the evaluation. Regardless of the charge, if reimbursement is only cost or less, the feasibility of the program is limited. The same would be true in relation to bad debts. If other programs in the institution were financially strong, more consideration might be given to a marginal program, assuming other benefits were identified. Growth potential for the program or by-products of the program (patient admissions) represents yet another consideration.

A program can produce multiple by-products. These may include additional related admissions; good public relations, which might produce unrelated admissions; and use of additional equipment to produce other income. Each of these factors should be considered in the evaluation. Once the program has been determined to be feasible financially, its impact on the department, the organization, and the community must be considered. The model for strategic management should be applied. Environmental analysis and evaluation of health care in relation to the program would be important.

Planning for the program would include the analysis and evaluation as well as the direction determined to be appropriate for the program. Any changes necessitated by the decision would be accomplished, and objectives could be developed. Planning for a new program will require determination of resource requirements (done to some extent during the financial feasibility study) and phases of implementation. Renovation or construction of facilities will require time frames and very careful planning. Involvement in planning of the personnel who will run the program is essential to the success of the program. Development of policies and procedures should be accomplished prior to implementation.

Once decisions are made and planning is complete, implementation may occur. Continual monitoring of progress is important. Feedback related to the objectives, including problem identification, financial status, and resolution, will determine the program's success. Evaluation after a predetermined time will hopefully provide the measurement of success.

TOMORROW'S STRATEGIES

Strategic management is a process for thinking, planning, and implementing that can be applied to all areas of health care organizations, including nursing. The process is relatively simple and requires a systematic approach. While it is generally sequential, it may overlap and several of its phases may occur simultaneously. The model for strategic management (see Fig. 8–1) illustrates the steps utilized in development of strategies and in their implementation and evaluation.

Key to the process is the analysis of the internal and external environments and the evaluation of issues and trends. The nursing administrator must be keenly aware of the continually changing environments, issues, and trends as well as the varying impact of each on nursing and on health care organizations. Preparation for such changes can only occur when one is aware of them, and a willingness and ability to change as necessary are important components in the system. Inability to be flexible can be extremely detrimental. A problem solving approach is the basis for the model, with consideration for each step a critical element in success. Success of an organization may be dependent on how well the strategic management process can be followed in planning and thinking for the future.

References

Ackoff, R. (1982). Our changing concept of planning. *JONA*, *12*(10), 35–40.

Andrews, K. (1980). *The concept of corporate strategy*. Homewood, IL: Jones-Irwin.

Ansoff, H., Declerk, R., and Hayes, R. (1976). *From strategic planning to strategic management*. New York: John Wiley and Sons, pp. 1–12.

Bopp, K., and Hicks, L. (1984). Strategic management in health care. *Nursing Economics*, *2*(2), 93–101.

Cain, C. and Luchsinger, V. (1978). Management by objectives: Applications to nursing. *JONA*, *8*(1), 35–38.

Drucker, P. (1974). *Management: Tasks, responsibilities, policies*. New York: Harper and Row.

Fox, D., and Fox, R. (1983). Strategic planning for nursing. *JONA*, *13*(5), 11–17.

Freeman, R. (1984). *Strategic management: A stakeholder approach*. Boston: Pitman Publishing, Inc., pp. 91–95.

Georgoff, D., and Murdick, R. (1986). Manager's guide to forecasting. *Harvard Business Review*, *64*(1), 110–120.

Gluck, F., Kaufman, S., and Walleck, A. (1982). The four phases of strategic management. *Journal of Business Strategy*, *2*(3), 13–15.

Hofer, C., and Schendel, D. (1978). *Strategy formulation: Analytical concepts*. St. Paul: West Publishing Co.

Kolderie, T. (1983). Government in the eighties: Shifting roles and responsibilities. *Journal of Health Administration Education*, *1*(1), 91–96.

Levinson, H. and LaMonica, E. (1980). Management by whose objectives? *JONA*, *10*(9), 22–30.

Lukacs, J. (1984). Strategic planning in hospitals: Application for nurse executives. *JONA*, *15*(9), 11–17.

Naisbitt, J. (1982). *Megatrends*. New York: Warner Books, Inc.

Ryan, J. (1975). The nursing administrator's growing role in facilities planning. *JONA*, *5*(9), 22–27.

Steiner, G. (1979). *Strategic planning*. New York: The Free Press.

Waterman, R. (1982). The seven elements of strategic fit. *Journal of Business Strategy*, *2*(3), 69–73.

FINANCIAL MANAGEMENT

INTRODUCTION

The health care administration of yesterday was primarily concerned with providing high quality health care services to the public. That responsibility was of primary importance and has been reflected in the non-businesslike posture found until recently in many of the health care organizations in the United States. However, statistics for the early 1980's have shown continual rises in health care costs to those figures for 1985, in which the American economy spent roughly $425 billion. This occurred despite the cost containment incentives, low demand for inpatient care, and moderate inflation that reflected the health care environment post-prospective payment (Dolkart, Freko, and Li, 1984). In newspapers and journals across the country, health care professionals, consumers, and regulating bodies question the costs of health care, the reason behind those costs, and what is being done about it. Regardless of the cause for the costs associated with health care, nursing administrators need an in-depth understanding of financial management in health care. As never before, sound financial management is not merely important, it is essential for the successful operation of any health care institution.

A number of factors have influenced the rising costs of health care. Equity in access to health care, a demand for which Medicare and Medicaid was presumably the answer, was one factor that drove the costs for health care up (Schramm, 1984). This attempt to provide accessibility for the elderly and the poor population removed many of the economic constraints of the system. This reimbursement system also encouraged a freer expenditure for higher technology for diagnosis and treatment of patients, demanded by both physicians and the public in general. The combination of expectations by the populations (for access, technology, and quality), high technology for medical practice, and the economic climate resulted in the high costs for health care (Schramm, 1984).

The health care environment will continue to be influenced financially in the future by several factors (Furst, 1981). Continued efforts by the federal and state governments to reduce health care spending represent one such factor. These efforts will probably include continued revision of the prospective payment reimbursement system to include physician payment, revision of controls for capital expenditure and revenue, and encouragement toward alternative financing mechanisms such as HMOs. The growth of HMOs and other alternative delivery systems is yet another factor that will continue to influence the health care environment. Reduction in hospitalization and health care costs may result from these alternative delivery systems. Finally, the environment of health care may be influenced by the increase in hospital chains or mergers of individual hospitals offering shared services, better access to capital, and expertise unavailable to individual hospitals.

Concern about the rate of increase in health care costs has been shared by private insurers, governmental bodies, and consumers. The factors that have and will influence those costs have been recognized and are hopefully being dealt with or planned for. Many of these factors are financial or affect the financial structure of the organizations: reimbursement, duplication of services, low productivity, equipment expenditures. In order to adequately address these financial issues, the nursing administrator must have a basic understanding of financial management.

The major role of the financial manager is to maximize the worth of the owner of the institution (Furst, 1981). The owner may of course be a group of stockholders (private institution) or the community (county, city, or state facility). Three functions have been identified as essential in the role of the financial manager: cash flow, investment, and financing functions. Basically, this means the financial manager must be sure that financial obligations can be met, that resources are invested in suitable assets, and that capital can be obtained at a minimum cost. While this sounds simple, it is somewhat complex.

This chapter will have as its focus financial management of health care institutions. It is not intended to be a comprehensive study, but rather a basic guide to financial management. Basic concepts of financial management will be introduced. This will include analysis of financial statements, including income statement and balance sheets. Reimbursement and allocation concepts will be explained. One section will also be devoted to budgeting. Various types of budgets will be discussed, and the prerequisite and process for these will be addressed. Analysis of budget variance will also be included. Planning for financial management is another section and will include forecasting and rate setting. Management of working capital and analysis of capital expenditures are additional sections. Capital financing and rate setting will also be addressed in this chapter.

BASIC CONCEPTS IN FINANCIAL MANAGEMENT

The financial decision making necessary for successful management is a basic process applicable to any organization. The basis for the decisions related to finance is the goal or mission of the organization, the financial focus of which is maximization of wealth for the owner (including the community). The supportive tools for this goal include analysis, planning, and control (Petty, Keown, Scott, and Martin, 1982). Decisions regarding improving the financial position of the health care institution must be based on an understanding of these tools and their relationship to the overall financial operation of the institution.

Financial Statement Analysis

Analysis of the financial statement of an institution must include review of three specific statements: income statement, balance sheet, and changes in financial position. Table 9–1 is an example of an income statement.

INCOME STATEMENT

Also called the statement of revenue and expense, the income statement of a health care institution generally will identify three major sources of

TABLE 9–1
Income Statement
Your Hospital
Statement of Revenue and Expense
Period Ending August 31, 1985

	Current Month					YTD				Last YTD
	Actual	Budget	Variance	% Variance		Actual	Budget	Variance	% Variance	Actual
Room Revenue	1,135,000	1,099,000	36,000	3.3+	12,064,000	12,236,000	172,000–	1.4–	12,240,000
Total Inpatient Ancillary	3,210,000	2,725,000	485,000	17.8+	35,549,000	31,348,000	4,196,000	13.4+	32,000,000
Total Outpatient Ancillary	701,000	550,000	151,000	27.5+	6,482,000	5,986,000	496,000	8.3+	5,975,000
Total Patient Revenue	5,046,000	4,374,000	672,000	15.4+	54,090,000	49,570,000	4,520,000	9.1+	50,215,000
Other Operating Revenue	36,000	40,000	4,000–	10.0–	380,000	436,000	56,000–	12.8–	435,000
Total Gross Operating Revenue	5,082,000	4,414,000	668,000	15.1+	54,470,000	50,006,000	4,464,000	8.9+	50,650,000
Deductions from Revenue										
Provision for Bad Debts	612,000	410,000	202,000–	49.3–	5,908,000	4,646,000	1,262,00–	27.2–	4,500,000
Charity	208,000	73,000	135,000–	184.9–	1,084,000	815,000	269,000–	33.0–	810,000
Contractual Allowances	590,000	838,000	248,000	29.6+	11,543,000	9,499,000	2,044,000–	21.5–	9,500,000
Total Deductions For Revenue	1,410,000	1,321,000	89,000–	6.7–	18,535,000	14,960,000	3,575,000–	23.9–	14,810,000
Total Net Operating Revenue	3,672,000	3,093,000	579,000	18.7	35,935,000	35,046,000	889,000	2.5	35,840,000
Operating Expenses										
Salaries Expense	2,955,000	2,355,000	600,000–	25.5–	28,032,000	26,861,000	1,171,000–	4.4–	26,750,000
Depreciation	177,000	152,000	25,000–	16.4–	1,641,000	1,668,000	27,000	1.6+	1,650,000
Insurance	94,000	81,000	13,000–	16.0–	888,000	894,000	6,000	0.7+	850,000
Interest Expense	40,000	91,000	51,000	56.0+	573,000	995,000	422,000	42.4+	950,000
Total Operating Expenses	3,266,000	2,679,000	587,000–	21.9–	31,134,000	30,418,000	716,000–	2.4–	30,200,000
Net Operating Income	406,000	414,000	8,000–	1.9–	4,801,000	4,628,000	173,000	3.7+	5,640,000
Non-Operating Revenue	118,000	34,000	84,000	247.1+	1,067,000	376,000	691,000	183.7+	400,000
Net Income (+)/Loss (–)	524,000	448,000	76,000	17.0+	5,868,000	5,004,000	864,000	17.3+	6,040,000

revenue: patient care, operations not directly related to patient care, and non-operating sources. These sources of revenue are generally broken down further. For example, patient care revenue might include room revenue, inpatient ancillary revenue (often broken down by department), and outpatient ancillary revenue. Revenue from operations not directly related to patient care might include office space rental, cafeteria, transcript fees, gift shop revenue, rental of television, or fees from educational programs. Gifts or donations, grants, sales of equipment, and income from taxation (state or county supported institutions) might be considered non-operating revenue.

ADJUSTMENTS

Another section of the income statement is referred to as "adjustments and allowances" or "deductions" from income or revenue. Three major components compose this section: bad debts, charity, and contractual allowances. Bad debts refer to loss of revenue caused by those who are able to pay their bills but do not. This may include, for instance, individuals who have moved. Bad debts are sometimes referred to as uncollectible accounts. Charity refers to the amount of deduction or allowance for the care of patients who are unable to pay. This includes care for indigent patients or those who are wards of the government. Finally, contractual adjustments are considered deductions from revenue. The amount deducted from charges (or anticipated revenue) because of the type of reimbursement or payment by the insurance company or third party payer is another definition of contractual adjustment. This is calculated to adjust revenues to meet requirements for reimbursement. For instance, if the allowable payment for insurance company X is 80%, the remaining 20% would be a contractual adjustment, which must be deducted before the organization would know what its net revenue would be.

An example is necessary to adequately explain contractual allowance. A major part of a hospital or other health care institution's revenues are obtained from those patients who pay "allowable costs" rather than billed charges (Furst, 1981). Medicaid, for example, generally will pay only allowable costs rather than what is charged. Contractual agreements, then, exist to determine which costs are allowable. The percentage of revenue from cost-based payers must be determined to complete the formula. Table 9–2 illustrates the formula to determine the contractual adjustment.

Assume that the financial requirements from patient revenues are $54,000,000 and that $3,000,000 in bad debt and charity and $1,000,000 set aside for an expansion project are not allowable costs. Once these are deducted, there is an allowable cost of $50,000,000. That is multiplied by the percentage of cost-based payers (75% at your hospital) to determine the revenue to be obtained from cost-based payers. That leaves $16,500,000 to be obtained from the other 25% of patients, or the charge-based payers. If the $16,500,000 is divided by the .25, the result is the total amount of billed charges needed to obtain the gross patient revenue, or $66,000,000. Deduct-

TABLE 9–2	
Contractual Adjustment Determination	
Financial requirements (patient revenues)	54,000,000
Deduct bad debts, charity	3,000,000
Deduct other non-allowable costs	1,000,000
Allowable costs	50,000,000
Multiply by percentage of revenue from cost-based payers	× .75
Equals: Revenue from cost-based payers	37,500,000
Subtract revenue from cost-based payers from total required patient revenue	54,000,000 −37,500,000
Equals: Needed revenue from charge-based payers	16,500,000
Divide by percentage of revenue from charge-based payers	÷ .25
Equals: Total billed charges (gross patient revenue)	66,000,000
Deduct required patient revenue	−54,000,000
	12,000,000
Deduct bad debt, charity, other non-allowable costs	− 4,000,000
Equals: Contractual adjustments	8,000,000

ing the required patient revenue of $54,000,000 and the $4,000,000 in bad debt, charity and other non-allowable costs, the contractual adjustment is determined ($8,000,000).

This illustration should explain how contractual allowances are figured. It is important to realize that these determinations may be obtained on a per patient day basis and in many cases are based on a ratio of the estimated total allowable costs to total charges (Furst, 1981). Frequent audits by the payers' insurance companies (Blue Cross, for example) are performed to ensure accuracy. Those may be done annually or more often. For example, if the estimated ratio of costs to charges is .95, that figure is applied to the charges billed to the patient. The resultant figure is the reimbursement received by the hospital. Example: The patient's bill is $2,800 multiplied by .95 = $2,660 paid to the hospital.

OPERATING EXPENSES

Operating expenses refer to those expenses that are necessary for the day to day operation of the health care institution. Salaries, supplies, equipment repair, minor equipment, depreciation, insurance, and interest expense are examples of such expenses. Interest expense is included by most health care institutions as an operations expense, unlike many other businesses who determine interest as a separate expense item figured after net operating income is calculated.

Many institutions break down expenses by department and/or by division. With most computer systems, the break-down may be done as desired to provide the most useful information to department managers and administrators. Again, monthly and year-to-date (YTD) figures are common and are helpful in determining the financial status of a department.

NET INCOME

Net income or loss is determined by subtracting expenses from income. Although this appears simple, it is made more complex by the contractual adjustments and other deductions and by the addition of non-operating revenue after operating income has been determined (see Table 9–1). Because of the connotations associated with the word "profit" in not-for-profit institutions, this section is often referred to as "excess of revenue over expenses." Income statements are usually generated on a monthly basis and reflect monthly and year-to-date (YTD) data as well as a comparison of actual to budgeted revenue and expense. Variance is generally reflected, and some institutions add a comparison with the previous fiscal year as well. Comparison with previous fiscal years may be generated only at year end or monthly as "last YTD."

BALANCE SHEET

A balance sheet is the second financial statement of the health care institution that should be analyzed. Standard accounting systems are generally in use in many health care institutions today, replacing fund accounting previously used. The balance sheet generally looks at two items: assets and liabilities. Fund balances are still maintained by most health care institutions since donations must be properly accounted for and may legally be restricted (Table 9–3).

ASSETS

Generally, assets may be classified as current assets (occasionally referred to as liquid assets), which may be converted to dollars within a brief period (usually one year). Fixed assets are those that are long term, such as property, equipment, and buildings. Current assets will include cash, accounts receivable, inventories, prepaid insurance and expenses, reserve from self-insurance (if such exists), and investments. Accounts receivable is generally the largest of the current assets, since it includes money to be collected from insurance companies or public insurers. Investments may include insurance escrow accounts, funded depreciation, and various funds into which the institution has placed money as an investment. These funds are to be differentiated from the unrestricted funds noted later on the balance sheet.

Fixed assets include the building, property, plant, and equipment. Accumulated depreciation must be deducted from the plant and equipment assets. Other assets that might include unamortized bond issue expense may be listed separately. Total assets are noted at the bottom of the section on assets.

LIABILITIES

Liabilities are figured in much the same way as assets. Current liabilities are listed first and include accounts payable, accrued and payable salaries and wages, as well as the taxes or retirement pay that is payable. Monies

TABLE 9–3
Balance Sheet
Your Hospital
Balance Sheet
Period Ending 9/30/85

Assets

Current Assets			
Cash		$ 503,000	503,000
Accounts Receivable	8,757,000		
Less Bad Debt Reserve	2,245,000	6,512,000	
Due from Medicare		1,921,000	8,432,000
Inventories			858,000
Prepaid Insurance			115,000
Investments			
Insurance Escrow		22,000	
Funded Depreciation		11,750,000	
CD		350,000	
Other		8,634,000	20,756,000
Total Current Assets			30,664,000
Fixed Assets			
New Additions		3,209,000	
Building		396,000	3,605,000
Plant and Equipment		16,682,000	
Less Accumulated Depreciation		1,100,000	15,582,000
Total Fixed Assets			19,187,000
Other Assets		78,000	78,000
Total Assets			$49,929,000

Liabilities

Current Liabilities			
Accounts Payable		1,826,000	
Accrued Payroll, Taxes		1,008,000	
Due to Medicare		1,241,000	
Other Current Liabilities		1,782,000	
Total Current Liabilities			5,857,000
Long Term Liabilities			
Bonds Payable		19,256,000	
Mortgage Payable		20,000	
Total Long Term Liabilities			19,276,000
Total Liabilities			25,133,000
Unrestricted Fund Balance			24,796,000
Total Liabilities and Fund Balance			$49,929,000

due to Medicare may also be listed. Current portions of any long-term debt are often listed under current liabilities.

Long-term liabilities include land mortgage, revenue bonds, and notes payable. If an amortized discount is given on the bonds payable, this is deducted from the liability. Liabilities are totaled before the unrestricted fund balance is added. The unrestricted fund balance is the difference between the institution's total assets and total liabilities and reflects the equity or net worth of the institution. Finally, the total liabilities and fund balance are noted as a total under the liabilities section of the balance sheet.

TABLE 9–4
Statement of Change in Financial Position
Your Hospital
Statement of Change in Financial Position
Period Ending 9/30/85

Sources	
Net Income (Loss)	5,868,000
Donations to Institution	575,000
Depreciation of Fixed Assets	1,641,000
Increase in Liabilities	838,000
Reduction in Assets	
Accounts Receivable	14,000
Other	1,934,000
Total Sources	10,870,000
Uses	
Increase in Assets	
Cash	18,000
Inventory	168,000
Other Assets	2,822,000
Fixed Assets	2,793,000
Decrease in Liabilities	
Accounts Payable	251,000
Accrued Payroll/Taxes Payable	518,000
Revenue Bonds	4,300,000
Total Uses	10,870,000

Balance sheets give an overview of the assets and liabilities of the institution. Total assets must equal total liabilities plus fund balance. Although balance sheets may only reflect the current year, last year's figures may also be added for comparison. This is another useful tool in analysis of the institution's financial status.

STATEMENT OF CHANGE IN FINANCIAL POSITION

The final financial statement for review is called the statement of change in financial position. This sheet summarizes the sources and uses of funds for the previous reporting year. The balance sheet and income statement are used to determine these figures. Table 9–4 illustrates this statement of change in financial position. Net income (loss) is taken from the income statement ($5,868,000). Donations to the institution may be added to the source column ($575,000). Depreciation of fixed assets is considered another source of funds ($1,641,000). Amortization is not included here. Increase in liabilities may be determined by subtracting last year's amount due to Medicare or other current liabilities from this year's column. The difference is an increase in liability over last year ($838,000). A reduction in assets is figured similarly by subtracting this year's assets from last year's. A reduction of the asset this year from last year would be reflected on the statement ($14,000 + $1,934,000). All sources could then be totaled ($10,870,000).

Uses of income are noted likewise. Increase in assets is determined in each category listed. Others may be added. A reduction in liabilities is determined in the same manner. Total uses are added to derive the figure $10,870,000.

Ratios in Financial Statement Analysis

Analysis of financial statements is important to the nursing executive. She must have a clear understanding of these statements and the data contained therein. Having an understanding of the institution's financial position is essential if she is to make rational and educated decisions in relation to her departments. Use of ratios is a common practice in the analysis of the financial position of businesses, including health care institutions. These will be discussed only briefly. The four ratios most commonly used include: asset management, liquidity, profitability and leverage ratios.

Asset management ratios measure the effectiveness of the business in handling its assets. Several ratios may be utilized in this category. Days of available supplies in inventory, turnover of fixed assets, and days of charges in accounts receivable are examples. Days of charges in accounts receivable is also called the average collection period and is one measurement of productivity in the business office. It should be noted, however, that a number of factors, including physician medical record completion, may also influence this figure. The average collection period (ACP) is determined through use of a simple formula:

$$ACP = \frac{\text{Average Net Accounts Receivable}}{\text{Average Daily Net Patient Revenue}}$$

When the average net accounts receivable is divided by the average daily net patient revenue, the ACP can be determined in days. Monitoring this number is useful in determining improvement in cash flow.

If these figures or others are analyzed, it is important to remember that they are comparative figures. Improvement within an institution is more important than simple comparison with other institutions. Many variables may be influencing the ratios in management of assets.

Liquidity ratios measure an institution's ability to meet current financial obligations. Current, quick, acid test, and days cash available ratios are examples. The current ratio may be determined by dividing current assets by current liabilities:

$$\frac{\text{Assets}}{\text{Liabilities}} = \text{Current Ratio}$$

This figure helps to determine the liquidity of the institution by determining the ratio between current assets and liabilities.

The quick ratio is like the current ratio except that inventory and other current assets are subtracted from total current assets before the formula is used. The acid test ratio looks only at cash and marketable securities divided by current liabilities. Days cash available ratio is another measurement that helps determine the adequacy of cash balances by comparing cash balance with daily cash needs.

Profitability ratios examine at least four factors to determine profitability of the institution. Return on assets is one ratio to determine the ability of the organization to generate a return on its total assets regardless of the type of financing available. It is figured by dividing total assets into net operating income before interest has been deducted. The patient revenue margin evaluates the patient revenues that the organization actually obtains from gross charges. To calculate this number, the net patient revenue is divided by the gross patient revenue.

Net operating and net profit margins are utilized to examine the overall profitability of the organization. Although these are similar, they are calculated a bit differently. The net operating margin is a measure of the organization's ability to generate profit from its operating revenues. It is calculated by dividing net operating income by total operating revenue. The net profit margin is computed by dividing the net income, including non-operating income, by the total operating revenue. Net operating income does not include non-operating revenue. For this reason, the net profit margin measures total profitability. The following formulas may be used:

$$\frac{\text{Net Operating Income}}{\text{Total Operating Revenue}} = \text{Net Operating Margin}$$

$$\frac{\text{Net Income}}{\text{Total Operating Revenue}} = \text{Net Profit Margin}$$

Leverage ratios are a group of ratios that measure the debt of the organization in relation to funds from equity. Two such ratios that are helpful in analysis of the financial position are debt/equity ratio and debt/total capital ratio. Debt/equity ratio is figured by dividing long-term debt by the unrestricted fund balance. The debt/total capital ratio is computed by dividing total debt by total assets or capital.

Use of ratios in business is common practice, and several organizations compute average ratios. This provides a standard by which organizations may compare themselves. Health care institutions have not developed much history in the use of ratios, but the American Hospital Association does collect data that are published quarterly in *Hospitals*. Because data are not readily available to establish a standard, each institution should look at its own historical data and review its progress as compared with previous years.

Finance Functions

There are three major functions of the finance manager necessary to meet the goal of maximizing the wealth of the organization: liquidity, investment, and financing. Ensuring that cash is available to meet financial obligations is known as liquidity. Use of liquidity ratios helps monitor the organization's liquidity. Appropriate investment is another essential responsibility for the finance manager. This may be accomplished through maintenance of good accounts receivable balances and wise investments. Finally, the finance manager must be able to obtain funds for the institution at as low a cost as possible. Reducing the cost of capital (money) requires determining the best mix of equity sources, long-term liabilities, and current liabilities (Furst, 1981). The nurse executive should have an adequate understanding of the responsibilities of the finance manager so that she may utilize his expertise as she plans her department's budget and makes sound decisions related to the institution.

Definitions

Several definitions are needed before continuing to the process of budgeting in the next section. Explanations will be given when necessary to further define a term.

Expenses are separated generally into one of several categories that may be reflected on income statements or may be utilized in the budget process. *Capital* expenses refer to those expenses that cost over a predetermined amount ($500.00, for example) and/or will last a long period. The time period and dollar limits will be determined by the health care institution. *Operating* expenses are those day to day expenses such as supplies, minor equipment, salaries, and utilities. These generally will vary with the number of patients. Another expense related to operating expenses is *variable* expense. This expense fluctuates with patient census or procedures. It might include RN salaries or patient supplies. *Fixed* expenses are those that will not vary with patient load. For example, the head nurse and unit secretary may be working whether there are 10 or 50 patients. Maintenance, administrative costs, and mortgage payments would be considered fixed costs as well. *Direct* expenses are costs that are assigned directly to a cost center or department. These can be easily identified and include salaries, supplies, and equipment. *Indirect* expenses are those costs that are often difficult to assign and are allocated to a specific department based on some proration or calculation. For example, square footage in a department may be utilized to allocate housekeeping costs.

ALLOCATION

Allocation of costs is another term that is of interest to nurse executives. Allocation of costs may be accomplished by one of several methods. Direct or indirect costs may be allocated. It is common to allocate costs because of cost based reimbursement methods (reimbursement based on costs rather than on charges). There are generally three types of allocation utilized in health care institutions: (1) Direct distribution of costs is accomplished by allocating costs only to revenue centers; (2) Stepdown allocation is frequently used by hospitals and refers to the method by which the costs of a cost center are allocated to all other cost or revenue centers and then that cost center is closed; (3) The most accurate method of allocation is double distribution, which allocates each cost center's costs to all other cost/revenue centers. The direct or stepdown method is then used to complete the process.

Allocation is performed for several reasons. It helps health care institutions to identify full cost information as a basis for establishing rates. It may also provide data to be utilized in negotiation for reimbursement contracts (Finkler, 1985). Table 9–5 differentiates the three methods of allocation. Explanations for each step are included in the table. It is interesting to note that, depending on how the allocation is done and the order in which it is done, allocations may be significantly different. The direct method particularly can result in severe distortions. While this cannot always be controlled by the nurse administrator, it is important that she is aware of the method used in order to justify variances over which she may not have any control. Another important fact related to allocation methods is the effect on reimbursement. It has been noted that the order for stepdown allocation is important. For example, since every department has depreciation, depreciation should be one of the first departments listed so that allocation to all other departments may occur. Reimbursement ceilings or restrictions may inhibit allocation of costs into a particular center. As a final point, one purpose of allocation is maximization of reimbursement. This can be accomplished because ancillary departments are often fully reimbursable whereas per diem charges are limited. Therefore, allocation of costs to the ancillary department rather than to nursing units may be advantageous.

An understanding of finance terms and the processes utilized by the finance department has never been more important to the nursing administrator. In order to justify changes in organization or to ensure financial viability of programs or services, the nursing administrator must have a good working knowledge of the financial operation of those departments for which she is responsible, as well as for the overall institution. Accounting ratios are helpful in making these determinations. Maintaining and studying the financial records are beneficial in controlling a major resource—finances— and the many other resources to which finances are tied.

BUDGETING

The process of budgeting has gained importance in recent years because of the rising health care costs and the emphasis on cost containment. Use of

TABLE 9–5
Allocation of Costs

Type of Allocation	Cost Centers (Non-Revenue)		Revenue Centers		Total Costs	Explanation
Direct	1	2	3	4		
Direct Cost	100	200	1000	2000	3300	Total Costs in All Centers
Allocate Cost Center #1 35%/65%	−100		35	65		Cost Center #1 Allocated 35% to #3, 65% to #4 (Non-revenue to Revenue)
Allocate Cost Center #2 40%/60%	—	−200	80	120		Cost Center #2 Allocated 40% to #3, 60% to #4
	0	0	1115	2185	3300	Total Costs After Allocation Equal Total Before Allocation
Step Down						
Direct Cost	100	200	1000	2000	3300	Total Costs in All Centers
Allocate Cost Center #1 30%/ 20%/50% to Other Centers	−100	30	20	50		Allocation to All Cost Centers After #1 as Noted: 30% to #2, 20% to #3, 50% to #4
	0	230	1020	2050	3300	
Allocate Cost Center #2 *New Total* to #3 and #4 50% and 50%	—	−230	115	115		Allocation of *New Total* to All Cost Centers After #2 as Noted: 50% to #3, 50% to #4
		0	1135	2165	3300	New Total Equals Old Total
Double Direct						
Direct Cost	100	200	1000	2000	3300	Total Costs in All Centers
Step 1						
Allocate Cost Center #1 60%/ 10%/30% to Other Centers	−100	60	10	30		Allocation to All Cost Centers After #1 as Noted: 60% to #2, 10% to #3, 30% to #4
Allocate Cost Center #2 25%/ 50%/25% to Other Centers	50 50	−200 60	100 1110	50 2080		Allocation to All Cost Centers Besides #2 as Noted: 25% to #1, 50% to #3, 25% to #4
Step 2						
Allocate Cost Center #1 60%/ 10%/30%	−50 0	30 90	5 1115	15 2095		Allocation of New Amounts of Cost Center #1 as Noted to #2, 3, 4
Allocate Cost Center #2 40%/ 60%		−90	36	54		Allocation of New Amounts of Cost Center #2 as Noted to #3 and #4
		0	1151	2149	3300	New Total Equals Old Total

data from budgets to guide decision making is important for every level of manager in the health care system (Hillestad, 1983). It is extremely important that budgeting be accomplished in such a way that it facilitates goal achievement.

A budget is a tool for planning, quantifying the plans and controlling costs (Finkler, 1984). A budget generally represents expected revenues as compared with anticipated expenses. The process of budget preparation is based on specific concepts of financial management, which will be discussed. There are numerous types of budgets, several of which will be defined and explained. Each institution has a specific and different process for budgeting. However, the basic steps in the process will be described, and examples will be utilized to clarify the steps.

Most health care institutions use historical data to develop budgets (Hoffman, 1984). In an *historical budget*, the previous year's expenses are used as a basis for expenses for the next year. *Forecast or statistical budgets* are related somewhat in that they are developed by establishing a level of anticipated activity based on historical and other data (such as loss or gain of specific programs). Once a level of expected activity is established, the budget is developed from that activity level. (Forecasting is discussed at some length in the next section of this chapter.)

Fixed versus variable budgets refer to those components of the budget that will or will not vary regardless of changes in the patient census or number of procedures (unit of activity). These were referred to briefly in the previous section. A *flexible* type of budget utilizes these budgetary components to determine how the budget should fluctuate, based on those changes in unit of activity.

A *trended budget* is one that is developed based on the previous years' expenditure patterns. If a specific percentage of expenses occurs in a particular month (e.g., July—8.5%, Aug.—6.2%), the budget will be developed using those trends to spread expenses.

A *zero-based budget* is one that does not utilize any historical data to determine activity level or expenses anticipated. All expenses are justified based on expectations or desires for the upcoming year (Hoffman, 1984).

Before the actual process of budgeting can occur, several prerequisites should be met (Furst, 1981). Because the budget is a tool for planning, the objectives or goals must be known. There must be an organizational structure to support the plan. Each individual who will have responsibility for the budget must also be involved in its development if commitment to the goals and budget is desired. It is also essential that the budget process be fully understood by new managers. Even managers who have had previous budget experience will need an orientation to the format or process utilized in the specific institution. Such an orientation or refresher class is beneficial not only to the managers but also to the process itself. Data must be available to facilitate forecasting or projecting activity. The accounting system must be able to identify cost centers and accumulate the data by cost center. The budget period must be clearly defined. Finally, feedback must be available to department managers during the year to measure and guide their performance.

The use of data management systems that are quite sophisticated or simple personal computers with the budgeting software available can significantly reduce the workload at the time for annual budgets. Computer literacy becomes a valued capability and serves to reduce the stress often associated with the budget process. Such data management throughout the year is also an aid to budget monitoring and control.

Budget Process

Assumptions related to the budget must be known and utilized throughout the process. The rate of inflation that will impact upon the price of supplies is one example of an assumption. Wage increases related to merit or adjustments to remain competitive are other such assumptions. Probably the most important assumptions are those related to workload. Anticipated occupancy or volume for the next one, five, or ten years will certainly have a significant influence on budget preparation (Finkler, 1984). The more data that are available, the better the manager will be able to plan. Input by department managers is important when assumptions are made, but the assumptions must be uniform and coordinated organization-wide. For example, if the OR is planning for 500 open heart cases, the open heart ICU should plan for that number as well.

Once assumptions are made, the next step in the budget process is prioritizing the goals of the organization. This is necessary because, especially in the long range plan, the program budget, and the capital budget, there are generally more items to be purchased than money available. Prioritizing helps to discern which goals are most important and which are affordable within a specific time frame. When programs are being considered, coupled with finite resources, emphasis on examination of all programs for efficiency and effectiveness becomes essential. This permits prioritization of programs as well as goals or objectives. This obviously must be accomplished before the capital and program budgets are prepared, unless a battle over specific items is desired. Power games are frequently played during the budget process. Use of prioritizing early in the process can help minimize the playing of these games. (Refer to Chapter 14, Games and Political Strategies.)

Keeping in mind the goals and objectives of the department and organization, the process for budgeting can begin with the development of the forecasted units of activity or occasions of service. With nursing inpatient units, this occasion of service or activity is usually patient days. However, this varies with the department. Table 9–6 lists several departments with their usual unit of activity. Once the units of activity have been predicted, other budgets may be developed. (See section on forecasting for detail in projecting activity.)

At the same time the statistical budget is being prepared to develop the

TABLE 9–6	
Unit of Activity for Selected Departments	
Department	**Unit of Activity**
Nursing Unit (inpatient)	Patient Days
L and D	Number of Deliveries
Pharmacy	Medications/IV's Processed
Lab	Number of Tests Performed
OR	OR Case Hours
Anesthesia	Anesthesia Case Hours
Housekeeping	Square Feet Cleaned
Emergency Department	Visits
Home Health	Visits
Laundry	Pounds Processed
Radiology	Procedures
GI Lab	Procedures

These are samples and may vary from institution to institution.

operating budget, the capital budget can be prepared. Cost control has had a significant impact on capital budgets at the same time that physicians' and patients' demand for technology has been high. Review of priorities will identify those areas where capital expenditures are most important. Input from the medical staff and board in relation to the capital expenditures is wise. Besides the cost involved, the long range effect on the institution of many capital expense items will require support of these groups. Each department will need to develop a list of capital expense items. It is important to remember that each institution develops its own definition of capital equipment. Generally, capital equipment meets requirements of cost and time for use. Once the list is developed and items are prioritized by whether the need level is urgent, needed, or desired, the list from all departments can be combined. A sample worksheet for capital items is seen in Figure 9–1.

Operating Budget

In determining the operating budget, several factors must be considered besides unit of activity. These factors may determine, for example, the hours of care to be budgeted for each patient day or for each procedure. Productivity goals, today more than ever before, are one such consideration. Productivity is addressed at length in Chapter 10. Productivity, defined as the relationship between goods or services produced and the factors that contribute to production, is used as a measure to determine whether the worker is producing as much as possible. Improvements in productivity may help produce more service with the same or less resources. With cost containment such an important issue, productivity becomes increasingly important.

In 1957 the National League for Nursing identified a number of other factors that today still may determine budget needs for nursing departments. The type and acuity of patients are factors that should be considered in

Department _____ FY_____

Capital Item/Equip	Justification of Need	Priority	Cost	Purchase Date Required	Relation to Goals/Objectives

Priority: 1 - Urgent   2 - Needed   3 - Desired

FIGURE 9–1. Sample worksheet for capital expense items.

preparing the operating budget. The types of services or procedures available in a hospital or unit will affect the budgetary needs for a department. Physical layout and the method for grouping patients (e.g., orthopedic versus neurological) can also influence the needs of a department. Speciality units will have specific needs as well. The mode of care delivery and the percentage of professional staff are influencing factors. How procedures are performed, record-keeping requirements, and types of equipment available can affect the requirements for staff. Support services, affiliation with medical and nursing schools, and personnel policies may all influence the needs for staff to be reflected in the operating budget.

REVENUE

There are two primary portions of the operating budget. One portion is revenue, and the other is expense. In figuring the revenue side, projected units of activity are utilized by the department. Units of activity projected for the year are multiplied by charges per unit of service to determine the expected revenue. It is important to understand that this calculation does not reflect what the hospital receives, but the charge. Refer to the income statement and balance sheet to note the deductions from revenue related to charity, bad debts, and contractual adjustments. Because of the reimburse-

TABLE 9–7
Determining Revenue Budget from Projected Procedures

Total Procedures Budgeted:			10,000
200 Procedure A	@ $200	=	40,000
300 Procedure B	@ $500	=	150,000
2500 Procedure C	@ $ 50	=	125,000
4000 Procedure D	@ $ 45	=	180,000
3000 Procedure E	@ $100	=	300,000
Total Revenue:			$795,000

ment for health care services, calculation by other methods is not always feasible for the health care institution.

In determining the charge per unit of service, one must consider whether one or multiple types of procedures or rates for room and board apply to the department. For example, on a medical nursing unit, there may be projected 7300 patient days. On the unit, there may be 20 semi-private rooms at a daily charge of $100.00 and 10 private rooms at a daily charge of $150.00. Assumptions regarding how many of the projected 7300 patient days will be in private versus semi-private rooms will be necessary before anticipated revenue can be calculated. If it is assumed that 40% of the days will be in private rooms and 60% in semi-private rooms, the revenue anticipated would equal $876,000. If, however, 50% of the days were projected to be in private rooms and 50% in semi-private rooms, revenue would equal $912,500.

In determining revenue for cost centers where procedures are done, the process involves calculating how many of each procedure are projected and the total revenue resulting from that projection (Table 9–7). In the example, the average charge per procedure equals $79.50, which is a wide variation from $45 to $500. Thus, it is significant how the figures are derived. Statistical information and program plans must be carefully analyzed in order to accurately determine the revenue budget.

When calculating revenue budget, it is also important to consider any charge increase before determining the budget. If the percent increase is known, actual charge can be determined by multiplying the percent increase times the current charge and adding the amount obtained to the current charge.

Because of the shift to prospective payment, much of the calculations utilized today may have to be combined with a different mechanism to determine more accurately projected revenue. Revenue for patients under DRG's will be predetermined and will not be based on patient days. Instead, the calculation will be for the number of patients discharged within a specific DRG. To further complicate this matter, some patients may be reimbursed through prospective payment, whereas others will continue to be paid per day. Table 9–8 is an example of a method for determining the revenue projection for such a unit.

EXPENSE

The expense budget is separated into two categories: (1) supplies and (2) salaries and wages. The supplies budget will be addressed first. Historical

| TABLE 9–8 |
| Revenue Budget Calculation for Patient Unit |
| with Mixed Reimbursement |

	Number of Patients Discharged	Imaginary Reimbursement	Revenue
DRG 125	50	1000	$ 50,000
DRG 126	100	1500	150,000
DRG 127	125	1200	150,000
DRG 128	75	2000	150,000
DRG 129	80	2500	200,000
			$700,000

Additional Patients (Per Diem Reimbursement)	ALOS	Room Rate	Revenue
580	× 3.2 ×	$425.00 =	$788,800
		TOTAL REVENUE:	$1,488,800

data are most frequently the basis for expense budgets. Consideration must also be given to whether the expense should be fixed, variable, or semi-variable. Those items that are fixed are probably easier to determine. Examples of fixed supplies may include office supplies and equipment maintenance or service contracts. Semi-variable supplies might include minor equipment (since, if the patient census were down, the equipment might not need replacement). Variable supplies include nourishments, medical supplies, monitoring supplies, and chart forms.

Another factor that might influence the supply expense budget would be changes in procedures or new programs. For example, although in the past monitoring supplies equaled an average cost PPD (per patient day) of $.13, that cost may increase significantly when the number of monitored beds available doubles. Another example might be the added expense for a disposable non-patient charge item such as disposable rectal temperature probes versus reusable items. Justification for such changes should always accompany expense projections. Supportive data may be needed as well to validate the need for changes.

Changes in the types of patient care on a specific unit may also affect the expense in a particular line item of the budget. For example, if a larger number of patients on a medical-surgical unit were to be surgical patients, there might be an increase in the amount of medical-surgical supplies and in nourishments (force fluids). Such considerations are important.

Figuring the budgeted expense for line items on the budget is not particularly difficult if patient day projections are utilized in addition to other information. An example of a worksheet that can be used to assist the process is found in Table 9–9. In the example used, data from the current fiscal year are utilized to determine the supply expense per patient day. This is accomplished by dividing the total patient days for the period into the total expense for that line item for the period. This figure is then multiplied by the projected patient days for the budget year. This new figure is multiplied by the inflation factor plus 100% to reach the total projected expense for the line item. This method can be utilized for variable items. If

TABLE 9–9
Supply Expense Budget Worksheet (Example)

Department <u>ICU</u>　　　　FY <u>1988</u>

Expense Line Item <u>Monitoring Supplies</u>

Current FY (to date)	Total Expense 2400	÷ Total Patient Days 3000	= Cost per Patient Day .80
Cost per Patient Day .80		× Projected Patient Days 3500	= Projected Basic Expense 2800
Projected Basic Expense 2800		× (Inflation Factor + 100%) 1.10	= Total Projected Expense $3080

Note: Inflation factor should be specific for the item where possible. For example, general inflation may be 5%, but monitoring supplies are anticipated to climb 10%.

an item is fixed or semi-variable, specific amounts may be determined based on estimated (and justified) needs. For example, under "Brochures," the addition of a brochure may significantly increase the budget amount over last year and would require explanation.

Salary budgets are a bit more difficult to determine. Because these budgets represent the greatest expenditure within the cost center and because they are the part of the budget over which the nurse manager has the most control, much care should be taken in their development. Several methods can be used to identify the needed staff for a specific unit. These methods are dependent on considerations already identified in this section.

Use of a patient acuity system is helpful, especially in light of increased acuity being experienced throughout the country. Determining workload is simplified if an acuity system is in place. Multiplying average daily census by acuity will determine workload. That number can then be multiplied by the targeted hours of care per workload unit to determine needed hours of care per day. This figure converts into FTE's, or full time equivalents (number of staff when all worked hours are added together and divided by hours worked by one full time person).

If an acuity system is not in place, other data may be used to determine the workload: patient mix, age, procedures, programs. In the absence of an acuity system, many hospitals utilize an average number of hours of care for the specific patient population. For example, oncology patients in hospitals within the VHA system (Voluntary Hospitals of America) may average 7.15 hours of care per patient per day (HPPD). The figure 7.15 might be used as the total HPPD. Direct versus indirect hours must be considered, since each unit may have different care requirements and different constant staff. The major drawback in use of this type of data is the danger of comparing units that, although both have similar patients by diagnosis, may vary significantly in age mix, acuity, etc.

Figure 9–2 provides a worksheet for the staffing budget. This worksheet may help the nursing manager calculate her needs in terms of staff. The top portion of the sheet can be easily completed once projected activity has been determined. Projected percent occupancy is determined by dividing total

Department: Stepdown Unit FY: 1990

Bed Capacity: 16 Projected % Occupancy: 75

Projected Patient Days: 4380 Projected ADC: 12

I. Direct Hours

A. 3.0 (Average Acuity) × 3.8 (Target Hours per workload) = 11.4 (Direct HPPD)

B. 11.4 (Direct HPPD) × 4380 (Pt. Days) ÷ 2080 = 24.0 (Direct Productive FTEs)

II. Indirect Hours

A. 53.7 (Hrs worked by Indirect staff in 24 hrs.) ÷ 12 (Projected ADC) = 4.48 (Indirect HPPD)

B. 4.48 (Indirect HPPD) × 4380 (Pt. Days) ÷ 2080 = 24.0 (Indirect Productive FTEs)

III. Non-productive FTE Calculation (Replacement Staff)

A. 5000 (Total paid Non-Productive Hours) ÷ 50,000 (Total paid Productive Hours) = .10 (% (Portion) Non-Productive Paid Hours)

B. .10 (Portion Non-Productive Paid Hours) × 24.0 (Productive FTEs) = 2.4* (Non-Productive FTEs)

*Direct only

FIGURE 9–2. Worksheet for staffing budget.

possible patient days (all beds filled every day of year) into projected patient days. Projected ADC (average daily census) is determined by dividing projected patient days by 365 (or 366 for leap years).

Direct hours may be calculated in the second section by multiplying average acuity and targeted hours per workload if a patient acuity system is utilized. If direct hours are pre-determined without the acuity system, one can begin the calculation at step I-B. Direct hours should be multiplied by patient day and divided by 2080 (worked by each FTE each year) to determine direct productive FTE's. (See example in Figure 9–2.)

Indirect hours should be figured separately. Unit secretaries, monitor technicians, and the head nurse or unit coordinator are usually constant staff, and their numbers will not usually vary with census. These calculations can be made using the formula in Part II-A and B of Figure 9–2. For example, if there is a unit secretary and a monitor technician on each shift each day,

TABLE 9–10
Calculation for Orientation

		RN	LPN	Other
Currently filled positions		13	7.2	——
× hours orientation (average)		120	120	——
× turnover rate		.25	.25	——
=	(1)	390	216	——
Currently unfilled positions		1.4	0	——
× hours orientation		120	0	——
=	(2)	168	0	——
Total orientation hours	(1) + (2)	558	216	——
× orientation replacement percentage		.5	.5	——
÷ 2080		2080	2080	2080
= FTE's		.13	.05	——

that would equal 48 hours worked in the 24 hour period. The head nurse's hours must also be figured. However, she generally has 24 hour, 7 day per week responsibility, so her hours per week must be divided by 7 days, and the 5.7 hours obtained would be added to the 48 other hours to total 53.7 hours. These hours would be divided by the average daily census to determine constant HPPD, which is then multiplied by patient days and divided by 2080 to determine constant productive FTE's.

The last section of the worksheet is a calculation for non-productive or replacement staff. This calculation will figure coverage for holidays, vacation, and sick time. Payroll records should be able to provide the data needed to calculate these FTE's. Non-productive and productive paid hours are necessary components for this formula. Each unit's portion of paid time that is non-productive will be different, since the tenure of employees may vary significantly from unit to unit. This non-productive time may be calculated separately for direct and constant staff or together, depending on the manager's ability to separate and plan her budget appropriately. It generally is simpler to calculate the two separately. It should be noted that this calculation does not account for the non-productive time of those staff members who make up the replacement staff.

Another consideration in the development of the staffing budget is the addition of budgeted FTE's and dollars for orientation and education (Kirby and Wiczai, 1985). Since staff are functioning at a significantly lower level of productivity during orientation and cannot generally perform at the same level as a regular staff member, the nurse manager may be able to justify budget dollars for orientation or at least part of it. Table 9–10 may be useful in calculating FTE's needed for orientation. Assuming that the orientee averages 50% productivity, covering 50% of her orientation time might be realistic. If coverage can be obtained for 75% or 60% these percentages could be plugged into the formula at "orientation replacement percentage." The number obtained would be divided by 2080 to obtain FTE's. Although the worksheet has columns for RN, LPN, and other, the same formula would apply for any category of personnel. Similarly, education hours might be

TABLE 9–11				
Staff by Shift and Category Worksheet				

Core Staff—FTE's

Constant	7–3	3–11	11–7	Total
HN	1.0	—	—	1.0
US	1.4	1.4	1.4	4.2
MT	1.4	1.4	1.4	4.2
				9.4 Subtotal (1)

Direct				
RN	6.5	4.7	3.2	14.4
LPN	2.9	2.2	2.1	7.2
NA	1.4	1.0		2.4
				24.0 Subtotal (2)

SVH Replacement FTE's		Orientation FTE's	
HN	0	RN	.13
US	.42	LPN	.05
MT	.42		.18
RN	1.44		
LPN	.72		
NA	.24		
	3.24		

Total Replacement 3.2 SVH   FTE's
                   +.2 Orientation
                   3.4 FTE's

Total constant (1)	9.4
Total direct (2)	24.0
Total replacement	3.4
Total FTE's	36.8

added for staff members. Realistically, in the current economic environment, this may be one of the first parts of the budget to be cut.

The next step in the staffing budget process is the breakdown of staff into categories and by shift. The manager may begin by looking at the percentage of staff he desires for each shift and the desired mix of RN's to other staff. Table 9–11 may be useful in determining staffing needs and placement of staff. In the example, data are used from previous worksheets. The manager of this unit has a mix of 60% RN, 30% LPN, and 10% NA direct care givers. He also has determined that he needs 45% of the staff on day shift, 33% on evenings, and 22% on nights. As a result, he has the total budgeted FTE's of 24 direct care giver FTE's broken down as shown.

Replacement for sick, vacation, and holiday (SVH) time has been figured at 10% in the example, and the orientation time was calculated by the formula in the worksheet in Table 9–10. Replacement FTE's may consist of staff who work parttime to cover paid days off for regular core staff, or overtime by core staff to cover each other. This should be projected as much as possible to ensure accurate dollar figures. Subtotals for direct, constant and replacement FTE's may be totaled to determine FTE's needed for unit.

Once staffing figures by shift and category are determined, these must be converted to dollars. A worksheet similar to that in Table 9–12 may be helpful in converting FTE's to dollars. Each employee is listed by name, and data related to the employee are completed. Differential hours with corresponding dollars are calculated. If an employee rotates shifts two days per week, for instance, 40% of the total worked hours would be differential hours. Differential amount per hour may be a dollar figure or a percentage of hourly wage. If a position is vacant, the FTE and anticipated dollars must still be filled in. If the nurse manager knows that he will utilize his regular staff to cover SVH time and that this will result in overtime, he must estimate the amount of overtime. The bottom of Table 9–12 includes calculation of total dollars and includes anticipated merit increases. If general increases are anticipated, these should also be included. FICA, retirement, and insurance costs to the institution are also added. In some institutions, these final calculations, including merit increases, FICA, etc., are done by the Finance Department.

Once the total staffing budget by unit has been developed, it is important to review the total budget for accuracy and to determine whether the organizational goals have been met. For example, if the percentage of excess revenue over expenses is not met by the projected budget, it might be necessary to adjust the budget by increasing revenue and/or decreasing expenses. Since increasing revenue is very difficult because it is related to predetermined calculations of activity, it usually is reduction of expenses that must be addressed (Finkler, 1984).

Reduction of expenses should be considered after evaluating various programs and equipment priorities, projected personnel needs, and efficient use of supplies. The process of negotiation can then be used to accomplish needed reductions (Finkler, 1984). Of major importance in the process of expense reduction is the impact of the reduction. Each manager is ultimately responsible for not only the budget but also for support of the organizational objectives and budget. Included in that responsibility is the responsibility to keep top level management informed in relation to the effect of budget cuts. If, for example, cutting the budget by 5% would mean that a particular program would be required to be eliminated, that information would be important for administration in the decision making process.

It is helpful when cuts in budgets become necessary or when planning to request increases in nursing hours that the nurse executive understands the effect such changes could make. More and more, the top level nursing administrator is expected to be able to calculate and explain the financial impact of such changes. By thinking through the previous steps used (see Fig. 9–2) to calculate FTE's from acuity and target hours, a formula can be devised to calculate the impact of an increase or decrease in nursing hours. If, for example, the nurse executive wishes to increase nursing hours by 0.1 NHPPD (nursing hours per patient day) and the projected patient days are 7500 for that unit, this formula could be used to calculate FTE's:

TABLE 9–12

Conversion of FTE's to Dollars Worksheet

Unit _____ FY _____

Name	Category	Shift	Hourly Wage	FTE's Worked	Annual Salary	Differential Hours	Differential Amount/Hour	Total Differential Dollars	Total Annual Dollars	Additional OT Dollars
M. Smith	RN	1	10.32	1.0	21,465	—	—	—	21,465	—
J. Doe	RN	3	9.30	0.6	11,606	1248	.93	1161	12,767	—
Vacant	RN	½	9.85	1.0	20,488	832	.98	815	21,303	—
N. Johnson	LPN	2	5.90	1.0	12,272	2080	.59	1227	13,499	850
							Totals	$ _____	$ _____	$ _____

Total Annual Dollars $ _____

Total OT Dollars _____

Merit Increase Dollars _____

Other Employment Costs _____

FICA _____ % _____

Retirement _____ % _____

Insurance _____ % _____

Total $ _____

$$0.1 \text{ NHPPD} \times 7500 \text{ Pt. Days} - 2080 = .36 \text{ Prod. FTE'S}$$
$$.36 \times .1 \text{ (Non-productive Percentage)} = \underline{.036}$$
$$\text{Total FTE's} = .396 \text{ or } .4$$
$$.4 \times \$12.00 \text{ (Average salary)} \times 2080 = \$9984.00 \text{ plus Benefits}$$

This calculation indicates the financial impact of the change by 0.1 NHPPD if patient days equal 7500. Similar calculations can provide the cost of changes in NHPPD of any amount or changes in patient days. In reverse, calculations may be used to determine how much less care patients will receive with cuts.

To summarize the process of budgeting, the organizational goals and priorities must first be known and understood as they apply to the budget. Assumptions must be known, including those projections for patient days, procedures, etc. The revenue budget is developed first from the projected days. The supply expense and personnel expense budgets are then developed. Finally, there is review of the budgets to ensure accuracy and compliance with profit or revenue over expense projections.

Analysis Of Variance

Budgets are guidelines that are based on specific projections for such units of activity as procedures or patient days. While flexible budgets may vary with changes in these units of activity, there must generally be an analysis of variance in the budget. Basically, this refers to an evaluation of where variance has occurred between what was planned in revenue or expense items and what actually occurred. This variance may or may not be justified, but should be analyzed and explained. Without appropriate analysis of variance, budgets would lose their purpose for control.

In some instances, expense variance occurs related to increases in patient days or procedures. This should be calculated to determine if the percentage increase in expenses is justified by the percentage increase in patient days or procedures. Increases in salary dollars may be related to increases in cost per hour worked or increases in hours worked caused by different factors. Expense variance may also be related to unbudgeted expenditures that were approved and necessary. For example, a cardiac monitor might unexpectedly require total replacement, calling for an expenditure that was not budgeted. Analysis of variance necessitates that the manager examine and think through the budget, and ensures maintenance of control as a purpose for budgeting.

In analysis of variance, the nursing administrator must first know if he is operating under a flexible budget. True flexible budget systems will show increases/decreases in budgeted amounts, varying as units of activity increase or decrease. For example, if a nursing department has projected 300 procedures for the month with anticipated revenue of $30,000, salary expense of $10,000, and other operating expense of $5000, revenue over expense would

			TABLE 9–13			
			Flexible Budget Analysis			

Month A					Month B	
Budget	*Actual*				*Budget*	*Actual*
300	300	Procedures	Procedures		300	400*
30,000	30,000	Revenue	Revenue		40,000*	40,000
10,000	10,000	Salary expense	Salary expense		13,333	15,000
5,000	5,000	Other operating expense	Other operating expense		6,667	6,000
15,000	15,000	Revenue over expense	Revenue over expense		20,000	19,000

*Note: Budgeted revenue in flexible budgeting is based on actual number of procedures (patient days or other unit of service) rather than on original number projected. In the example, 300 procedures were projected with projected revenue of $30,000, but 400 were done. Expected revenue for 400 procedures is $40,000.

be expected to be $15,000 (Table 9–13). If the department does have 300 procedures, $30,000 revenue, salary expense of $10,000, and other operating expense of $5000, the department has met budget. With the flexible budget, increases may be noted as actual units of activity rise. In month B in the example, there were 400 procedures. Budgeted revenue then rises to $40,000, and budgeted expenses increase correspondingly. In the example, actual salary dollars were greater than the flexible budget figures and other operating expense as well as revenue over expenses were less than should have occurred with the change in number of procedures.

In analysis of non-flexible budgets, it is not as simple to determine cause for variance. The "easy" answer is to blame variance on changes in units of activity, but this may be inaccurate. To determine whether costs have increased per hour worked or per product purchased, or whether more hours were worked or more products purchased, simple calculations may be used. For payroll costs, the manager will need to divide man-hours into dollars to determine the cost per man-hour. Comparison of budgeted with actual expense will demonstrate whether costs per man-hour have increased (Furst, 1981). For example,

$500,000 ÷ 50,000 Hours = $10 Cost per Man-Hour

Comparison of hours budgeted with hours worked will determine variance there. A combination of these factors may influence variance. All variances may be analyzed similarly.

FORECASTING

Forecasting is the process of predicting the future. In health care, forecasting is the process utilized to predict or project activity on which budgeting is based, programs or ventures are planned, and even new directions are taken. Forecasts or predictions should be considered as part of data collection. The accuracy of forecasting is dependent on numerous factors, which will be discussed.

It has been emphasized throughout previous chapters and will be emphasized in following chapters that change within the health care system is rapid. Nursing administrators, like all managers, are confronting many uncertainties and many new realities (Georgoff and Murdick, 1986). These factors influence to varying degrees the current activities and future plans of the nursing administrator. Many techniques have been developed that may assist any manager in evaluation of the factors that influence the future success of the business or organization.

Regardless of the technique used, crucial assumptions must always be made, historical data have questionable value during the changing times, and the economy is tenuous at best. Each technique available for use in forecasting also has limitations, such as data needs, time, costs, and competencies (Georgoff and Murdick, 1986). The decision regarding the type of forecasting technique to use and under which circumstances is a difficult one, even for professional forecasters.

There are at least 20 methods of forecasting currently in use. Because of the diversity of programs and ventures in which health care institutions are involved, nearly any method may find a place in forecasting for a health care institution. The complexity of some methods prohibits their use except in large, sophisticated organizations. There are four types of methods described by Georgoff and Murdick (1986) into which the 20 methods may be categorized (Table 9–14).

In deciding which type of method or which specific method to use, the manager should examine several dimensions about each method considered. In relation to time, it is important to determine the span of time the forecast will cover, how quickly it is needed, and how often it would need to be updated. Limitations on quantitative skills, computer capabilities, and financial resources would be important considerations as well. Availability and fluctuation of past data, significant changes in environmental variables or management decisions, and shifts in variable relationships are input concerns the manager must be able to address. In terms of desired output, considerations might include level of accuracy, turning points reflected, and detail.

In evaluating these factors, Georgoff and Murdick (1986) have developed a rather detailed chart that may be useful to those managers who wish to devote much research to forecasting methods. However, they offer several pointers that may be beneficial to all nursing administrators. Attempting to generate a forecast for an extensive period is frequently a mistake in light of the rapidity of change in health care. Use of a computer to generate forecasts is a sophisticated method. However, the level of discomfort of the manager with computers may result in this technique being wasted. There must also be trust in the forecast since future plans are necessarily based on the prediction. Cost/benefit analysis of a technique is helpful before a great deal is spent on an unsatisfactory technique. Since accuracy is so important,

TABLE 9–14
Forecasting Methods

1. Counting Methods:
   A. Market testing—representative responses to new programs or products, tested to estimate future response.
   B. Consumer market survey—representative attitudes and intentions data.
   C. Industrial market survey—fewer, more knowledgeable subject sampling.

2. Time Series Methods:
   A. Moving averages—recent values averaged to predict future outcome.
   B. Exponential smoothing—weighted combination of recent outcome and previous period estimates.
   C. Adaptive filtering—derivation of weighted combination of actual and estimated outcomes; reflects pattern changes.
   D. Time series extrapolation—future extension of least squares function.
   E. Time series decomposition—prediction of outcome from trend, seasonal, cyclical and random components.
   F. Box-Jenkins—complex, computer-based iterative procedure.

3. Judgment Methods:
   A. Historical analogy—based on elements of past events analogous to present.
   B. Delphi technique—successive series of estimates utilizing group results in each step.
   C. Naive extrapolation—simple assumption about economic outcome or simple extension of current results.
   D. Sales force composite—compilation of estimates of dealers, adjusted for expected changes.
   E. Jury of executive opinion—consensus of group of "experts."
   F. Scenario method—description of assumed future expressed in narrative and as sequence of time frames.

4. Association or Causal Methods:
   A. Correlation—predictions of values based on historic patterns of covariation.
   B. Regression models—estimates produced from predictive equation.
   C. Leading indicators—generated from one or more preceding variable.
   D. Input-output model—indicates effect of one industry's demand change on other industry.
   E. Econometric models—outcomes forecast from integrated system of simultaneous equations.

From Georgoff, D., and Murdick, R. (1986). Manager's guide to forecasting. *Harvard Business Review, 64*(1), 110–120.

combining techniques may improve the forecast. Finally, judgment, as always, is crucial, as long as it is applied in a structured manner.

Process of Forecasting

There are four basic steps identified by Finkler (1984) for forecasting: data collection, graphing of data, analysis, and development of formulas for projection. Data collection is basically historical collection. If projections are to be made about numbers of patient days or procedures, collection of historical data about those activities would be needed. Appropriate time periods should be utilized in forecasting. It is better, for example, to review data by month rather than only annual numbers, since review of monthly numbers enables the manager to see trends or patterns with specific areas or departments. Review for a period of time back is certainly more helpful

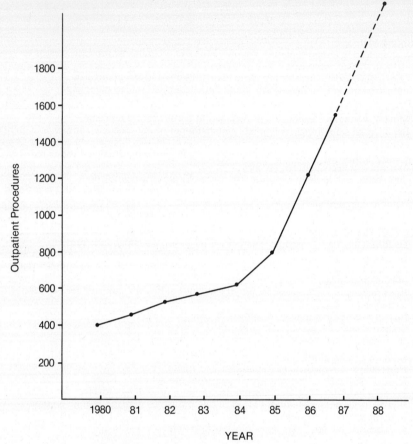

FIGURE 9–3. Graph of patient procedures.

than review of only one year, since it permits a view of several Januarys, several Februarys, etc. A three to five year backward look is often suggested. Consideration must be given to recent changes or predictable changes affecting the projections.

The second step in the forecasting process is graphing of data. Time is generally plotted on the horizontal axis, and the data desired to be predicted is plotted on the vertical axis. The purpose of the graph is to provide a picture of trends or patterns. Figure 9–3 demonstrates use of a graph.

Once data are graphed, they must be analyzed. Patterns or trends can be noted over the years. In looking at the example in Figure 9–3, one can see a gradual increase in procedures until 1985, when the rate of increase changed sharply. Graphs can show seasonal changes and variations when done on a monthly basis or may indicate lack of predictability. For example, a monthly graph may show that January procedures are up one year and down another.

The final step in the process of forecasting is use of available data to develop a forecast. Selection of a technique occurs at this point, based on the factors previously discussed. Use of historical data is characteristic of health care institutions and, for many nursing departments, is relatively simple. Use of seasonality is helpful in making predictions by month. One must consider, however, that the factors influencing seasonal variations may vary from month to month. For example, if near drownings usually occur during the hottest month and instead of August, that month was July, data and therefore predictions may be distorted.

Flexibility is necessary as forecasts are prepared. Consideration given to needs, time factors, desired outcome, and availability of data may influence the forecast. In any case, a manager must recognize that a forecast is hopefully an educated prediction upon which future plans may be based. The accuracy of that forecast, therefore, is very important and could spell the success or failure of a particular department (Golden, McDevitt, and Bloch, 1981).

RATE SETTING

Forecasting is one step often necessary before rate setting can occur. The institution's legitimate financial requirements are met through the rates that are set by the institution. It is, therefore, very important for rates to be sufficient to generate adequate cash flow and to maintain the financial viability of the institution (Furst, 1981).

There are three major steps in rate setting. *Financial requirements* must be determined first. *Allocation* of the financial requirements to revenue producing departments must then occur. *Rate setting* must be accomplished in such a manner as to generate adequate cash flow. Each step is dependent on the previous one, and each step is important to the process.

The financial requirements of health care institutions include operating expenses and capital needs. These requirements may be subdivided into current requirements and an operating margin. The current requirements result primarily from provision of patient care and are the primary determinants of the rates necessary to be charged by the institution. Other factors that must also influence these requirements are bad debts and charity. Research and educational programs not covered by grants, tuition or other sources are also included. An operating margin sufficient to cover capital expenditures must also be earned by the institution. These expenditures include equipment needs (discussed in section on capital expenditure analysis) and major renovations, expansion, or plant replacement. The operating margin must also be adequate for any increases in working capital and cash balances that are needed. The last determinant for rates is the return on equity for those institutions that are investor owned. Additional discussion related to capital, capital expenditures, and external control of rates is covered in later sections of this chapter.

Once the financial requirements have been identified, it becomes necessary to allocate these requirements to the revenue producing departments (Furst, 1981). All budgeted direct expenses are allocated as required or permitted by third party payers. These include planned expansion, research, education, net working capital requirements, charity care, and bad debts. Once these have been allocated, the rates currently in effect are used to determine revenue that could be obtained in each revenue center. A comparison of the financial requirements with the revenue that could be obtained with current rates will demonstrate a variance that can be used to set new rates by department.

The final step in setting rates is to determine which revenue center requires rate adjustment. For example, if the majority of bad debt and charity expenses is allocated to the maternal-child nursing units because that is where the expense occurs, those units may require the largest adjustment. It is important to realize, however, that an institution may feel it is unreasonable to substantially increase rates in those departments and may prefer to shift the cost difference to other departments. Cost shifting, while not uncommon, can create significant problems with reimbursement for the institution.

Several methods may be used in determining the rates of individual revenue centers. *Surcharge* methods are based on the cost of supplies plus an amount (percentage usually) tacked on. *Relative value* is another method and is determined by the relative value of a procedure or room to other procedures or rooms. *Hourly charges*, common to operating rooms, are a third method for setting rates. Each of these methods determines the rate by comparing financial requirements for the department with the costs of the supplies or service. For example, if the financial requirements for Department A are $115,000 and the total costs are $100,000, the ratio is 1.15 to 1. This ratio can be multiplied by the costs for a particular procedure to set the new rate. Occasionally, an institution sets its rates by checking with another institution and setting rates accordingly. While it is wise to remain competitive, this method used alone could be disastrous for an institution.

MANAGEMENT OF WORKING CAPITAL

Each institution must optimize the investment of its working capital if it is to be successful as a business. This means that working capital must be managed in such a way that invested funds are planned and controlled (Furst, 1981). Included in this is management of current assets that are used to support the revenue producing activities of the organization. It is important to note the difference between working capital and net working capital. Working capital refers to current assets, and net working capital is current assets minus current liabilities. There are four major areas that will be discussed: cash management, accounts receivable, inventory, and current liabilities.

Cash Management

The cash budget is a summary of the projected cash flow and examines whether more cash flow is needed, how much, and when borrowed cash flow could be repaid. It also looks at excess funds. The cash flow cycle is needed in order to develop the cash budget. This cycle is determined by identifying sources of collections (such as third party payers) and looking at the time lag from discharge of patient to payment. This is used to determine the cycle for collection and can be identified by type of payer.

Once the cycle is determined, it can be applied to revenues billed to project revenue received each month. For example, if one assumes revenue billed of $300,000 and one knows that 25% will be received in the month billed, that would mean $75,000. If another 50% is received the following month, that would be $150,000, etc. When this is done for each month's projected revenue, cash flow and the cash budget are determined. The cash budget generally subtracts bad debt allowance before projecting expected receipts.

Excess cash balances, even for short periods, are invested in order to earn additional income. Treasury bills, certificates of deposit and money market certificates are several options for short term investment. The rates of return vary with the type of certificate, the time period invested, and the economy.

Accounts Receivable

Accounts receivable are the largest category of current assets. Depending on the collection period, cash flow may be significantly affected by the amount of accounts receivable. Particular attention must be paid by the finance manager to the collection period so that it can be shortened if necessary. One method for reducing the collection period is to improve processing within the institution. This impacts on the medical and nursing staff, since it often requires chart completion and signatures on dictated forms. Pre-admission interviews are also helpful in identifying early those patients who may need alternate sources of assistance to pay bills. Write-off of bad debts may also be done in a more timely manner to improve this collection period (Furst, 1981).

Inventory

Management of inventory is another method for managing working capital. This involves ensuring that inventory levels are maintained at reasonable levels. Maintenance of a safety stock and determination of par levels are important in inventory management. Factors that influence these levels include usage, availability, time between order and delivery, and absolute necessity of the item.

Current Liabilities

There are two sources of current liabilities that should be managed in controlling working capital: trade credit and short term debt. Permanent assets are usually financed with equity, long term debt, or trade credit. Often, discounts for early payment will be given to the institution by companies. This is referred to as trade credit. Failure to take advantage of this discount costs the institution. By the same token, institutions should not pay until the bill is due, since use of the money (or investment of the money) until it is due earns income. Short term debt is usually in the form of loans from banks and may require a compensating balance (a minimum amount left on balance and not usable), may or may not be secured with accounts receivable, or may be associated with a line of credit offered to the institution by the bank.

CAPITAL EXPENDITURE ANALYSIS

Capital budgeting was discussed earlier in this chapter. The purpose of this section is discussion of the analysis of capital expenditures through the techniques of net present value analysis and cost/benefit analysis. Net present value analysis can be compared to compound interest. With compound interest, the interest is paid on the principal and accumulated interest. With net present value analysis, the opposite process occurs. Instead of adding the interest, there is a discount from the ending amount. If payments, for example, are to be received at some end point, the discounted percentage is subtracted to determine the current value.

Another type of analysis is cost/benefit analysis. This may be utilized with multiple capital expenditures. A piece of equipment, for instance, may be purchased to replace a fully depreciated older model. Although the older model works, its operating costs are significantly higher than the new model, resulting in an overall savings even after annual depreciation on the new model. Salvage value of old equipment or the income from sale of old equipment may be deducted from the costs of new equipment before it is depreciated. Additional considerations in analysis of capital expenditures include indirect benefits, such as additional obstetrical admissions because a neonatal ICU is available, and non-monetary benefits such as improved public relations.

In decision making related to capital expenditures various rankings may occur. Equipment may be ranked depending on its life saving potential, for example. Other rankings may occur, such as sorting equipment by its necessity in maintenance of operations, cost savings, or revenue producing ability. Because of the high cost of capital expenditure and the criticism of the high costs associated with health care, analysis of capital expenditures in some systematic manner is important.

COST OF CAPITAL

Defined as the "rate of return that must be earned on capital investment to leave unchanged the economic value of the institution," cost of capital is an important financial term (Furst, 1981, p. 149). The financial requirements of the institution, discussed earlier in this chapter, include revenues over and above costs of operation. The institution must earn a rate of return on investments that at least equals the cost of capital. The methods of financing primarily used by hospitals, debt financing and equity financing, may vary from each other by several percent. To provide for rational decisions related to investments and to ensure that the rate of return on investments covers the cost of capital, a weighted average cost of capital can be figured. This figure is important for the manager. For example, if the institution uses 25% debt financing and 75% equity, these weights would be multiplied by the interest rate to determine the weighted cost. For example:

Debt 25% × Interest Rate 10% =   2.5%

Equity 75% × Interest Rate 16% =   12.0%

                                       14.5%

There are several uses for "cost of capital" figures. Rate setting is dependent to some degree on these figures, and as health care becomes more regulated, these figures may be important in determining operating margins (Furst, 1981). In any case, the nursing administrator must be knowledgeable about what the costs of financing are.

CAPITAL FINANCING

Sources of financing for capital expansions have become more scarce in recent years. Philanthropy has declined as a source of financing but through the development of foundations may increase in importance once more. Government grants and appropriations are another source that can provide significant amounts of funds for such expansions or projects. Debt financing, however, is the major source of funding for renovation or construction. It should be understood that the major forms of debt financing available to health care institutions include conventional mortgages, tax-exempt revenue bonds, and FHA insured mortgages. The advantages and disadvantages of such financing must be considered before decisions are made.

Before capital financing occurs, the health care institution must be evaluated, as are other borrowers, in several key areas. The financial history of the institution is important. Income statements and balance sheets will be reviewed. Support from the community will be another key factor. The certificate of need (CON) process requires approval from state agencies prior to certain expenditures. These CON's generally will be included in the evaluation. Certainly, the quality of the management and the quality of the medical staff will be factors that may be given consideration in the evaluation.

The financial feasibility of a project will also be reviewed before capital financing is undertaken. Rate of return, debt to capital ratios, and cash balance at the end of the period of construction or renovation would be included in the study to ensure that undertaking a project would not prove detrimental.

PROSPECTIVE RATE SETTING/EXTERNAL CONTROL OF RATES

Under DRG's (Diagnosis Related Groups), hospitals are reimbursed at a set rate by diagnosis regardless of the costs or charges for the care provided. Currently, Medicare patients fit into this reimbursement category and other third party payers are considering it for the future. The basis for prospective payment is incentives to shorten length of stay and reduce costs. The system has been phased in, and changes may soon involve physician payment and capital equipment.

Rates set by the prospective payment system change the focus of management toward reduction of length of stay and costs. These rates are externally controlled and result in many cases in cost shifting to other payers. The results of such cost shifting or rate control have a short term rather than a long term effect.

TOMORROW'S STRATEGIES

Three major factors have been identified by Furst (1981) as influencing the financial management in health care institutions. Each of these factors may significantly affect the future of health care as it exists. The nurse administrator must be prepared to respond to the changes that occur.

First, government spending is being reduced annually. No longer will health care institutions be able to rely on such reimbursement to operate. Prospective payment is anticipated to spread to physicians and skilled nursing facilities as well. Insurance companies are encouraging development of PPO's (preferred provider organizations), HMO's, and other discounted rates with specific providers. Competition among health care institutions is also likely to produce price wars in the institutions.

Growth of hospital chains is occurring and provides incentives to single institutions to join the ranks. Large organizations can provide economies of scale, consultation, and investment opportunities unavailable to smaller, independent hospitals. As chains of hospitals grow, the pressures from the prospective payment system and discounted rates will force smaller, independent facilities to close.

Finally, HMO's and PPO's are abounding. The shift of the health care dollars in this direction will negatively impact on many of the smaller insurance companies, since the larger companies will expand their efforts in these directions. The development of Medicare HMO's, previously considered very likely, is questionable because of the lack of government commitment.

These developments provide growth opportunities and challenges to the nursing administrator as well as to other managers. Each of these changes reflects the concern for rising costs in health care. The emphasis on financial management has never before been so important. It is vital for the nursing administrator to be prepared by understanding and using information discussed here in her future financial planning. (Refer also to Chapter 13, Health Care Environment.)

References

Dolkart, D., Freko, D., Li, W. (1984). First quarter trends: Changing environment. *Hospitals, 58*(15), 37–38.

Finkler, S. (1984). *Budgeting concepts for nurse managers.* Orlando: Grune and Stratton.

Finkler, S. (1985). *Seminar on budgeting for nurse managers.* Atlanta, Ga.

Furst, R. (1981). *Financial management for health care institutions.* Boston: Allyn and Bacon, Inc.

Georgoff, D., Murdick, R. (1986). Manager's guide to forecasting. *Harvard Business Review, 64*(1), 110–120.

Golden, C., McDevitt, C., Bloch, K. (1981). Good forecasting builds good budgets. *Hospital Financial Management, 35*(8), 18–26.

Hillestad, E. (1983). Budgeting: Functional or dysfunctional? *Nursing Economics, 1*(3), 199–201.

Hoffman, F. (1984). *Financial management for nurse managers.* Norwalk, CT: Appleton-Century-Crofts.

Kirby, K., Wiczai, L. (1985). Budgeting for variable staffing. *Nursing Economics, 3*(3), 160–166.

National League for Nursing. (1957). *Nursing Service Budget.* Publication No. 22.

Petty, J., Keown, A., Scott, D., Martin, J. (1982). *Basic financial management.* Englewood Cliffs, NJ: Prentice-Hall.

Schramm, C. (1984). Can we solve the hospital-cost problem in our democracy? *New England Journal of Medicine, 311*(11), 729–732.

PRODUCTIVITY MANAGEMENT

INTRODUCTION

The health care environment has entered a path of change, and the course it takes has serious consequences for all health care providers. The evolving methods of payment for health care services are based, of course, on financial incentives to encourage cost control and foster competition. The potential impact of this redirection on health care providers and recipients is enormous (Arthur Anderson and Co., and American College of Hospital Administrators, 1984). The movement of health care institutions from a service orientation to an economic orientation is a very real one. Survival has become the primary motivating factor. The conflicts that face hospitals complicate the picture even more as consumers demand cost control *and* high technology, high access, and high quality of care. Providing that quality remains a goal but one that is tempered with the realities of limited resources. It will be the efficient use of those limited resources that provides the key to the high quality, cost effective health care services that spell success for the health care institution.

Productivity management has taken on new importance in the uncertain economic environment, and improvement in productivity has emerged as a key strategy for cost containment. Hospitals and most other health care

10

institutions are very labor intensive with salaries and benefits for employees composing 50 to 60% of expenses. Reduced Medicare reimbursement, reduced Medicaid funds, increased regulation, and pressures for rate control from insurance companies and businesses combine to reduce revenue. With all these factors playing key roles in the amount of revenue for these health care institutions versus increased costs for supplies and equipment, malpractice insurance, and salaries, it is easy to see the impact they may have. Unable to control the revenue sources through pricing alterations, health care institutions must instead critically evaluate how productively human and material resources are being used. The nursing administrator, as every top level manager, will need to realize that productivity management is not a one time solution to a problem but a continuous, conscientious integration of multiple management activities toward efficient delivery of quality health care services. Determining what those activities are and how to integrate and control them is productivity management.

Productivity has been defined as the relationship between quantities of goods or services produced (outputs) and quantities of the factors that contribute to the production (inputs). Productivity management is aimed at varying the relationship between the outputs and inputs to achieve one of several positive outcomes within the organization: (1) increasing output, decreasing input; (2) increasing output, keeping input constant; (3) increasing output more rapidly than input increases; (4) keeping output constant, decreasing input; and (5) decreasing output more slowly than input decreases (Kaye and Utenner, 1985). Any one of these relationships could be used to improve productivity.

Productivity alone does not determine an organization's performance. Effective operation, employee satisfaction, quality of output, efficiency in use of supplies, financial stability, and even image may be considered in evaluating an organization's performance. However, productivity can pull together at least some of these factors to improve overall performance of the organization. By managing the ratio between inputs and outputs, the health care manager can effectively help to contain costs, therefore meeting a major objective of the health care institution.

This chapter will discuss productivity management as it is impacted by the environment. How nursing departments fit into the system will be emphasized. Factors that influence productivity will be discussed, and specific methods to improve productivity will be identified. Finally, a management program for productivity will be explained, and strategies will be described.

PRODUCTIVITY MANAGEMENT

The changing health care environment, which has led to the emphasis on productivity, will continue to influence health care institutions in significant ways. Competition among providers of health care continues, as multi-hospital, for-profit chains grow and grouping of not-for-profit hospitals becomes more common. HMO's and PPO's will offer alternative health care delivery, and business ventures will be sought to provide non-traditional revenue sources. Rapid technological change, changing work ethics, and professional accountability can be expected to influence these organizations (Kaye and Utenner, 1985). As demands for more health care technology, services, and access with the same or less resources become more common-place, productivity management will become an even more important responsibility of every manager. Creative and innovative approaches to improving productivity will be welcomed.

Concerns for Nursing

How nursing fits into this system for productivity has produced concern and challenges for nursing administrators. A number of reasons for concern have been identified. Nursing is a profession that provides multiple services to consumers. Each service may require multiple skills or education to perform. Details of procedures or interventions may be developed, and there may be an expectation that such details are consistently followed. However, many aspects of nursing care entail professional discretion. The assessment, planning, and evaluation of care, for example, do not fit into categorized or step by step procedures. Comprehensiveness, timeliness, and intensity defy specific categorization. Attempts at quantification of one's judgment and communication may complicate matters even more. Even more difficult to fit into a mold is the lack of sequential pattern that characterizes most nursing interventions (Haas, 1984).

Fiss and White (1977) analyzed productivity measurement in nursing and described other concerns. They identified that much of what nursing does is intermediate, not resulting in a final outcome that is measurable. Quality of care, which is always an issue, is difficult if not impossible to measure objectively. Inputs in nursing are diverse and constantly changing, while outputs are heterogeneous and unstable. Just distinguishing nursing contribution to the output from the contribution of others (the physician, therapist, or even patient) is difficult.

Ruh (1982) found that measuring productivity in service type organizations was difficult because "once the service is performed, the evidence disappears." The intangibility of the outcome or output casts doubts on productivity management programs. Especially when follow-up is sporadic, selective, or absent and when outputs are poorly defined, measuring nursing productivity is complicated. The addition of the word "acceptable" to the measurement of outputs has not really helped either, since "acceptable" has varying definitions to different people (Haas, 1984). It is because of such debates that measurement of nursing productivity is met with concern by nursing administrators. Making chief executive officers understand these

TABLE 10–1
Factors Influencing Productivity

Reimbursement
Pre-admission certification
Demands for specific services
Manager effectiveness
Outpatient services
Resources available
Function of equipment
Motivation of employees
   Compensation, working conditions
   Participation in decision making, challenges
Communication
Flexibility, authority
Facility layout
Practice patterns of professionals
Documentation
Number and type of procedures performed
Systems

concerns is an important responsibility for the nursing administrator, if she is to reasonably defend the costs for nursing services. To ensure efficient delivery of care, the nursing administrator will be required to comprehensively control the care delivered to patients through use of a classification category or some other mechanism (Kirk and Dunaye, 1986).

Factors Influencing Productivity

A number of internal and external factors may influence productivity (Table 10–1). Those external factors, which are controlled very little or not at all by health care institutions, may affect productivity in varying degrees. Certainly, the reimbursement available may influence the pressure on health care institutions to emphasize productivity to a higher degree. More directly, changes in reimbursement and pre-admission certification may affect the number of admissions and lengths of stay, resulting in fewer patient days (often the output in the productivity equation). Certain demands for services may be such that cost efficiency and, therefore, productivity cannot be improved. For example, demand for extracorporeal shock wave lithotripsy may occur from a new urologist on staff at a facility. While the number of patients with diagnoses requiring the procedure (or invasive surgery) might justify the purchase of the unit, the ability to schedule the procedures in a timely sequence and the lack of training of other urologists in the procedure could negatively influence productivity.

Internal factors that influence productivity are numerous. Productivity management cannot be successful without a clear understanding of these factors. The chief influence on productivity comes from the management group (Kaye and Utenner, 1985). These individuals are the ones who manage all the hospital's resources each day. If they are well educated to effectively manage in the current and changing environment, productivity improvements may be possible. However, failure of these managers to effectively manage can be detrimental to the organization. Incentives to encourage improved productivity can be a valuable investment for the organization.

The change to outpatient care is yet another factor that may influence productivity by shifting outputs from one service to another or by reducing overall patient days. This particular factor may be external, as in changes in consumer demand or in third party payer pressures, or may be internal forces to improve efficiency and quality of service.

Resources available to facilitate getting the job done is another factor that affects productivity. Unavailability of the right tools or supplies not only may slow down procedures but also may produce frustration on the part of employees. If equipment works poorly or inconsistently, productivity can be significantly reduced. Associated with this factor is the procedure itself. How efficiently the procedure is in meeting the desired outcome is variable. Examination of procedures may reveal unnecessary or missing steps that complicate or unnecessarily lengthen procedures. The "better mousetrap" or improved method of accomplishing the task can improve productivity, too.

The worker himself can have a tremendous impact on productivity. Motivation of the employee to improve performance is often tied to incentives. Fair and equitable compensation, good working conditions, and benefits are certainly part of the incentive. Other factors, however, can be just as important. A sense of belonging and participation in decision making are two such factors. Employees need to feel they are part of the organization. They usually respond positively to challenges and increased responsibility if they are allowed to participate in the decisions that affect them. Each of these factors affects the morale of employees. Morale is directly related to motivation. When morale of employees is good, they are motivated to perform at a higher level of productivity.

Communication channels are another factor that influences productivity. It is important to maintain open and clear lines of communication so that necessary changes can be initiated and understood. Communication breakdown can adversely affect productivity when it affects flow of services, supplies, or equipment. Good communication is essential to ensure that everyone involved in input is working as well as possible toward the goal desired.

Flexibility that is allowable within an institution can have an effect on productivity. If a manager is to be effective, he must have the authority to handle problems independently and the flexibility to adjust resource utilization to need. For example, he must be able to send staff home or adjust schedules to meet work demand. If the manager lacks this authority and flexibility in managing the department, accountability for results cannot be reasonably expected.

The physical layout of a facility may impact on productivity as well. Inconveniently placed treatment rooms or difficult access to needed equipment slows down procedures and results in reduced productivity. Long hallways, requiring extensive time for trips to and from patient rooms, reduce efficiency as well. Crowded conditions in departments that are too small may result in an inability to adequately store supplies and equipment. When this necessitates extra trips to retrieve needed supplies or equipment, productivity falls.

Practice patterns of physicians or other professionals influence productivity. Professionals who require an extensive period of time to perform procedures that are accomplished in briefer times by others can impact on productivity in a very negative way. Similarly, if a professional is repeatedly late in beginning procedures, he delays others and reduces productivity. Maintaining schedules as much as possible is important to maintaining and improving productivity.

The number and type of procedures performed by a group of employees are another factor that influences productivity. Generally, the larger the number of procedures an employee can perform, the more flexibility there is and the greater the potential to improve productivity. The more diverse the number or type of procedures, the more difficult it is to switch from one to another. Related procedures are not particularly difficult as compared with unrelated procedures, but performing unrelated procedures can result in reduced productivity. Concentration is disturbed and time is lost when the employee switches from one type of task to another.

Documentation is yet another factor that influences productivity. Quality is often very difficult to quantify. Measuring quality through the use of standards is an attempt to quantify quality. Documentation serves to provide some measurement that the standards are being met. Through documentation, it may be determined that specific actions have occurred that provide the basis for quality care (output) (Boyer, Corbett, and Jansen, 1986).

Managing Productivity in Health Care

Health care is an industry that has many intangible and even more unmeasurable outcomes. Even more of a problem is determining who had responsibility for an outcome when several persons may be involved in care of the patient. Patients may leave a health care institution without being "well." Lack of follow-up also prevents measurement of outcomes. Complications or other illnesses may also occur, which may interfere with outcome measurements (Haas, 1984).

Although it is easier to measure inputs in health care institutions, there is still some question about separating the input from various sources. The input of equipment versus supplies versus other employees against, for example, the nurse's input is difficult to separate and measure. The work environment and all that the environment entails, then, may significantly influence input.

Creating an environment for productivity is essential if a nursing

administrator desires to manage productivity well. The first step in creating
the environment for productivity is self-evaluation. The nursing administrator must carefully examine her feelings about productivity and her style of
leadership. She must be able to coordinate the efforts of her health care team
to obtain the maximum productivity from that team. A leadership style that
considers not only the system but also the people and the effects of each on
productivity will produce the best motivation and the best productivity.

Once the nursing administrator has evaluated how she fits into the
scheme of productivity, she must examine the factors that influence productivity. Identified in the previous section, these factors may have varying
levels of impact on productivity. Understanding this is essential for an
environment for productivity.

The nursing administrator must also involve team members in the
planning for a productivity program. The team members, in the case of the
nursing administrator, may include the entire nursing staff. If involvement
of the staff at the planning stage is not feasible, nursing managers and
representatives from the staff may be involved to maintain the level of
communication important to the program. Involvement of team members
not only improves communication but also is a source of valuable information
that can be used in establishing a productivity management program.

In creating the environment for productivity management, the nursing
administrator must communicate to staff the importance of the program, the
role of all individuals in the program, and the concern and interest she has
in each of the staff members. Cooperation and enthusiasm for any change
may not come quickly. However, good communication breeds good understanding, and an understanding of the reasons for management of productivity in the health care environment is essential for success.

A PROGRAM FOR PRODUCTIVITY MANAGEMENT

A productivity management program is an organized way in which a
health care institution may approach the management of productivity. Such
a program may meet several important objectives. One objective of any
productivity management program should be the education of department
managers and employees about productivity. Motivation theory has shown
that individuals who know what is expected of them are more likely to
produce than those whose goals are vague or unclear (see motivation section
in Chapter 5, Foundations for Leadership). Additionally, department managers will need to understand productivity management and to develop
skills necessary to accomplish the goals of the program.

Another goal of a productivity management program would be development of indices for objective measurement of productivity. Through the

use of historical data as well as statistics from other institutions, indices of workload may be identified by department. In nursing, for example, patient days and acuity may be employed to provide workload units to be used as a measurement of overall workload on a specific nursing unit. Procedures, case hours, or visits are other examples from nursing.

Identification of improvements in systems, procedures, traffic flow, or even geography might be another objective of a productivity management program. Since productivity may be influenced by such factors as resources, equipment function, and facility layout, improvements in any of the procedures, facilities, or systems could enhance productivity. Another objective of such a program would be development of a mechanism to monitor productivity and to balance workload with staffing based on this monitoring. A reporting system that provides data related to actual workload compared with actual staff and needed staff is an important tool for management in controlling productivity.

Steps in Development

Before a program for productivity management can be developed, a committee composed of top management and administration should be selected and should be involved in determining the guidelines for the program. Because nursing has the largest number of employees in nearly every health care institution, there should be good representation from nursing. Initial steps in program development include education for the committee and for other departmental managers. The goal of the committee initially is the development of productivity measures and targets for each department. Ideas for improving productivity may also be generated.

In developing the productivity measure for a department, several questions must be answered. The scope and organization of the department are characteristics that may affect productivity and would therefore be important. Staffing and scheduling, department layout, equipment, and any unique policies or procedures might influence productivity as well. The working relationships between departments and the systems used within a department are other characteristics that would need to be identified as measures for productivity are considered. Department managers are generally able to identify other characteristics within their departments that could adversely affect productivity. They should also be encouraged to identify those characteristics that might positively influence productivity. Within nursing departments, characteristics that might negatively affect productivity could include: delays in transport of patients, delays in cleaning rooms for transfers, admissions, inconvenient admission times, practices of physicians in rounds, procedures, equipment breakdown, excessive overtime or extra shifts resulting in fatigue, performance of other departments' procedures after hours, and full time to part time staff ratios. Those characteristics that could positively influence productivity might include: cross-trained personnel, level

TABLE 10–2	
Comparison of Two Workload Measures	

A. Patient Days

$$\frac{840}{\substack{\text{Patient Days}\\\text{For Month}}} \times \frac{5.0}{\text{HPPD}^*} = \frac{4200}{\substack{\text{Earned Worked}\\\text{Hours}}}$$

B. Weighted Patient Days

$$\frac{840}{\substack{\text{Patient Days}\\\text{For Month}}} \times \frac{5.0}{\text{HPPD}} \times \frac{1.2}{\substack{\text{Average}\\\text{Acuity}}} = \frac{5040}{\substack{\text{Earned Worked}\\\text{Hours}}}$$

*This is usually a budget or pre-authorized average HPPD (hours per patient day).

of education among staff members, rapid response time by support services, exchange cart systems, flexible staffing systems, modular geographic units, and adequate part time staff.

Once the characteristics of a department have been identified and evaluated, an appropriate measure of workload must be selected. Several alternatives may be available, and selection may be made on the basis of data available for review or the ability to compare data with those of other hospitals. The department manager, of course, must be involved in the decision. Lack of statistical information may predetermine the selection. Examples of workload measures include procedures performed, visits, case hours, patient days, weighted patient days (patient days times acuity), weighted visits or procedures, calendar days, hours of care, and number of employees. The selection of a workload measure is the most critical factor in managing productivity. The difference between patient days and weighted patient days could impact significantly on the percentage of productivity. For example, on two nursing units a comparison may be made. One unit may use patient days as the workload measure. Patient days multiplied by average hours of care per patient day equals hours to be worked by staff. It can easily be seen that, when an acuity factor is also included in the multiplication, an increase in the hours to be worked by staff would occur (Table 10–2). There are advantages and disadvantages to each workload measure, and there are workload measures that are appropriate or inappropriate. It would not be appropriate to use calendar days on a nursing unit, since the level of workload varies so much with the census or occupancy of the unit. (Refer to Table 10–3 for advantages and disadvantages of specific measures.) Once a method of workload measurement is selected, historical data for the department can be collected and graphed to determine the current level of productivity. (Refer to Chapter 17, Patient Care Management, for discussion of patient classification system selection, which can be very important in development of workload measures.)

During collection of data related to workload, the department manager may also generate ideas about improving productivity. Often this is referred to as a wish list—"I could improve work performance or efficiency if...." Ideas may include those over which the department manager has no control.

TABLE 10–3		
Examples of Workload Measures		
Workload Measure	Advantages	Disadvantages
Procedures performed	• Better indicator for departments that are procedure oriented or have in- and outpatients • Easy to calculate	• Does not consider complexity of procedures
Visits	• Better indicator for departments that are oriented to and operate by visits • Easy to calculate	• Does not consider number of procedures/tasks in a visit (i.e., complexity of visit)
Case hours	• Considers complexity of cases, which alter workload	• Does not consider numerous factors impacting on case length • Difficult to calculate
Weighted procedures/ visits	• Considers complexity of procedures or visits, which alter workload	• Changes in complexity of a procedure or type of visit may not quickly be identified • Difficult to calculate
Calendar days	• Ideal for areas where workload is relatively constant • Easy to calculate	• Does not consider variations in workload for causes other than more worked days
Hours of care or patient days	• Easy to calculate • Better for departments that have continual patient contact	• Does not consider acuity or variations in workload based on severity of illness
Weighted hours of care or patient days	• Considers workload variations based on illness acuity • Better for departments that have continual patient contact	• Difficult to calculate

For example, reducing turnover time for operating rooms might improve productivity for the Surgery Department, but the OR manager may be unable to get the rooms cleaned faster by Housekeeping. Ideas may also be controllable, given specific resources. Use of a specific type of prep tray may improve the productivity in the cardiac catheterization laboratory, for example.

When historical data have been collected and reviewed, a determination may be made about whether the productivity is acceptable or could improve. Often administration will set all goals to reach a specific percentage improvement. It should be considered, though, that some departments are functioning maximally or in fact are overworked. Careful analysis should precede target determination. Targets should be negotiated between administration and department managers. Targets are the amount of hours of work needed for the workload generated. This should be a reasonable time value per unit volume. This may be converted to FTE's if desired. Table 10–4 is an example of a report generated each pay period. On this specific unit, targeted hours are by acuity level. In the example, the patient days for each level are multiplied by target hours to reach a total that is compared with worked hours.

TABLE 10–4
Productivity Management Report

Unit _____   Pay Period _____

Patient Days
Level I Patients   _____ × 2.0 HPPD = _____
Level II Patients _____ × 4.0 HPPD = _____
Level III Patients _____ × 10.5 HPPD = _____
Level IV Patients _____ × 18.5 HPPD = _____

Total A. _____ Hours Earned
B. _____ Hours Worked
C. _____ (A ÷ B)
_____ Productivity Ratio
(C × 100%)

Implementation of the productivity management program should occur as soon after initial introduction as possible, given that all steps have been carried out. The reason for this is to maintain the momentum and enthusiasm. When implementation is delayed, interest is reduced and questions are raised about the importance of the program. Computer assistance in generating the reports is important, although not essential. The major data needed for comparison are actual workload and targeted hours of work to compare with actual hours. Targeted hours are also referred to as earned hours, as in the example found in Table 10–4. Reports may be generated manually by filling in statistical data. Reports may be generated by pay period or by month. Monthly reports are more difficult to generate because exact hours worked data are generally available by pay period (usually two weeks) rather than by month. Formulas are available to estimate with a great deal of accuracy the data for monthly reports. Although different institutions may tailor their reports to meet their needs, there are key elements that should be reported. These include the volume or workload for the reported period, the time value per unit of volume (goal or target), the required or earned hours, and the actual hours worked. Variances may be reported, as well as the productivity ratio or percentage.

Evaluation of data produced is the next step. Since selection of productivity measures and targets is often difficult, this step is needed to determine if selection was reasonable. Variation from a normal range (determined by the institution but generally between 90 and 110%) should be analyzed carefully. The variation may be understood or may be totally unexpected and not understood. Targets may need revision if they are obviously significantly out of line. Several pay periods or months of data may be needed for review.

Ongoing monitoring of productivity is essential for a good productivity management program. Continual monitoring of productivity by various mechanisms is very important. Monthly or bimonthly formal reports should act as a summary of productivity, but they cannot serve to correct productivity problems in as timely a manner as is desirable. Nursing departments

TABLE 10–5
Example of Productivity Calculation

Unit 10 West—Oncology   Date 8/31/86

Patients

Level I	6	×	2.0 HPPD =	12
Level II	12	×	4.0 HPPD =	48
Level III	10	×	10.5 HPPD =	105
Level IV	4	×	18.5 HPPD =	74

Total __32__ Patients   Total = __239__ Hours Earned

Divided by 8 hr/Shift   __29.9__ Shifts Earned

Multiply by:

    50% Staff 7–3 = __14.95__ # Staff
    30% Staff 3–11 = __8.97__   # Staff
    20% Staff 11–7 = __5.98__   # Staff

Staff Permitted: 15 on 7–3
                    9 on 3–11
                    6 on 11–7
                   30 Total

Staff Scheduled: 15 on 7–3
                    9 on 3–11
                    7 on 11–7
                   31 Total

Disposition: 1 staff member on 11–7 will be reassigned or sent home

---

may determine levels of productivity by day or shift if good patient classification tools or other workload measures are available. For example, a manager may calculate the hours of care needed for the number and type of patients on the unit at the time. From this calculation, the manager may determine the number of staff needed to provide care for those patients. Adding or deleting staff based on the calculations (done by shift if necessary or desirable) is an excellent method for controlling productivity. It is important to remember that there are three shifts when calculations are done based on HPPD (hours per patient day). Table 10–5 demonstrates a method for the calculation and its impact.

Changes in any of the factors influencing productivity may result in changes in productivity. If these changes occur, it is important that they be recognized and addressed. Goals or targets may require revision for various reasons. Actions to improve productivity may result in the target being met consistently. To motivate even better productivity, the target may be revised. Reports generated during the program should be utilized by managers to enhance efficiency and productivity. Reports can, for example, determine if measures to improve productivity have been successful or not. They also permit comparison of productivity with that of other departments and other institutions. Productivity management programs such as the one described are important to improving productivity (VHAMS, 1985). Table 10–6 summarizes the steps in developing a productivity management program.

| TABLE 10–6 |
| Steps in Development of Productivity Management Programs |

1. Education for managers and steering committee
2. Identification and evaluation of department characteristics
3. Selection of measure of workload
4. Collection of historical data
5. Development of ideas for improving productivity
6. Analysis of data
7. Negotiation of target for productivity
8. Implementation
9. Evaluation—review data produced
10. Revision of targets
11. Ongoing monitoring for control

Improving Productivity

Improving productivity does sometimes require creative approaches. The first person who must be involved is the manager. The manager must be involved in selection of the workload measure if maximal support for the productivity program is desired. Such involvement provides incentive for the manager to meet the targets for productivity. Mutual agreement on the target between the manager and administration is also necessary for optimal support. Incentives of various types are used by some managers to enhance productivity (Pointer, 1985). Examples include recognition, awards, or monetary rewards. Education for managers and non-management employees is another means to improve productivity. Associated with these personnel related measures is another one—employee involvement programs. Support of these type programs has been shown to be effective in improving productivity, just as manager involvement has been successful.

Implementation of systems to measure and control productivity has a positive effect. People perform better if they know someone is watching. It is also very helpful to implement improvements in systems and methods or procedures. Work simplification, finding an easier way to do the job, may include elimination of unnecessary steps in procedures or improving cooperation between departments and may significantly impact on productivity. For example, if a particular procedure requires cooperation between departments, the procedure should be streamlined to divide responsibilities and not allow duplication of any tasks if unnecessary. Clear-cut responsibilities prevent extra work and confusion as well as improve productivity. Accountability for outcome should be established, not as a mechanism for punishment but for reward. If one is rewarded (even through a pat on the back), one is likely to perform better. Managers should use performance evaluation to control performance, handle performance problems, and produce efficient workers (Lachman, 1984). Through the use of performance evaluation for accountability, productivity can also be positively affected.

Analysis of all types of systems, design or layout of departments, and organizational structure is another tool that may result in improved productivity. Examples of layout, design, or other similar problems that impact on productivity may include location of utility rooms and supplies; lengths of hallways; assignment of patients; disorganized supply or equipment storage, resulting in difficulty in finding supplies; and disorganization by a staff member making rounds. Data identified during the analysis may be useful in redistribution of resources. There are obviously some problems over which a manager may have little or no control. For example, the manager cannot very well change hall length. However, a number of creative ideas may be used to address other problems. Utility rooms or supply storage problems may be identified that are subject to change or adaptation. The location of substations down lengthy hallways, the use of supply carts, or even the use of supply baskets for most frequently used supplies would be useful in resolving or minimizing the issues of design or layout problems and could improve productivity by reducing travel time and steps for the staff members.

Assignment of staff as reasonable to rooms in close proximity to one another is another important point. Organization, too, plays a very significant role, not only in keeping supplies and equipment easy to locate, but also in keeping the staff members working without frequent or unnecessary interruptions in work flow. For example, before beginning rounds, the nurse should organize her thoughts and the needed materials to carry with her. If it is likely she will need to discontinue or restart an IV in route, she may carry alcohol wipes, IV catheters, or start sets with her. If the nurse knows she will have to change Mrs. Smith's dressing while there, she should be prepared to do so. In making rounds with physicians, similar preparation is needed. Prescription pads, stethoscope, suture removal sets, etc., may be needed, for example. This type of organization is a big time saver.

In looking at organizational structure, work assignments may also be evaluated to determine if the correct worker is performing the task or if a different employee is needed. Substitution of one level employee for another may be considered, but it is unwise to make this type of change without fully evaluating the impact. A less costly staff cannot necessarily function at the same level, so that the loss in capability may not actually prove to be more productive, but rather may be less productive (Herzog, 1985).

Mechanization or use of computers or other technology may be considered and may, in fact, improve productivity. Streamlining paperwork or record keeping may be quite successful. This computerization may even include computer documentation of nursing care plans, nursing actions, and treatments. The time saving varies with the system but is often substantial once the initial time involvement for training occurs. Herzog (1985) recognized this method and two other less common methods for improving productivity. Selection or careful choice of an employee was one of these other two methods. As candidates for positions are more numerous, selection of the best candidate may enhance the productivity. Job consolidation is another such method. It involves combining the tasks of two or more positions. If similar skill levels are present in the positions, this may be helpful.

This may be similar to yet another method—cross training. Cross training of personnel to cover one another's functions has long been recognized as an effective method to improve productivity. An example would be the home health nurse who draws blood for the lab, runs an ECG, or gives a respiratory therapy treatment. Cross training provides a worker who becomes more valuable because he can perform multiple functions.

Improving productivity should be the responsibility of every employee. Employees who know what is expected, who receive feedback for good and for poor performance, and who are rewarded for good performance will help enhance productivity. It is the responsibility of the manager to see that this occurs.

STRATEGIES FOR TOMORROW

The nursing administrator of today must prepare for tomorrow by developing several strategies to assist in maintaining a productive nursing service. Nurses are the only health care employees who are with the patient around the clock. Future productivity will require good decision making continuously. There must be collaborative working relationships among physicians, nurses, and administration to ensure that this decision making can occur (Herzog, 1985).

Maintenance of quality care is another factor in future productivity. Although fewer patients and shorter lengths of stay may occur, those patients will be certainly sicker. If quality of care declines, readmission and longer stays may result. Quality will be necessary to put the best care into the shorter stay. It is therefore imperative to monitor and emphasize quality of care as a critical factor in productivity. One example of how this may impact on overall hospital productivity may be seen in a patient admitted to an ICU. Because of emphasis on reduced costs and shorter length of stays, there may be attempts to transfer the patient from the ICU earlier than optimal. Because of such an early transfer, the patient may develop complications. On the other hand, keeping the patient longer in the ICU may result in better education, closer observation, and fewer complications, reducing the overall length of stay. Continual monitoring of the quality of care, however, is necessary to ensure that desired outcomes are achieved for patients through adherence to prescribed standards of care.

Improved technology, including computerization in nursing, although costly, can help to improve the productivity of the employee in the future. However, that employee will need to be better trained and to have more skills and expertise. The nursing administrator should be planning for this. Maximizing the nursing resources through position consolidation, flexibility in staffing and in role or function, and reduction in the fragmentation of job design will be important.

Computerization in nursing will continue to advance beyond current capabilities, which permit care planning and documentation. Future strategies should include capabilities to document performance, monitor quality, evaluate productivity, and maintain documentation retrievable by an individual nurse. Computer software will be needed to correlate the relationship of quality to productivity as well as to performance. Information systems already have many of these capabilities, and enhancement of these will provide significant improvement for productivity in the future (McAlindon, Silver, and Edwards, 1986).

The key to productivity in nursing for the future is likely to be linking motivation to productivity. The nursing administrator who can successfully manage this will have a nursing department that is highly productive. This may be accomplished by enhancing staff participation in understanding and developing productivity programs (Dahl, 1986).

Motivating employees to perform at specific levels will challenge the future nursing administrator, since many factors besides staff participation may influence that motivation (see Chapter 5, Foundations for Leadership). Development of a committee of staff members to monitor productivity and develop strategies for enhancing it is one mechanism that may be helpful, although perhaps difficult for managers to accept.

On the input side of productivity, strategies may be developed that may provide improvement. Services that may be contracted may provide such a strategy. For example, in a home health agency, there may be a need at times for an enterostomal therapist. The home health agency may hire such an individual, who then operates at less than optimal productivity. If the home health agency were able to contract part time services of the enterostomal therapist, department productivity could be improved.

There are numerous factors that will continue to have an impact on productivity. Evaluation of these factors will be no less important as a future strategy than it is now. Improved productivity for nursing in the constraining environment of health care will be a tremendous challenge for every nursing administrator.

References

Arthur Anderson and Company and American College of Hospital Administrators (1984). *Health care in the 1990's: Trends and strategies.*

Boyer, N., Corbett, N., and Jansen, R. (1986). Tracking productivity: An easy, quick and useful way. *Nursing Management*, 17(1), 35–42.

Dahl, T. (1986). Crisis in productivity. *Healthcare Forum*, July/August, 17–19.

Eastaugh, S. (1985). Improving hospital productivity under PPS: Managing cost reductions. *Hospital and Health Services Administration*, 30(4), 97–111.

Fiss and White (1977). Productivity in nursing. *Topics in Health Care Financing*, 4(2), 85.

Haas, S.A. (1984). Sorting out nursing productivity. *Nursing Management*, 15(4), 37–40.

Herzog, T. (1985). Productivity: Fighting the battle of the budget. *Nursing Management*, 16(1), 30–34.

Kaye, G. H., and Utenner, J. (1985). Productivity: Managing for the long term. *Nursing Management*, 16(9), 12–15.

Kirk, R., and Dunaye, T. (1986). Managing hospital nursing services for productivity. *Nursing Management*, 17(3), 29–32.

Lachman, V. (1984). Increasing productivity through performance evaluation. *JONA*, *14*(12), 7–14.

McAlindon, M., Silver, C., and Edwards, H. (1986). Computer software for nursing. *Computers in Nursing*, *4*(1), 17–26.

Pointer, D. (1985). Responding to the challenges of the new health care marketplace: Organizing for creativity and innovation. *Hospital and Health Services Administration*, *30*(6), 10–25.

Ruh, W. (1982). The measurement of white collar productivity. *National Productivity Review*, Autumn, 416–426.

Selbst, P. (1985). A more total approach to productivity improvement. *Hospital and Health Services Administration*, *30*(4), 85–96.

VHAMS, (Voluntary Hospitals of America Management Services), (1985). *Productivity management program—project description*. Bay Medical Center, Panama City, Florida.

MARKETING FOR HEALTH CARE

INTRODUCTION

Increasing competition among providers of health care services has resulted over the last few years in tremendous changes in strategies to meet the new challenges. Among the strategies identified for survival of hospitals and other health care institutions is increasing the market share for the organization (Coddington et al, 1985). This particular strategy requires application of the principles of marketing and an understanding of the importance of marketing to any business.

There has been, prior to the mid 1970's, an aversion by health care organizations to "marketing," which can be attributed to the concept that health care is a service and that health care professionals should not "sell" the service (Roberts, 1985). Whether or not health care institutions recognize or accept the concept of marketing, they have and do engage in it to some degree (Clarke, 1984). By the mid 1980's, health care organizations realized the necessity of marketing the services offered, and generally were attempting to address the need. The approaches utilized by health care organizations

11

TABLE 11–1
Functions of Marketing
Information
Equalizing/distributing
Centralized exchange

as well as by many other businesses in addressing the need for marketing have not always been based on marketing principles and certainly have not always included a good understanding of the concept of marketing.

As in any business, in health care services the customer is key to success. Managing the relationship between the institution and the customer is the key to marketing of health care services. A full understanding of how this really works is important to the successful business operation of any health care organization. This chapter will define the concept of marketing, including the differentiation from "selling." Principles of marketing will be discussed, and the ethical/legal implications for health care institutions will be addressed. Methods for identification of the market in health care will be included as well. Various products to be marketed, including the development of new programs, will be addressed. Implementation of the market plan, with sections on pricing, advertising, and distribution, will be discussed. There will be another section on marketing strategies for health care and on evaluation of the effectiveness of those strategies.

CONCEPT OF MARKETING

Marketing has been defined by the American Marketing Association (1960) as the "performance of business activities that direct the flow of goods and services from producer to consumer or user." The theory that underlies marketing is one of motivation. Certainly, Maslow's motivation hierarchy or other similar theories such as those discussed in Chapter 5, Foundations for Leadership, serve to explain how demand for something can change or even be present (Maslow, 1954). Gratification at any level is important as a basis for marketing through the meeting of the customer's needs or desires. Matching the product to the consumer and transferring ownership of the product from producer to consumer are the basic activities involved in marketing (Eliopoulos, 1985). These basic activities, which result in the exchange of services or products for something of value, are made more efficient through three essential functions performed by marketing: information, equalizing and distributing, and centralized exchange (Table 11–1). This total system of distributing goods or services to consumers is referred to as macromarketing (Cunningham and Cunningham, 1981).

The information function of marketing serves to provide the business or organization with information related to the needs and desires of the consumer. In health care institutions, the information would be related to patients and their perceived needs or desires related to health. It would be important, for instance, for the hospital to know that potential obstetrical patients would want an alternative of rooming in for infants and mothers as opposed to traditional nursery care. Accuracy and timeliness of information would obviously be important as well to maintain a competitive environment.

Equalizing supply and demand is another function in macromarketing. Production of a product and provision of services greater than the demand can result in excess expense that could be detrimental to a business. The function of marketing is to determine the supply needed for the demand and to create ways of keeping extra services available until the demand rises to meet that supply. The cost of providing a heart surgery program in a hospital is quite high. Demand initially may be a bit low, and actual costs per procedure could be tremendous. However, as the program becomes more popular, the demand would increase and the costs would be reduced. The program might eventually expand to a point at which additional surgeons, operating rooms, and ICU beds might need to be added to provide the supply of services desired. Marketing's function is to equalize that supply and demand as much as possible.

Centralization for products or services is a third function for marketing. Centralized exchange of services or products in return for payment improves the efficiency of the system (Cunningham and Cunningham, 1981). An example of this function may be seen in the centralization of cardiovascular services in a hospital. Electrocardiogram, echocardiogram, thallium studies, stress testing, and cardiac catheterization may be centralized under one umbrella. By reducing the number of exchanges and/or interactions, the efficiency of operation can be significantly improved.

Marketing goes beyond the three functions identified under the subheading of macromarketing to a process of developing strategies that enable the health care institution or any business to earn a profit. The necessity of profit to any business has been discussed in an earlier chapter (Chapter 7, Business Concepts). Micromarketing involves product development and distribution and begins with determination of the demand.

Demand can vary from none to an overfull demand. The state of demand for services or a product is one of the most crucial factors related to marketing within an organization (Kotler, 1973). Five states of demand that exist in the marketplace have been identified: no demand, latent demand, faltering demand, full demand, and overfull demand (Table 11–2). Each state is associated with a specific approach to achieve the desired demand.

If a service or product has no demand, there could be one of several reasons. A totally new service, a service that is very common or readily available, or one that has no value at the location it is offered are three such reasons. Dependent on the cause of no demand, the market may need to be stimulated to create a demand. An example of a service in health care that previously was faced with no demand was hyperbaric chambers. The use of hyperbaric chambers at any location away from coastal areas was thought to be absurd. Today, through the use of several marketing techniques applied

TABLE 11–2
Levels of Demand in Marketplace

Level	Approach
No demand	Improve techniques to increase demand
Latent demand	Develop product to meet demand
Faltering demand	Market service to improve demand
Full demand	Hold on to market
	Stabilize demand
Overfull demand	Increase supply
	Reduce demand

consciously and subconsciously, hyperbaric chambers can and are utilized in numerous non-coastal areas. One such technique for improving demand is education. Providing information about the multiple uses of hyperbaric chambers, not related to diving accidents, stimulated the demand in the example.

A latent demand for a product or service occurs when there is a significant need not being met by other means. The development of the service or product to meet that need is the task of marketing. An example of a latent demand is seen in the need for cost effective emergency care in more convenient locations than the few hospitals within a locale. The development of urgent care centers was one resultant service to supply what consumers had identified as a need.

When the demand for a service or product begins to waiver, it may be referred to as a faltering demand. Remarketing requires evaluation of the market to determine whether the service or product still has sufficient demand and then developing strategies for the product or service if justified. Faltering demand is frequently seen in programs that were initiated with great enthusiasm following publicity of sorts, only to lose much of their attraction after the publicity was gone. Such was the case with many cardiac rehabilitation programs in areas that faced faltering demand. Remarketing was needed to build the demand for the service.

Full demand occurs when the supply is equal to the demand for a desired product or service. Even this state of demand requires a marketing task—maintaining the demand. The demand for the service may change as perceived needs change. Competition may produce a greater supply of the product or service.

When the demand for a service or product exceeds the supply, an overfull demand state exists. Increasing the supply of the service or product is one solution. However, this may not be possible or desirable, so marketing can be used to reduce the demand or demarket the service or product. This can be accomplished in a variety of ways, which may include promotion of other services, reduction in service, or price hikes.

Principles of Marketing

A product orientation, while important in business, is too narrow a focus for health care institutions. It fails to consider the other necessary ingredients for success. A product orientation concentrates on selling a product or service. A market orientation begins and ends with customer needs. Marketing the product or service is the important step.

Philip Kotler (1977) identified a number of major differences between selling and marketing. These are critical points for those marketing health care services. The businesses that have a sales orientation tend to concentrate on occupancy, volume, and the products or services of today. Those with a marketing orientation consider profit planning by service, customer mixes, and marketing mixes to achieve the desired market shares. Long run trends and opportunities are considered in marketing strategies. Analysis of markets with consideration of superior value to customers and customer needs/desires being of primary importance is another major difference of institutions with a market orientation. Each of these demonstrates a major factor in the concept of marketing—importance of the customer. This and other concepts have been identified by Cunningham and Cunningham (1981).

Customer satisfaction is a major concept of business and certainly of marketing. What the customer wants should be considered even as a service is developed, as it is delivered or sold, and after it has been used. Continual consideration of the needs and desires of the consumer is one major principle of marketing.

Broadening the definition of the organization's mission is another principle important in marketing. Hotels, for example, provide rooms for the night. However, if they are to successfully market themselves, these hotels will market themselves as "a home away from home" or some similar term to engender more than a room. Hospitals, then, must broaden the definition beyond "caring for the ill" to providing a range of services including preventive care and community education programs.

Another concept for marketing is the understanding that products and services become obsolete. Services can be displaced overnight or over long periods of time. Failure to consider this possibility could prove disastrous for some health care institutions. As patient admissions decline, for example, plans for other services must be made to maintain a successful business.

Researching the needs of the consumer is an important part of the marketing concept. Although consultants may be helpful in determining this information, those individuals who will buy the service can best determine what the need is.

The key management person of an organization is responsible ultimately for the success of the organization. One principle of importance to successful marketing is the acceptance by the top management official of the place of marketing within the organization. This individual will determine whether the marketing concept can be implemented within the organization.

A focus on profit versus sales is a final principle necessary to the marketing concept. Profit is necessary for survival. Sales do not necessarily equal profit. Concentration on profit, then, is actually concentration on survival. For health care, profit can no longer be a dirty word, but must become a primary objective as it is with any business.

Legal/Ethical Implications of Marketing

Controlling the flow of goods and services from producer to consumer, as most other activities, is regulated by law. Antitrust legislation, in the form of four major laws, was passed to provide for free and open competition. The Sherman Antitrust Act of 1890 prohibits monopolies and provides a penalty for those who would restrain trade. Both the Federal Trade Commission Act and the Clayton Act of 1914 gave the federal government authority to address the problem of monopolies. This included prosecution. The Celler-Kefauver Act of 1950 was passed to prevent mergers that would reduce competition or lead to monopoly. These pieces of legislation, while restricting some business activity, were all aimed at maintaining competitive business.

Another legal issue that impacts on marketing is price fixing (Cunningham and Cunningham, 1981). Price fixing refers to predetermining a price for the sale of a product or service. Such price fixing may be horizontal (between two competing businesses or organizations) or vertical (between a wholesaler and retailer). Price fixing may occur for several reasons. Price wars over similar products in competing businesses could lower prices until profits in the industry dropped dangerously low. Price fixing could prevent this. Oversupply of a product or service could result in a similar price war to improve the percentage of business of one company over another with a resultant reduction in profit. Price fixing provides a solution to loss of profit/ loss of business for competing firms. Also related to price fixing are fair trade acts, which prohibit sale of services or products for different prices to different customers except under specific circumstances, such as changing market conditions, cost justification, or meeting competition. Price fixing and fair trade concerns apply to the health care industry. An example of price fixing in health care might be seen in a situation in which competing hospitals got together and decided to offer mammography at a particular fee at both hospitals to prevent loss of customers (and of profits) at either hospital. As an example of unfair trade, a health care institution could be accused of violating fair trade acts if customer A were charged one fee for a particular lab test while patient B was charged a different price for the identical test under the same type of circumstances on the same day. There is the potential for these activities to occur if supervision by management is not adequate.

Four P's of Marketing

There are generally four factors in marketing that must be taken into account when developing a marketing program for the health care institution. Called the "four P's" (Table 11–3), these factors may influence the outcome of the marketing program (Kotler, 1976). Product, price, place, and promotion

TABLE 11–3
Four P's of Marketing

Product
Promotion
Place
Price

must be given consideration before planning can occur for marketing a health care service, a program, or the institution.

The *product* is, of course, what is offered for use by the consumer. Services, ideas, programs, or specific items are included. Health care organizations may offer education; health care services for palliation, cure, or prevention of health care problems; and ideas such as "wellness" or "cost effective alternatives." Whatever the product, the content and packaging of that product will contribute to its success by conveying the advantages of the product to the consumer (Stanton, 1985).

The *price* the consumer pays for the product is another factor that will influence the success of the marketing program. Consumers want quality products and services at a fair and competitive price, and the price includes not only the dollar amount but the non-monetary costs. These non-monetary costs may include energy, convenience, and opportunity, or the total gain for the price paid.

The *place* in marketing generally refers to accessibility, or how easily the consumer can get to the product offered. Health care institutions may not be able to improve accessibility to some of the products offered, but other products may be offered in locations with improved accessibility. Additionally, the reduced accessibility may be outweighed by some other benefit offered.

Finally, the factor of *promotion* must be considered. Health care has an advantage over many businesses because of the broad interest in health among the population. Promotion of health related products (including services) draws a large audience. The image of the organization and the enthusiasm and public relations of the employees are important to the ultimate satisfaction of the consumer (Stanton, 1985).

PLANNING THE MARKET STRATEGY

Strategy has been defined as the plan for achieving objectives. This plan is based on the desired direction of the organization and considers the limitations the organization may have, as well as the policies of the organization. (Refer to Chapter 8, Strategic Management.)

In the development of a market strategy, the overall direction and goals of the organization are important. It is equally important that realistic, specific, honest objectives be understood. The strength of the organization and the marketing strategies may be undermined if objectives are too vague (Eliopoulos, 1985). An example might be the difference between the objective "to meet the obstetrical needs of the community" and the objective "to improve the private pay to indigent obstetrical clientele ratio." To prevent misdirection of marketing efforts, the second example is a more clear objective.

Analysis of the Market

Organizations and businesses cannot effectively plan market strategies until they are able to analyze the market position of their products. Called strategic positioning, this type of market analysis looks at the product-market attractiveness and competitive position of each market (Cunningham and Cunningham, 1981). The anticipated growth rate of products (or services) is the method for measuring the attractiveness of the products. The market may be called a growth market if it will be growing at a rate equal to or faster than the economy.

Market share is the term used to describe the organization's or business's competitive position as compared with other like businesses. Improving one's market share or share of the total market is considered profitable, based on an assumption that providing more of the product or service (to a point) will reduce the cost per unit. This should generally be true, since more efficient operation is associated with increases in production.

Hall (1978) identified four strategic positions in which businesses may find themselves. These are based on the attractiveness of the product and its competitive position in the market. The low potential/low position product is one that is not attractive and is unsuccessful. This type of product can be disastrous and will generally be dropped or sold at drastically cut costs. In health care, an example might be the use of alcohol to stimulate appetite for the malnourished elderly in a strongly conservative community.

The low potential/high position product is one that is selling very well but whose market has better potential for growth. Stabilization of the price structure and maintaining the market would be important for the organization with this type of product. The opposite position, high potential/low position, is much more difficult. In this situation, the market for the type of product is strong, but the organization's product is not attractive to the consumer. An example might be fitness programs that are potentially strong. One health care organization's program, however, may be too costly in terms of convenience, monetary costs, and/or other costs than a competitor's similar program. In situations such as this, change in the program could improve the competitive position of the product.

The best product market in which an organization may find itself is high potential/high position. In this position, the organization has a large market share and has potential for maintaining that share and increasing it as well.

This type of strategic position has positive effects on the organization's profit level.

Identification of the strategic position is an important step in analysis of the market through evaluation of the organization's market share. This should not, however, minimize the need for the health care organization to look carefully at the consumer it serves. Part of the analysis is to identify the needs and desires of the consumer in relation to what the organization has to offer. This requires that the customer first be identified. Health care organizations can count among its customers not only patients, but also physicians, families, other organizations, visitors, and the community. Each of these groups may be consumers of the services of a health care organization.

Knowing what the customer wants or needs is part of the analysis stage in marketing. Some of this information may be known from past experience, but market research may be needed to collect sufficient data for appropriate marketing plans. Market research through demographic analysis may be used to sample specific populations in relation to specific services, programs, and ideas. Market research can be done by the organization, by health care consultants, or by marketing consultants. In each case, the aim is the same—what does the customer want/need and what does he like that he has? Market research can also assist in determining the profile and size of the market. Numerous techniques may be used for determining the market for a product or service. Brainstorming, community forums, Delphi techniques, simple surveys, or complex interviews can contribute data for market research.

Once the customer is identified, health care organizations must more specifically determine what the product is that is to be sold. Included in that determination are those factors that the customer considers when making the purchase—the additional benefits or advantages of a particular service. For example, a maternity program may offer prenatal childbirth classes and delivery plus an infant car seat, a newsletter, various bumper stickers, discount coupons for infant furniture and clothing, an infant shirt with the hospital's name, a toy, and more; or the program may offer only prenatal childbirth classes and delivery. The product is the total package.

Health care institutions are extremely diversified. Instead of the hospital care offered in the past, health care institutions offer a wide variety of services and programs. Diagnostic studies on an inpatient and outpatient basis are certainly one aspect of the services. Surgical procedures are no longer limited to inpatient status. Wellness programs, including classes, exercise sessions, and other therapeutic activities (sauna, whirlpool, etc.), may be available. Emergency services have expanded to urgent care facilities. Outpatient therapy is available for various types of rehabilitation—occupational, physical, speech, and hearing. Educational programs cover a variety of topics and reach out to a range of customers, from the general public to medical, nursing, or allied health personnel. Consultation is yet another service offered for sale through health care organizations. Even within the health care organization, nursing units may market their specialty to certain of the customers, e.g., physicians.

Once the customer is identified and the product has been determined, planning the market strategies can occur. Planning means assessment, identifying alternatives, and choosing the best alternative to meet the need. The principles of marketing must, of course, be considered in the plan. Development of the product's marketing mix is the final portion of this planning stage. This is the consideration given to the four P's identified previously, as they interact with one another. The product and the price seem relatively simple. The major factor to be considered in these is competition. Selling at the lowest price is not always best. This is dependent on how different the specific product is from similar products. Pricing will be addressed in more detail in a later section of this chapter.

How the product will be distributed must be considered as well in the development of marketing strategies. Communication regarding the product must also play a significant role in the decisions related to marketing mix. Because the price, product, promotion, and place interact with one another, the impact of one on the others is important.

There are other considerations to be made in developing the marketing plan. Several uncontrollable environmental variables may affect the outcome of the plan. The level of inflation will affect the price of the product. Since consumers react to inflation by buying less, substituting cheaper products/ services, working more, or using savings, the purchase of certain health care services can be seriously affected (Cunningham and Cunningham, 1981).

Demographic shifts in the population—employment, population growth patterns, and migration of population groups—change the market for the organization. The size and type of the market may change dramatically if unemployment drives groups to other locations or increases the elderly population of an area, for example.

The confidence of consumers in the products or services sold is probably a more significant environmental factor than any other as far as health care is concerned. The image of a health care institution to the public is important. Health is valued by the public, and any business that deals in that commodity is scrutinized by the public. Consumerism, another uncontrollable environmental variable, is aimed at giving consumers more power in relation to the products sold or bought. With health care, this is certainly important and may be used to advantage with the right market approach.

Once the variables have been identified and their impact on the health care organization has been evaluated, the plan can continue. Strategies must be developed to improve the market share of the organization in relation to one or more of the products of the organization. Several strategies may be incorporated to achieve this purpose (Goldsmith, 1980). Consumers are more directly involved in decisions regarding health care, but physicians maintain control for most hospital admissions. A strong physician network for referrals and consultation is important. Market efforts, however, must be directed to the consumer as well. Feeder systems such as clinics, urgent care centers and alternate delivery systems such as PPO's or HMO's are other alternatives for marketing.

IMPLEMENTATION OF MARKETING

Once the product and the market are identified and the plan to sell the product is developed, implementation becomes important. This may be accomplished in a variety of ways. The most difficult task facing health care institutions may be overcoming the reluctance to market the product. Many health care professionals continue to perceive marketing as conflicting with their values (Eliopoulos, 1985). There is much concern among those professionals that the consumer will be the loser in the competition created by some marketing strategies (Wilson, 1985). Marketing strategies relate product to consumer, even creating need for a product at times. This is one of the concerns identified by some health care professionals. The biggest problem seems to be in the area of advertising.

Advertising is the paid promotion of the product being sold. It is *not* related to personal selling, because face-to-face communication is not included. Of course, advertising's purpose is to inform the audience about the product and the business that is selling the product. It uses persuasion to convince the audience that the product of this organization is better than the competitor's product. While advertising varies from business to business, advertising in health care has tended to be less aggressive. This may change as competition becomes stiffer.

Advertising may be used for several reasons. It may make the consumer aware of the organization and the products/services it offers. It can communicate price—not necessarily the dollar amount, but the added benefits of the service offered as compared with that of the competition. Advertising can even create and increase the demand for the products.

Pricing is another aspect of implementation. The functions of pricing include comparison, stimulation, and rationing. Price can be a critical concept for marketing, but price alone does not influence significantly the market share of an organization (Cunningham and Cunningham, 1981).

Comparison of products can be accomplished through pricing. Consumers look at what they get for the price to be paid. The quality of the product is given consideration during the comparison. Because of the increase in revenues associated with higher prices, the price mechanism may act to stimulate the production of a product (or service). Finally, price may result in rationing. If a price becomes excessive, the result will be that fewer consumers can afford the product.

Pricing is based on a series of steps. Product decisions are related to distribution, communication, and pricing. Pricing objectives are determined by these product decisions, but generally they are related to return on investment. Pricing can produce a maximal return or a satisfactory return and still produce profit. Satisfactory return is a return that will remain competitive. This type return is more usual in health care, since competition is so fierce.

Cost-plus pricing is very common in businesses and is the practice of adding a percentage to the cost to determine the price. This permits firms to determine the percentage that is needed to meet the business' profit margin and to adjust the price, then, based on costs. As production costs drop, price can drop.

Price discounts for quantity, introductory offers, or promotional discounts are other pricing strategies that can be utilized in health care. For example, educational offerings may be priced at a reduced rate when three persons register together.

Distribution is another aspect of implementation that should be coordinated with those others identified to achieve maximal results from the marketing approaches planned. Knowledge of the availability and demand for a service can certainly be identified, but how it will be distributed can determine how successful the campaign is. For example, if a service is advertised strongly and the demand for the product/service is so great it cannot be met, the marketing campaign may result in a negative impact. (The organization can't deliver as advertised.) This may be more important with material products, such as clothing, than with services, but nothing seems to upset people more than to find an advertised product unavailable.

The marketing of services differs from that of other "products" in several ways, which become important as the marketing plan is implemented. Services are intangible. A product that is purchased becomes an asset, whereas a service does not necessarily become an asset. Services also differ from other products in their utility. If the utility is derived from an action or performance, a service is involved, as compared with a physical object.

Services have other characteristics that are important to understand when implementing the marketing plan. Services cannot be inventoried. Maintaining a standard in the performance of a service is often difficult even within an organization. The seller of the service is part of the service in many cases. Understanding these characteristics is important in marketing the services of the organization.

Strategies for Marketing Services

Cunningham and Cunningham (1981) identify four strategies for marketing services. Each of these four strategies is important in the health care setting. Examples of the strategy applied to health care will help to clarify the meaning of the strategy. The strategies include gaining the competitive edge, cutting costs, setting prices, and introducing a new program or service.

Gaining a competitive edge is essential for health care organizations in the health care environment faced today. Improving the profit margin by lowering production costs can be utilized in health care through group purchase of supplies. Another example might be provision of a nurse to supervise and care for a group of patients receiving IV therapy on an outpatient basis rather than several nurses in different areas providing a similar service. Product differentiation is yet another mechanism for gaining the competitive edge and refers to the observable differentiation between like products. An example of this differentiation is the women's services offered at one hospital as "a resource center" versus the services advertised as "complete diagnostic and referral services—more than a resource center."

Cutting costs in health care can be accomplished in several ways. Since health care is a service industry, most of its costs are labor costs. Automation may be helpful, and substitution of "cheaper" labor is an option. One consideration in cutting costs, however, is maintaining productivity. Utilizing messengers or transporters to run errands and transport patients can free nursing staff to better care for patients, for example.

Setting prices for services is very difficult because consumers believe "you get what you pay for." If prices are too low, consumers will shop elsewhere for services, fearing the quality is inadequate. Prices may often be set, then, based on what the market will bear. Customers for services may base what they are willing to pay on their perceived value for the service. Providing a health education program for free may draw fewer attendees than one priced at a relatively low cost.

Although market research is helpful, offering a new service to the market is always risky. Testing is difficult and often costly because of the start-up costs for any new program. New offerings also quickly become open services to competitors who wish to take advantage of the popularity of the service.

Other strategies that are useful in health care can improve overall productivity as well as improve the market share (Cunningham and Cunningham, 1981). Modifying the timing of demand is one such strategy. If the operating room has fewer regular inpatient cases on Friday, offering discounts for Friday outpatient surgery may improve utilization of the OR. Changing the expectation of the buyer is another such strategy. Hotels use this with express check-out, and hospitals may provide VIP discharges in a similar way. Involving the customer in the service is another method for improving productivity. Self-care units and rooming-in for new mothers are examples of such strategies.

EVALUATION

Evaluation of marketing efforts can be accomplished in many ways. Market research can determine not only needs but also accomplishments. Evaluation should begin with an analysis of how effectively the objectives of the marketing plan were met. If an objective was to improve inpatient admissions by 10%, that objective can be measured easily.

The cost of the marketing efforts can be measured and the cost/benefit ratio examined. Although there is no magic number in terms of these costs, recommendations for costs for marketing and public relations may be reviewed and analyzed.

How the objectives were met is another aspect of evaluation. It may be determined, for instance, that although use of the human resources director as the "director" for marketing worked, much of that manager's other responsibilities were not fully carried out. However, hiring a marketer to carry out and/or plan marketing strategies does not necessarily resolve all problems.

Each institution or organization will need to evaluate its needs for marketing and determine how best those needs can be met. Each marketing program will also need evaluation in terms of objectives. Quantitative and qualitative data must be analyzed to gain information about the total effect of the program. Adjustments or revisions in the market plan should be made after the evaluation is accomplished. Cost-effectiveness and utilization of resources may be analyzed and the results utilized to influence decisions regarding services or programs offered.

MARKETING NURSING SERVICES

Marketing nursing services is basically no different than marketing any other service, department, or program. The simple steps identified previously may be applied to the nursing program or service that the nursing administrator desires to market. Identification of the desired service is, of course, essential and may require survey of the client population. Once the demand for a service is known, the approaches identified in Table 11–2 can be utilized to reach the desired level of demand. Specific strategies may be developed to address the product, place, price, and promotion necessary to optimally market the program or service being offered. Allocation of resources in view of economic or other constraints will be a priority consideration for the nursing administrator during this phase. Other steps, which include development of objectives, program implementation, and evaluation, must also follow the sequence described previously in this chapter.

Nursing has a multitude of potential services and programs suitable for marketing. While the nursing department may need assistance from marketing departments to implement new services, there is no reason that nursing departments cannot successfully market not only services but also nursing itself. Although nurses have felt at times that marketing was contrary to the "service orientation" they were taught, several ideas over the years have surfaced to stress the need for nursing services. Those ideas identified by Eliopoulos (1985) include the fact that nursing is essential and has equal worth to other professions, that nursing is better able to provide certain services, and that nursing is cost effective. These facts, coupled with the economic climate of health care, necessitate an aggressive approach to marketing nursing to groups that include legislators, consumers, third party payers, boards of trustees and administrators. The image and functions of nursing, both current and future, are poorly understood, at least at times, to these groups. Marketing nursing actively may be essential to maintain or attain desired status and even viability for nursing. Nursing must even be marketed within an institution. The nursing department may be marketed for its ability to provide nursing services or to cost effectively provide what have grown to be non-nursing functions (for example, therapies).

Several strategies may be particularly suitable for nursing in marketing itself as a profession (Eliopoulos, 1985). Nurses must promote a positive image. Nurses must first be convinced of their worth and then sell the idea to others. The role of the nurse executive in this strategy involves positive reinforcement and recognition for the contribution of nurses to the health and welfare of the consumer. Education of the identified groups about nursing is another key strategy. This may be accomplished through a variety of methods, which include highlighting nursing activities and demonstrating the broad capabilities of nurses to the key groups. Development of and adherence to nursing standards are essential if nursing is to be viewed as a profession of worth. These are occasionally difficult, since they require monitoring of nursing activities and disciplinary action when standards are not met. However, if approached fairly and consistently, these difficulties will reap tremendous benefits through respect and knowledge that only high standards are acceptable. Gaining support for nursing is another important method for marketing of nursing. Building relationships through good communication, mutual problem solving, sharing of ideas, and negotiations is a reasonable approach to obtain support.

Innovations from within nursing, coupled with sound financial, personnel, and patient care management, provide recognition for the nursing administrator that can be invaluable in marketing the department. The strategies identified are important in producing the positive results that are the primary goal of marketing. Each of these steps forward, then, is helpful as nursing continually strives to develop and to implement new services or programs as part of an overall marketing plan. The future of nursing may depend upon the image of nursing and on the demand for nursing created through successful marketing (Eliopoulos, 1985).

TOMORROW'S MARKETING STRATEGIES

Marketing has an important role in health care organizations of today. Customers will exist without marketing, but to keep the customer or gain new ones, marketing is necessary. The process of marketing is similar to the problem solving process—assess, plan, implement, evaluate. Utilizing that process is necessary to have a well organized marketing approach.

Concepts of marketing apply to businesses that sell products or services. However, services have some special characteristics, which have been identified in this chapter. A number of environmental factors may also influence how well a product or service "sells." These environmental factors include inflation, consumerism, and demographic changes.

An understanding of marketing principles and concepts, characteristics, and influencing factors is helpful as marketing strategies are developed within health care institutions. The aim for marketing is unchanged, however, regardless of the approach or the "product." Providing a service the customer wants at a competitive and fair price when he wants the service is the key to a successful service. Marketing strategies should help to do just that.

As the nursing administrator plans her strategies for the future, she must first have an understanding of these basic principles and strategies for marketing. However, more importantly, she must apply those principles in her goal development and achievement. Now and in the future, marketing may frequently be the key difference between success and failure for nursing and for health care. The ability to identify the desired service, develop the service, market the service competitively, maintain the full demand for the service, and continually evaluate and update the service as desired will be one major and necessary characteristic of the nursing administrator of the future.

REFERENCES

American Marketing Association (1960). Committee on definition: Marketing definition. Chicago.

Clarke, R. (1984). The marketer and the miracle worker. *Marketing: The competitive edge*, Satellite Video Teleconference, AHA, pp. 18–25.

Coddington, D., Palmquist, L., and Trollinger, W. (1985). Strategies for survival in the hospital industry. *Harvard Business Review*, 63(3), 129–138.

Cunningham, W., and Cunningham, I. (1981). *Marketing: A managerial approach*. Cincinnati: South-western Publishing Co.

Eliopoulos, C. (1985). Selling a positive image builds demand. *Nursing Management*, 16(4), 23–26.

Goldsmith, J. (1980). The health-care market: Can hospitals survive? *Harvard Business Review*, September-October, p. 100.

Hall, W. (1978). SBUs: Hot, new topic in the management of diversification. *Business Horizons* (February), pp. 19–21.

Kotler, P. (1973). The major tasks of marketing management. *Journal of Marketing*, pp. 42–49.

Kotler, P. (1976). *Marketing management*, 3rd ed. Englewood Cliffs, NJ: Prentice-Hall.

Kotler, P. (1977) From sales obsession to marketing effectiveness. *Harvard Business Review*, 55(6), 67–75.

Maslow, A. H. (1954). *Motivation and personality*. New York: Harper and Row.

Roberts, E. (1985). The hard sell plays well in our hospitals. *Florida Trend* (November), pp. 100–105.

Stanton, M. (1985). Patient and health education: Lessons from the marketplace. *Nursing Management*, 16(4), 28–30.

Wilson, E. (1985). To advertise or not to advertise: Why doctors are divided. *Florida Trend* (November), 107–108.

ENVIRONMENTAL INFLUENCES

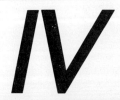

It is certainly no secret that the health care industry is in a continual state of change. Competition and changes in reimbursement have provided the incentives for changes in the delivery of health care to the American public. Several environmental forces have precipitated these changes facing health care organizations. Consumers, which include patients, third party payers, industry, and physicians among others, have recognized that the cost of health care is tremendous. The demand for greater access, more services and programs, and the "best" of everything is being replaced with a need to provide basic health care for less and with more consumer involvement. The impact of the realization that resources are finite has yet to be measured. The cry for ever increasing technology is being replaced by the need for high tech/high touch. The move toward increased competition between providers of health care has also produced change within health care organizations. A renewed interest in ethical decision making is yet another environmental force that continues to impact on the health care industry.

This section is devoted to the influence of the internal and external environment on health care organizations. Chapter Twelve, Change, addresses the major theories about change and discusses the various types of change. Emphasis is placed on planned change and the process of change. Resistance to change and strategies to overcome that resistance are also included. Evaluation and stabilization of change are additional sections of this chapter.

Health Care Environment, Chapter Thirteen, discusses in some detail the environment in which health care finds itself and the impact that this has on the delivery of services. The effect of consumerism, technology, ethical dilemmas, and the economy on health care is addressed. Strategies for dealing with these forces in the future are included in this chapter.

Chapter Fourteen, Games and Political Strategies, addresses the development of the informal organization within health care institutions. The development of game playing as a method for managing interactions is discussed. Various common games in health care are identified, and strategies for addressing the games are reviewed.

Risk management, more than ever before, has taken such a high priority that many states have legislation passed or pending that requires full time risk managers in each health care institution. Chapter Fifteen, Risk Management, discusses risk management and the environment that has produced this phenomenon. Elements of a risk management program and the prerequisites of a program are included. The relationship of risk management to quality assurance is emphasized in this chapter. The organization of a formal risk management program to handle liability issues and to "manage risks" is also addressed.

This section, in combination with earlier sections, provides the basis for the practice of nursing administration to be discussed in Section V. The importance of environmental influence and change on the health care institution is the emphasis of this section.

CHANGE

INTRODUCTION

Health care and nursing have undergone tremendous change within the last two decades. The continual changes in environmental forces affecting health care and nursing will result in even more change for these professions. Whether the nursing administrator is caught up in the change or manages the change may determine her success in managing her departments and may influence the success of the organization.

The role that change plays in the success of the organization is a rather complex one. Change may produce multiple crises, may influence productivity, may breed conflicts, or may affect morale (Spradley, 1980). The effect of change on morale, productivity, conflict, and crisis is frequently dependent on how that change is handled. Rather than awaiting the effect of change initiated by others, initiating change can help to place nursing administrators at the controls in health care. In order to accomplish change successfully, one must be able to fully understand it.

Change refers to an alteration or transformation and can include growth and maturation. The extent to which and over which change may occur is quite broad. Every individual and group is in some process of change

12

continually. Changes that affect health care may originate in individuals or in the multiple groups that play a role in influencing health care.

Toffler (1979) has identified changes that have and are currently influencing health care so dramatically as originating from five major categories:

1. Environmental factors
2. A focus on prevention of illness
3. Movement toward self-care and responsibility in relation to health
4. Consumer participation in health planning
5. Role changes in health providers

The influence on health care of each of these categories varies from year to year, although each category does continue to play a role. Since we continually attempt to maintain equilibrium, change might be considered as disruptive (Lancaster, 1982a). However, although adaptation is a mechanism to maintain balance, it can also be considered a change. Accomplishing change *does not necessarily* require action. Other forces can accomplish change. Accomplishing *specific* change requires assessment, planning, implementation, and self-evaluation—the problem solving processes.

This chapter will discuss theories of change, including types of change, elements of change, principles governing change, and requirements for change. The strategies for making change and the dynamics of successful planned change will be examined. The process for change, including its phases and the effect of pace on change, will also be addressed. In looking at the implementation of change, those factors that facilitate or obstruct change will be reviewed. The role of communication is another important aspect of change that will be included. Evaluation, maintenance, and stabilization of change will also be discussed. The impact of change on health care will be addressed throughout the chapter.

CHANGE THEORY

Much of the original work on change theory can be accredited to Kurt Lewin, who in 1951 described the basic steps in change as unfreezing, moving to a new level, and refreezing. Lewin considered unfreezing the necessary preparation for change to occur. He believed that the members of the group in which the change would occur must understand and accept the advantage of the change. When the various participants in change have enough data to develop a plan of action, the move to a new level described by Lewin can occur. Integration of the new behaviors is the refreezing identified by Lewin. This would, of course, require reinforcement of the behaviors, which is one aspect of the refreezing phase.

An example could be used to clarify Lewin's theory. Consider the prospective payment system. The process of unfreezing occurred as more and more people—consumers, legislators, third party payors—began to question the increasing costs for health care and the lack of incentives for cost containment. Moving began when the plan was tried and met certain objectives. Since hospitals have now been required to operate under this payment system, refreezing has occurred.

Others have developed theories of change since Lewin's work. In 1962, Everett Rogers adapted Lewin's original theory and expanded it to describe planned change as compared with any type of change. The unfreezing described by Lewin could be broken down into three steps—awareness, interest, and evaluation. One of the major differences in Rogers' theory lies in the reversibility of the change. He believed change was not such a simple acceptance and adoption of the behavior. He believed a trial period must occur, followed by adoption or rejection. This is similar to the moving and refreezing phases described by Lewin.

Another theorist, Lippitt (1973), defined change as an alteration in the status quo. He based his theory on Lewin's and further introduced the idea of a change agent into the specific steps of the process. The steps identified by Lippitt include diagnosis of a problem, assessment of the change agent's motivation and resources, selection of the appropriate role for the change agent, maintenance of the change, and termination of the helping relationship. Lippitt felt that change would occur regardless of circumstances and that the manner in which it was controlled was important.

Basic theoretical concepts in relation to change described by Lewin, Lippitt, and Rogers are based to a great extent on systems theory. Systems theory provides a basis for the interaction of elements or parts and the relationship of these to the whole (Bertalanffy, 1968; Auger, 1976). Systems are interdependent and will strive to restore equilibrium when homeostasis is interrupted. Change upsets the balance, requiring adaptation from system to system. Systems theory helps in the organization of material relating the parts to the whole, therefore avoiding a disjointed approach. The concept of driving forces and restraining forces was introduced by Lewin at the time of his early work (1951), and can parallel the physiological forces that determine the function of the body systems and their relationships.

Driving forces are considered those forces that influence the change positively or toward the desired direction. Restraining forces would be those forces that obstruct or block the process of change. The driving and restraining forces described by Lewin arise from the structural nature of the environment and from the interaction of individuals with the environment (Pierce and Thompson, 1976). Change cannot occur if the balance between these forces is maintained. Change will occur, however, if one set of forces is more powerful than the other. For the change to occur, an increase in driving forces and/or a decrease in restraining forces is essential.

One other aspect of systems theory that is important to change theory is the concept of maintaining the viability of the whole. If the structure and the interaction between systems are important in maintaining balance or adaptation to change, the achievement of objectives that will result in this goal of viability must be a part of that concept. In health care, the three implications of systems theory, i.e., structure, interaction, and viability of the whole, may be applied very easily. Health care organizations are very structured, and the multiple subsystems within the system are quite inter-dependent. Forces from within and without the systems are continually attempting to alter or change the various systems. The maintenance of viability of the system is dependent on whether the systems can interact successfully and whether an appropriate balance can be restored.

Greiner (1967) described patterns for organizational change in which it was emphasized that change occurs in organizations as a result of the forces therein. These forces may determine whether top level management makes major decisions regarding change or whether a group decision takes prece-dence. The approach used also determines the accountability for the change and certainly has an impact on how well the change is accepted. When top management announces a change determined unilaterally, the assumption is made that the change will be accepted and implemented because of the authority associated with the management position. Group involvement in decisions about change varies from identification of the problem to devel-opment of alternative solutions, with varying amounts of input into the decision for change.

Blake and Mouton (1978) have used the various change theories in application to organizations and managers. Although the terminology used throughout differs, the manner of change follows the basic steps described by major change theorists—Lewin, Lippitt, and Rogers. Blake and Mouton applied these theories in experiments and study to demonstrate the process of change. For example, change in an organization culture followed the steps of grid seminars (unfreezing, assessment), team building, intergroup devel-opment, ideal strategic model, implementation (moving, trial period), and consolidation (refreezing, adoption).

Principles Governing Change

There are a number of principles that govern the changes that may occur within the system. Systems may be open or closed. Closed systems have little interaction with the environment and are affected by the environ-ment minimally or not at all. Open systems, which apply most commonly to social organizations and health care organizations more specifically, have continual interchange of data, activity, etc. The open system may have interaction between its subsystems and may interact freely with other systems. There is certainly a great deal of potential for factors outside the system to influence it when it is an open system.

Homeostasis, or maintenance of balance within the system, is common to both closed and open systems. Restoration of the equilibrium is the goal of the system. Stability, then, is sought after any change to provide this equilibrium. When a change occurs, other changes may follow of necessity to return homeostasis to the system.

Systems must also have boundaries that define the limits of the system and separate it from the environment. The extent of exchange of information and resources is dependent upon the type of boundary. A boundary that is permeable to a large number or amount of inputs has a much greater interaction with the environment, but it will also be less predictable (Lancaster, 1982b). A boundary may serve as a filter to unwanted or unneeded input.

Systems are organized and structured to varying degrees. The subsystems of the system may appear to be systems themselves until the interactions are examined. Within the structure of the system, interdependence of the subsystems is evident and this interdependence is yet another principle that governs change. Interaction between subsystems and input into a system from outside its boundary will require energy exchange. Energy input is a part of the change and/or part of the process of stabilization, which will be discussed later.

Finally, the principle related to driving versus opposing forces is important in the discussion related to those factors that influence change. Change produces resistance, since it requires at least a temporary variation from the state of equilibrium. The driving forces then must be increased and/or the opposing forces minimized to effect the change. Restoration of the equilibrium would then follow.

Types of Change

Although many theorists have made significant contributions to the study of types of change, the work of Warren Bennis (1966) is especially important. Bennis described eight types of change, which vary in the deliberateness of change and participation in goal setting. *Coercive* change is described as one sided in both characteristics. *Emulative* change has no clear relationship defined but is associated with a formal organization. A deliberate type of change that has an imbalance of power but some mutual goal setting is called *indoctrinating* change. Bennis described *interactional* change as one with mutual and equal involvement but without deliberateness. *Natural* change is one that occurs without any plan or goal. *Planned* change is described by Bennis as one in which mutual and equal deliberateness and goal setting occurs. *Socializing* change is related to interactional change but involves society. Finally, change that results from collection and interpretation of data is called *technocratic* change. Because of the differences in goal setting and deliberateness, variation in resistance to change occurs.

Duncan (1978) and Sampson (1971) were other theorists who studied and tried to categorize change. The major focus of their work seems to have been in this categorization of change by specific characteristics. Whereas Duncan described change as haphazard or planned, Sampson felt change could be spontaneous, developmental, or planned. Duncan characterized haphazard change as random without preparation. Undesired change may certainly occur this way, but desired change may occur without deliberate efforts being made toward the change. Planned change, by contrast, is a result of specific planned actions taken to adjust to some situation. The other type of change identified by Sampson has been referred to as developmental change, characterizing change that occurs during the maturation process of a group, individual, or organization. Such change follows a sequence and is generally orderly in nature.

Elements of Planned Change

The elements of planned change were identified by Lippitt (1973) in his description of the process of planned change. He felt that planned change would involve a system, a change agent, application of knowledge, and collaboration. The change agent assists the process and monitors the progress.

Motivation for change is a requirement for success of any planned change. An openness to change and a willingness to break with the past are key ingredients in this motivation (Levenstein, 1979). Another requirement for change is action. Without action, the status quo is maintained and no change occurs.

PROCESS OF CHANGE

Successful planned change can be determined by five factors, according to Rogers and Shoemaker (1971). *Relative advantage*, or the perceived superiority of a new idea over an old one, is critical to the adoption of change. Actual advantage is not significant. Economic factors, time required, societal factors, and convenience may be used to judge the worth of the idea (Lancaster, 1982a).

The *complexity* of the proposed change is another factor that can determine success. The more difficult an idea or process, the more likely that it will not be adopted. Participants are very ego-centered when considering new ideas and may reject one because of their inability to understand it.

Compatible ideas are also more easily adopted, since they do not require any change in values or needs. If an idea is not compatible with existing ideas or activities, adoption may be delayed, if it occurs at all.

If results of the new idea are visible and *observable*, the idea will be more readily adopted. *Trialability* of an idea, i.e., testing on a pilot basis, is less risky than a massive change, and it too is more readily acceptable to participants in the change process.

The steps in the process of change are generally sequential and to a great extent follow the problem solving approach: assess, diagnose, plan, implement, evaluate. Spradley (1980) developed a model for planned change

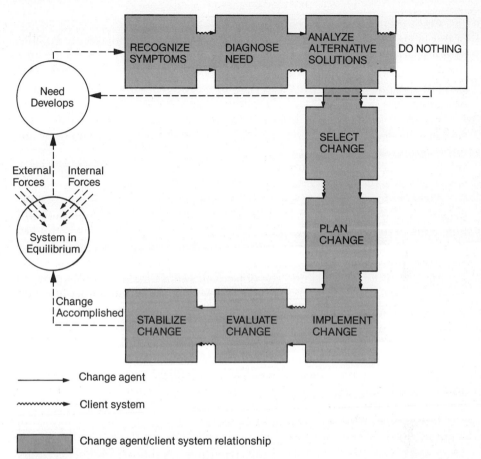

FIGURE 12–1. Planned change model. (Reprinted with permission from Spradley, B.: Managing change creatively. JONA 10(5):33, 1980.)

that can easily fit the process (Fig. 12–1). The process begins with the recognition of a need for change.

Recognition of a problem is often evidenced by the presence of symptoms of the problem. To avoid confusion and to prevent planning for an unneeded change, it is important that the symptoms be recognized and evaluated carefully. Proceeding to step two, *diagnosis* of the problem, will be determined by the results of the assessment.

Analysis of the symptoms will require data collection, identification of causal relationships, and investigation. Once these actions have been taken, an accurate diagnosis may be possible. It is critical that quick or rash conclusions be avoided. The role of the change agent in the process of planned change is obvious at this point in the process. Recognition of symptoms of a problem can be made by any individual or group. However, the required data collection and investigation are such important work that a well motivated individual, willing to make necessary changes, is essential.

Once the diagnosis is complete, the planning stage begins. One aspect of this stage is the *analysis of alternatives*. Although the responsibility belongs to the change agent, a group of individuals may be better able to develop the list of alternative solutions. The list may include no change or combinations of alternatives. The pros and cons of each potential solution should be examined.

Based on knowledge of the problem, its cause, and the alternatives, the *most appropriate alternative is then selected*. This often entails risk taking by the nurse administrator. Additionally, it is tempting to desire that all potential solutions be selected to ensure resolution of the problem. Such an approach is self-defeating and can certainly result in failure.

Planning for the change is usually the most difficult step in the process. Because of the details required to develop the plan, it may also be the most time-consuming aspect of the process. Development of objectives is the key portion of the plan. It is important to remember that the objectives are like any other objectives—they should be specific, measurable, and reasonable. Action steps for accomplishing the objectives and a timetable are part of the planning activity. The plan should also address requirements for resources— personnel or human resources, financial resources, administrative support. A plan for evaluation of the change and for maintaining the change is another consideration (Spradley, 1980). Recognition of those resisting forces and anticipation and management of the resistance may need to be planned for as well. Throughout the process, the input and participation of the entire affected group are important. Their feedback may be extremely important to the success of the plan.

Implementation of the planned change may be accomplished at once or through the use of a pilot project or phases, which is often more readily acceptable. The use of a pilot project permits modifications as necessary before a full scale change is implemented. Other advantages of piloting a program or project include reduction of anxiety related to unknown results and the use of a successful pilot to positively influence or "sell" the change to others.

Evaluation of the change is a necessary step in this problem solving approach, since it identifies the effectiveness of the change and the smoothness of the process. The objectives established early in the process may be utilized to determine the success of the implemented change.

Refreezing, identified by Lewin as a major phase of change, is applied to the process of planned change through *stabilization*. Positive reinforcement for desired change and associated behaviors is one method for maintaining the change to achieve the new state of equilibrium.

Application by the nursing administrator of this model for planned change can be illustrated with an example. A nursing administrator hears complaints of unfair workload and assignments. She also hears that the new graduate nurses are very upset about the reality of nursing practice, the expectations that exist and are different from what they envisioned nursing practice to be. These symptoms, she discovers on investigation, are related to the problem that the new graduates, after the usual orientation period, are unable to function at the level desired. This has created resentment by the experienced staff, who must handle their own work and assist with the new graduates' workload. The new graduates are frustrated with their inability to function appropriately. Discussions with the school of nursing faculty identify the limited clinical experience the students had during their educational process.

The diagnosis of the problem is made: limited clinical experience has resulted in inadequately prepared graduates. Several alternatives may be considered as possible solutions to the problem. One alternative requires the school of nursing to increase clinical time. The nursing administrator has no control over the school of nursing, and this alternative would address future graduates rather than current graduates. Termination of the new graduate nurses would be an alternative. Since the new graduates cannot function at the desired level, they might be replaced with more experienced nurses. This alternative would result in delays in staffing units, and money already spent for orientation would be wasted. An extended orientation with a preceptor approach would assist this specific group and could be applied at other times once it was established. This would have some costs for the department, but the end-result would be favorable. Implementing a program to allow students to work part time during school would increase clinical experience, but would not address the current new graduates.

The nursing administrator could select a combination of alternatives to include (1) additional orientation through the preceptor program and (2) allowing students to increase their clinical experience through part time work. The nursing administrator might wish to pursue further discussions with the school of nursing as well, but since she cannot control the outcome she will not select this as the appropriate change. The nursing administrator then plans for the change that has been selected. She chooses a group to assist in establishing the objectives and timetable and in actually implementing the change. Once the change is implemented, the nursing administrator evaluates the success through determining the satisfaction of the experienced and new staff members. If the change is successful, restoration of the equilibrium will occur as stabilization of the change occurs.

Resistance to Change

Resistance to change is a powerful opposing force that can, in fact, prevent successful change. There is always some resistance to change that must be addressed. The nature of the change and the perceptions about the change may engender resistance. Although communication may help to prevent misconceptions, understanding of resistance may be helpful in the implementation process.

Psychologically, individuals resist change because it creates at least temporarily a change from the status quo or a disequilibrium. Fear of failure,

TABLE 12–1
Concerns of Employees Related to Change

Effect of Change on:
Role in organization
Status
Power
Convenience of job
Restrictions of job
Content of job
Performance of job
Financial status
Promotional status

fear of loss of current satisfaction, fear of success, and reluctance to admit weaknesses have been identified as factors that might produce opposition to change. Ignoring and rejecting ideas may, in fact, be a protective mechanism utilized by individuals who fear they will lose what is comfortable for them or who fear they will be found to be lacking, since a change would imply an inadequacy of previous practices (Pierce and Thompson, 1976).

Barbara Stevens (1975) suggested the use of introspection, which could be utilized in anticipating the reaction to change. Such careful analysis could be used to determine the expected effect of the change on the organization. Workers would, of course, be interested in the effect any change would have in relation to their concerns (Table 12–1). Once the nurse administrator has attempted to consider the effect of the change on the employees, she may predict response through an understanding of the process through which resistance goes—identified by Stevens (1975) as the stages of resistance. From (1) undifferentiated resistance from multiple sources to (2) direct conflict between opposing sides to (3) minimal if any adversaries, the transition toward acceptance of the change occurs.

The resources available to implement change are varied, depending upon the organization, the nursing administrator, and the type of change. The use of persuasion, influence, or force may be perceived as necessary by the nursing administrator, depending on the situation. The method she utilizes may be dependent on the stage of acceptance of the staff. Those stages have been identified by Rogers (1983) as awareness, interest, evaluation, trial, and adoption. More persuasion may be necessary at the interest stage, for example, than during the trial period.

Acceleration and enforcement of the preferred behavior may be important tools for the nursing administrator during the implementation of change. However, these actions fail to permit time for acceptance and may prove detrimental to the success of the change. It is important to note that a specific behavior may be contrary to the beliefs of the individual. This cognitive dissonance, or conflict between belief and behavior, may actually result in a change in belief when the behavior is enforced (Stevens, 1975). This fact may be important to the nursing administrator who cannot or does not desire to await the change in attitude that occurs with the stages of acceptance.

Table 12–2
Why Resistance to Change Occurs

Inadequate preparation of staff
Lack of involvement of staff
Inadequate communication
Fear of failure
Lack of understanding of need for change
Misconceptions regarding change
Group norms violated
Increased workload concerns
Poor planning
Lack of consideration of potential problems
Change for wrong reasons

Resistance to change is a defensive mechanism produced to protect individuals or groups from the effect of the change. It occurs in response to the perception of a threat to security (Metzger, 1978). Reactions may range from apathy to aggression. The conditions under which the resistance occurs are related to those factors identified in Table 12–2. Each of the factors can be addressed separately.

Lack of preparation of the staff occurs when they have not been told of the change until it occurs. Fear of the unknown, noted earlier, is an example of the type of reaction that can result from inadequate preparation of the staff. There is fear of the alteration in role or power base for the individual. Concerns related to the effect on status of any change are also felt or expressed by staff members. Preparation for the change must include adequate explanations of the effect of the change on roles, power, and/or status of individuals or groups. Any alteration in responsibility, power base, or status produced by the change may still produce resistance, but these will be identified concerns that can then be addressed or explained on an individual basis and can be weighed against other positive factors occurring with the change.

When the staff members are not involved in the decision making regarding change, there tends to be much resistance. Involvement of staff, on the other hand, engenders a feeling of participation in decision making, which produces less resistance and more positive feelings toward a change. Buying into a change developed and planned by others is much more difficult than accepting change in which one has had input. Being a part of the decision making, even to a limited degree, will also enhance communication and encourage feedback.

Inadequate communication hinders understanding, magnifies fears, and encourages resistance. Distorted information or lack of information fosters suspicion and rumors, which then can threaten the success of a change. Good communication, then, is necessary to help each individual understand the impact of the change. Concerns shared during such communication may be very important, and knowledge of them may be essential to the success of the planned change.

Fear of failure is another significant factor in resistance to change. If a planned change is felt to be poorly planned or not adequate to meet the need, there may be resistance. Groups or individuals may feel that the planned change will fail and that there is not good reason to place much effort behind perceived failure. This fear of failure or inadequacy can be somewhat overcome by careful and detailed planning and by communication.

Occasionally, resistance is met because there is not a clear understanding of the need for the change. Change for the sake of change or for the wrong reason is generally considered poor reasoning. Many individuals may resist because they believe the change does not help or may actually hinder the group or organization. The reason for a change should be clearly stated and not masked or dressed up. Misconceptions related to change often result in similar reactions. The necessity of clear communication and adequate preparation is evident.

If group norms or values are ignored when change is planned, resistance is a natural result. Changing values and beliefs is a difficult process in itself. Making other changes that require changes in values of a group becomes a significant problem. Values are the basis of attitudes and actions and, as such, influence the change process to a significant degree. Consideration of group norms or values during the making of decisions regarding change can prevent or reduce resistance related to this cause.

The degree to which a change affects the workload of an individual or group is reflected in the degree of resistance exhibited by the individual or group. When the activities, content, or performance of a job will be affected, resistance results (Lancaster, 1982a). Minimizing the effects of the change on the workload or actual reduction of a workload through the change will also minimize the resistance to the change.

Poor planning is another cause of resistance. Inadequate assessment or diagnosis of problems, lack of information related to the change, inadequate preparation or communication, and lack of consideration of all alternatives may be factors in poor planning. Each of these or a combination of them may occur and result in resistance. Planning must include assessment, alternatives, preparation, communication, and consideration of potential problems and how to deal with them.

Regardless of the cause or reason for resistance to change, the process of change will require some degree of facilitation. Facilitating change during the implementation phase of the change process is the responsibility of the change agent. Responsibilities for the change agent include generation of ideas, development of an atmosphere facilitative to change, providing motivation for participation, and overcoming resistance (Lancaster 1982a). Change agents must also be involved in assessment, evaluation, and implementation of the change.

Rogers and Shoemaker (1971) identified six categories of adopters of change who play a role in this process of change. These adopters begin with the *innovators*, who are enthusiastic and work to bring about change. *Early adopters*, while less enthusiastic and more likely to avoid controversy, are generally supportive and are sought by others for advice. *Early-majority adopters* provide effective support in their acceptance of change just before the majority of the group. The group that is skeptical of change and accept it because of economics more than other reasons is called *late-majority* adopters. The *laggards* compose the group of individuals who discourage support of change and are generally negative. The most negative group of individuals are those who encourage rejection. These are called *rejectors*. Knowledge of these levels of adopters will be helpful to the change agent as she plans the process of change.

The change agent can provide the motivation, if the participants can be convinced that their contributions are valuable and that the change is non-threatening. In establishing a climate conducive to change, the change agent must listen to participants, gain cooperation, respect ideas, and delegate responsibility. Managing the change requires the cooperation and acceptance of participants, as well as support and recognition for the participants. The role of good communication by the change agent cannot be overemphasized in facilitating change.

Several activities by the change agent may serve to facilitate change. Some of these have been identified previously in other sections of this chapter, but it is useful to note them again. Assessment of the change for its value is a crucial first step. Knowledge of this will assist the change agent in later explanations. The analysis of the change and those driving or opposing forces will assist the change agent in predicting needed actions to provide support for the change. The resources available and needed for the change can then more clearly be delineated, and the actions for counteracting resistance can be planned.

In explanations regarding change, the change agent must be able to focus on the positive, plan for correcting deficiencies, and describe compatibility of the change with group norms. By providing solutions to questions, assisting the process, and serving as the major resource, the change agent can effectively manage the change. Positive reinforcement for those who expedite the process of change is an important mechanism in persuading participants to accept and promote change and should be utilized freely by the change agent.

Trust is a key element for the successful change agent. Accessibility to participants; honesty about goals, problems, and priorities; and listening are aspects of the trust relationship that must not be overlooked. The change agent then plays a key role in implementation of change. The role of the change agent may also continue during evaluation and stabilization phases.

EVALUATION OF CHANGE

Before the success of a change can be evaluated, the criteria should be developed prior to implementation. Several specific areas should be addressed in developing evaluation tools: efficiency, effectiveness, and satisfaction. A baseline for measurement should be identified in order to compare results after the change and accurately reflect the effect of the change.

Quantitative data should be collected and analyzed where possible, but all relevant indices should be included. The process of change, as well as the content, timing, resources utilized, cost, and complications, should be assessed. The level of resistance and the impact on the group or on individuals are all important variables in evaluation.

Evaluation of the change should occur only after a state of equilibrium has been achieved. This state of equilibrium may be recognized by the sense of balance that exists. This is a time when the change is not occurring but has in fact been completed as much as is possible to be observed. The effectiveness of the change—how well the desired outcome was achieved— may then be measured. Questions related to efficiency or the economical use of resources during the change would also be appropriate. The impact of the change on the job satisfaction of the group or of individuals and the general satisfaction with the change should also be considered during this evaluation.

There may be a desire to look at more specific data during evaluation, and this, too, may be important, depending on the type of change. Specifics such as factors that supported or obstructed the process would be an example of potential evaluation data. Those tools the change agent found to be particularly useful during the process would also be valuable in future changes within the group or organization. Effective strategies during implementation could be added to the desired data for evaluation.

STABILIZATION OF CHANGE

Because of the need to return to equilibrium, stabilizing and maintaining the change are nearly as important as any other step. This is Lewin's refreezing step. Reinforcement by the change agent and others of the use of new methods or of new behavior is key to this phase. Two way communication must continue to overcome or prevent any other resistance. Continued follow-up is necessary as well, to identify strengths and correct deficiencies encountered along the way.

Reinforcement and follow-up may be accomplished through several mechanisms. A continuing education program is one method for reinforcement and follow-up. It can be utilized to orient new staff members to the change and to keep the current staff continually reminded of the positive aspects of the change. Monitoring of the progress or status of the change provides a means for evaluation of the change. It would also provide feedback related to problems being encountered. Continued support for the change by management is certainly important, but maintaining support from the group and the individuals involved in the change is essential. Continued

	Table 12-3	
	Levels of Change Related to Difficulty	
Level of Change	Time Required	Level of Difficulty
Knowledge	Short period	Least
Attitudes	Moderately short period	Low
Behavior—individual	Moderate period	Moderate
Behavior—group	Long period	Most

(Adapted from Hersey, P., and Blanchard, K. H. (1982). *Management of organizational behavior.* Englewood Cliffs, NJ: Prentice-Hall, Inc.)

communication, then, is perhaps the most important follow-up and reinforcement technique available.

STRATEGIES FOR CHANGE

How easily change may be implemented can be affected by a number of factors, which have been described. Strategies for implementing change may be based on good planning, overcoming resistance, and excellent use of a change agent. There are perhaps other considerations in strategic thinking related to change. The level of change as identified by Hersey and Blanchard (1982) is related to the level of difficulty and time for accomplishment. Table 12-3 is adapted from the work of these authors as they describe a continuum of difficulty related to change.

Changes related to *knowledge* are the simplest and require the least expenditure of time. These changes are related to information—acquisition of knowledge. An example of this level of change would be teaching nurses about a new medication for treating heart disease. Because of emotions that are tied to *attitudes*, these changes are more difficult and more time-consuming. An example of a change related to attitudes might be in teaching staff members about contracting AIDS, since knowledge and attitude would need to be changed. Changes in *individual behavior* are the next most difficult to accomplish, because they frequently require change in knowledge and/or attitude first. Teaching the nursing staff about the proper care of AIDS patients would be an example. *Group behavior* is most difficult to change, since many individuals with varied levels of knowledge and varied attitudes must reach a level of acceptance before the change is successful. An example of this type of change might be seen in conversion of a nursing department from traditional care planning and documentation to a computerized care planning/documentation system.

Strategies for making changes must consider first the levels of change needed and then determine the effective approach (Table 12-4). Hersey and Blanchard (1982) describe participative and coercive strategies. Participative, by its nature, is descriptive of the activity desired of individuals—participa-

TABLE 12–4
Strategies for Effecting Change

Strategy	Described By	Characteristics
Participative	Hersey and Blanchard	• Alteration in knowledge and behavior • Long lasting • Most effective when participants well motivated • Produces commitment
Coercive	Hersey and Blanchard	• Use of force to improve change • Requires strong power base • Rapid • Works best with new situations and dependent participants
Application of power or force	Chin and Benne	• Use of force to impose change • Strong use of power • Rapid • Requires adherence to rules by participants
Empirical-rational	Chin and Benne	• Assumes participants are rational and will support what is advantageous • Fast, long lasting
Normative-reeducative	Chin and Benne	• Assumes participants are rational and intelligent • Assumes behavior patterns are supported by values, norms of group • Produces commitment

tion. Education is a key to this strategy and, if successful, will produce positive attitude changes toward the desired idea or activity. Motivation of the individuals is important if this strategy is to work. An example of this type of strategy can be applied to the example of computerized documentation and care planning. Education of the staff to the many advantages of the system is a basic first step. A demonstration of those advantages through a pilot unit with enthusiastic support of the involved staff then serves to motivate others to accept the change. Participation by affected staff at every stage of the process is very effective in gaining the needed support for the change.

Coercive strategy is the use of force to impose change. An example of this type of change may be seen in the mandate that if a nursing unit is short staffed, staff members from the off-going shift will be *required* to work over to ensure that the unit has good staffing. This type of coercion would often be associated with punishment for non-compliance. The potential for failure with this strategy is great, but if the leader has a strong power base, this strategy can be effective and can produce rapid change. However, the change may be short-lived or produce undesired effects such as low morale.

Chin and Benne (1976) describe three strategies for change: empirical-rational, normative-reeducative, and application of power. Empirical-rational strategy assumes that individuals and groups are rational. It is based on the belief that participants will cooperate with change that is advantageous to them. Therefore, emphasis on the positive aspects of change for the group can result in a successful change process. An example of this strategy would be a change in organizational structure that provides a transport team to assist in movement of patients throughout the hospital. This change frees other staff members to stay at the bedside as they desire.

The normative-reeducative strategy is based on the assumption that behavior patterns are supported by values and norms of the group and that change requires alteration in knowledge and attitude. A change that exemplifies this strategy would be a change in mode of care delivery from team to primary nursing. Such a change would require that the group value the continuity and accountability found with the primary nursing and that new information would have to be learned before the change could occur. Success with this strategy usually requires a longer period of time and produces strong commitments. Facilitative strategies fit under this category, since they are used to facilitate change through education and motivation.

Use of power or force as described by Chin and Benne (1976) is similar to the coercive strategy described by Hersey and Blanchard and requires considerable power for implementation. Dependent participants in new situations are most affected by this type of strategy.

SUMMARY

Change is a continual process that occurs with or without a plan. Planned change, which may be simple or complex, is most successful when a process similar to the problem solving approach is utilized and when consideration is given to the participants or those affected by the change.

Planning requires assessment, identification of alternatives, selection of an alternative, implementation, and evaluation. The opposing or restraining forces of change produce resistance, which varies significantly with the type of change, the preparation, the level of change, the degree of planning, the change agent, and the strategy used. Successful planning includes steps to minimize resistance and to facilitate the change process.

Stabilization or maintenance of the change is the final step in the process and is necessary to restore equilibrium and maintain homeostasis. Future plans for change should consider the success of a change within a group, as well as the multiple factors that influenced the success. Because change is inevitable and difficult at times, the management of change is an important tool for the nursing administrator who is building a department or an organization (Hoffer, 1986). How successful she is in this project may certainly influence her overall success in administration.

TOMORROW'S STRATEGIES

The mid 1980's were the epitome of change for hospitals and nursing service departments. A refreezing appears to be occurring to some extent.

Another major current of change can be expected. In anticipation of this, the nursing leader needs to be cognizant of the changes she initiates within her department. As mentioned earlier, change for change's sake is not justified. Owing to the tremendous changes that have just occurred, unnecessary change will do nothing to stabilize the system. The forces of change that have affected health care during the last decade have been reacted to in multiple ways, often at the expense of the employee. Health care professionals have sometimes worked against one another or at best may have worked independently of one another. This has created many problems that must yet be addressed. The nursing administrator of the future must be able to recognize the effect of such interactions and must be prepared to resolve the resultant issues. Reaction to the forces of change and to the changes that will occur will be necessary, but a proactive stance will also be important. This means broadening opportunities for nursing and a greater independence of practice. It also means conserving resources and rebuilding nursing departments for the future.

Such activity does not preclude change, however, and the nurse administrator will find it necessary to make changes. The important concept here is related to the rapidity of change. It will be essential for the nurse administrator to be able to change quickly, in anticipation as well as in reaction. Understanding the principles of planned change is essential, but having the expertise of accomplishing change in a timely and effective manner will be even more important.

Strategies for accomplishing change in the future, then, must have a basis in strategic management — thinking and planning for the future in an organized, problem solving manner. The successful future nursing administrator will continually operate in this way. This nurse executive will keep the nursing staff knowledgeable about plans for the future, to minimize education time when the need for a change arises. Maintaining good morale among staff members and a strong power base will also be important, as will communication and participation in decision making. Each step toward change that is already accomplished will improve the timeliness of change when it is needed or desired. The most important strategy for the nursing administrator in accomplishing change will be maintaining the direction of change so that it is viewed positively. How well the nursing administrator handles this may determine the overall effectiveness of the individual as a manager.

References

Auger, J. (1976). *Behavioral systems and nursing*. Englewood Cliffs, NJ: Prentice-Hall, Inc.

Bennis, W. (1966). *Changing organizations*. New York: McGraw-Hill Book Co.

Bertalanffy, L. von (1968). *General systems theory: Foundation, development, applications*, rev. ed. New York: George Braziller.

Blake, R., and Mouton, J. (1978). *The new managerial grid*. Houston: Gulf Publishing Co.

Chin, R., and Benne, K. D. (1976). General strategies for effecting changes in human systems.

In Bennes, W. G., Benne, K. and Corey, K. *The planning of change*, 3rd ed., New York: Holt, Rinehart, and Winston.

Duncan, W. J. (1978). *Essentials of management*, 2nd ed. Hinsdale, IL: The Dryden Press.

Greiner, L. E. (1967). Patterns of organization changes. *Harvard Business Review*, May–June, pp. 119–122.

Hersey, P., and Blanchard, K. H. (1982). *Management of organization behavior*. Englewood Cliffs, NJ: Prentice Hall, Inc.

Hoffer, A. (1986). Facilitating change: Choosing the appropriate strategy. *Journal of Nursing Administration*, 16(4), 18–22.

Lancaster, J. (1982a). Change theory: An essential aspect of nursing practice. *In* Lancaster, J., and Lancaster, W., editors: *Concepts of advanced nursing practice: The nurse as a change agent.* St. Louis: C. V. Mosby Co.

Lancaster, J. (1982b). Systems theory and the process of change. *In* Lancaster, J. and Lancaster, W., editors: *Concepts of advanced nursing practice: The nurse as a change agent.* St. Louis: C. V. Mosby Co.

Levenstein, A. (1979). Effecting change requires change agent. *JONA*, 9(6), 12–15.

Lewin, K. (1951). *Field theory in social science*. New York: Harper and Row, Publishers.

Lippitt, G. (1973). *Visualizing change: Model building and the change process*, LaJolla, CA: University Associates, Inc.

Metzger, N. (1978). *The health care supervisor's handbook*. Germantown, MD: Aspen.

Pierce, S., and Thompson, D. (1976). Changing practice: By choice rather than chance. *JONA*, 6(2), 33–39.

Rogers, E. (1983). *Diffusion of innovations*. New York: The Free Press of Glencoe.

Rogers, E., and Shoemaker, F. (1971). *Communication of innovations: A cross cultural approach.* New York: The Free Press of Glencoe.

Rowland, H., and Rowland, B. (1985). *Nursing administration handbook*, 2nd ed. Rockville, MD: Aspen.

Sampson, E. (1971). *Social psychology and contemporary society*. New York: John Wiley and Sons, Inc.

Spradley, B. (1980). Managing change creatively. *JONA*, 10(5), 32–36.

Stevens, B. (1975). Effecting change. *JONA*, 5(2), 23–26.

Toffler, A. (1979). Focus on the future. Keynote address, National League for Nursing Convention, May, 1979, Atlanta, GA.

HEALTH CARE ENVIRONMENT

INTRODUCTION

Change is inevitable. It occurs continuously whether it is desired or not, and it is often unnoticed. The cultural lag described by sociologists produces errors in behavior among the individuals of society because they have failed to notice or appropriately respond to the change (Levenstein, 1985). The changes occurring in the health care environment are so rapid and so great that understanding and preparing for them are extremely important to the survival of health care institutions.

Society in America has not fully evolved but is now in a state of flux and change, which will certainly be carried over into the future. The changes or trends occurring in society in general have a significant impact on the health care environment. The integration of health care into society and societal issues has never been so complete or comprehensive as it is today. Some of the societal trends identified by Naisbitt (1982) in *Megatrends* are quite specific for health care, whereas others are more general. Even the general trends, however, have a significant impact on the health care environment.

Naisbitt identifies one major trend as the movement away from industry and toward information as the base for jobs. The society of today is now based primarily on the creation and distribution of information instead of on industry. This means that the majority of jobs in America are related to

13

information in some way. Health care, of course, is an information and service profession. America is also part of a global economy and no longer operates in an isolated manner from other countries. The impact of this trend on health care may be overwhelming, as other countries turn to the United States more and more for help in addressing health care needs.

In the past, society generally ran by short term considerations. Now, long term emphasis has gained importance, and planning for the future is stressed in all areas of society. Innovations in planning and activities have become critical for all levels. No longer will centralization of thinking and planning, much less action, meet societal needs. Decentralization is the trend. As information can now be shared instantly through our media networks, society is demanding more direct involvement in decisions about itself. Americans have also discovered they no longer are forced to choose "either/or." Rather, multiple choices are open to them in every arena. All of these trends in society may impact on health care directly or indirectly (Naisbitt, 1982).

Many of the changes described were resisted by American society. Others occurred without resistance over time. As the issues and trends in health care are identified and discussed, the greatest challenge for the health care and nursing administrator is a change in perspective. This chapter will look first at those issues and trends in health care that were born of the social philosophy in America and that are more general in the impact they have on the health care environment. Access to care, quality issues, organizational structures, ethical concerns, and services will be included under this heading. Another section will be devoted to the environment related to legislation and regulation. Payment systems, risk management, and other regulatory mechanisms will be discussed. A section on economic and financial issues or trends related to health care will include issues of productivity, joint ventures, and capital acquisition. The changes occurring related to health care practitioners will be included in another section. Downsizing, shifts in resources, and selective hiring will be discussed in this section. Finally, the effect of technology on the health care environment will be addressed.

ISSUES IN HEALTH CARE

As the conflict between unlimited access and high quality care versus control of costs continues to surface, the real dilemma of unlimited versus minimal access in health care surfaces. While no one wishes, at least openly, to deny access to care to anyone, limitations on that access are being considered strongly. The major emphasis is on access to minimal care versus access to all care. Much of this is related to the change in life expectancy created by the advances in medicine and to the reduction in health care spending by the federal and state governments. In the United States, the changes in treatment of chronic diseases have continued to extend life to an expected life span averaging 74.5 years (Fries, 1986). This significantly increased the outflow of dollars from governmental payers to the point at which the health programs were endangered. Cutbacks and program changes were implemented through the prospective payment system to ensure longer survival of the programs and to provide incentives for reductions in health care costs. These reductions in governmental health care spending, however, are likely to affect the access to health care of medically indigent as well as Medicare and Medicaid patients (Anderson, ACHA, 1984). The costs for health care have been so great that the public has reacted and has also demanded that costs be reduced. The public will ultimately decide how health care dollars will be spent. Preserving an equity of sorts in allocation of health care will be the responsibility of that public (Friedlaender, 1986).

Quality of care issues have been raised as another significant factor in the health care environment. As concern for cost reduction has occurred, fears about reduction in quality have surfaced. Quality care costs in many ways. Value conflicts among health care professionals have sharpened in the environment of health care. In our nursing departments, we see these conflicts in staffing, discharge decisions, and planning. As acuity of patients has risen, emphasis on shorter lengths of stay has created these conflicts related to quality of care.

Patient acuity is one aspect of the environment that is directly related to the issue of quality. Several factors have influenced this trend in patient acuity. An aging population is one such factor. Those chronic diseases mentioned earlier have their greatest impact on the elderly consumers. Even the aging phenomenon is chronic and covers a variety of body systems. Elderly patients with multiple problems compose much of the consumers of health care. Current medical care is aimed at postponing the onset of chronic illness and preserving function (Fries, 1986). For many years, all surgery was performed in hospitals. As anesthesia techniques and technology improved, however, much surgery has moved to the outpatient arena. This reduced significantly the number of less acutely ill patients who were inpatients. As diagnostic studies, previously only paid by third party payers if done on an inpatient basis, moved to the outpatient arena, even fewer patients who were not very ill were admitted. As prospective payment, peer review organizations (PRO's), and preadmission certification have reached into hospitals, controlling inpatients' lengths of stay and admissions, patients have been admitted later and discharged sooner, resulting in the patient being hospitalized only when he is most ill. This trend has quite an impact on health care, as these critically ill patients fill ICU beds or must be cared for outside ICU's. Lengths of stay, which decreased for a time, have begun to level off, but the trend toward shorter length of stay is likely to continue (Goldsmith, 1986; Detmer, 1986).

This trend toward later admissions and earlier discharges has had yet another effect—on the location for health care delivery. Hospitals generally experienced declines in daily census and total occupancy as much of health care moved into other settings. Although occupancy has stabilized in many areas of the country, home health care has become more popular and has expanded its services to include care for more seriously ill patients. IV therapy, highly skilled nursing care, and complex therapies have found their way into home health care settings. Outpatient facilities for diagnosis and treatment have sprung up throughout the country. Ambulatory surgery, birthing centers, imaging centers, and outpatient laboratories have changed the focus of health care services. Wellness and health promotion centers, rehabilitation centers, and oncology centers have been added to the outpatient treatment facilities, which have pulled business away from hospitals (Moore, 1985). With this trend in a shift to outpatient services, it's not surprising that many inpatient facilities are expanding services to include many of the outpatient types of services identified.

Organizational structure changes are another trend noted in the health care environment of today. Corporate ownership of health care facilities of all types, including hospitals, has been on the rise (Shimberg, 1984). This has been recognized for several years now. It has even been predicted that there may be only investor-owned mega-corporations for health care in the future. Even not-for-profit health care institutions are grouping themselves into structures that facilitate increased competition. Although that trend is questioned by many of the experts, there is no doubt that business coalitions are purchasing health care services (Freedman, 1985). Health maintenance organizations (HMO's) and preferred provider organizations (PPO's) are also springing up everywhere to emphasize health promotion and preferred services. Health care institutions are aligning themselves with these organizations to improve patient referrals and compete effectively in the marketplace (Teitelman, 1984).

Competition and marketing are other trends identified in the health care environment that have had and will continue to have a significant impact on health care. Competition, perhaps always there, has never before been as strong. Competition has expanded from competition among hospitals to competition among all types of health care institutions, as the freestanding diagnostic and treatment facilities have grown in number and scope. Owners of many freestanding facilities are physicians, so that competition has occurred and will continue to occur between the physicians and the hospitals where the physicians continue to practice. Marketing of the various services being offered is another mechanism having a high priority in the health care environment today, as the need to compete strongly has risen. More is being spent on marketing, and marketing strategies have expanded greatly to effectively meet this need.

Although consumers certainly have many more choices today and use them, there still is much confusion about health care services. Third party payers are requesting or demanding second opinions on diagnoses and treatment choices. Choices are so diverse and multiple that patients often don't know what to choose. Costs for health care have risen so much that many consumers delay treatment because of costs. Increases in co-payment by the patients have also influenced the delays in treatment. Concerns for quality of care, access to care, and costs have raised yet another issue as well—ethical considerations. Dilemmas are facing consumers, who may be asked, for example, to decide between aborting a fetus and caring for a malformed child and exhausting their financial resources. The ethical dilemmas, however, extend far beyond the consumer to the health care practitioners, who may, because of cost reductions, be unable to provide a "needed" service. These ethical considerations are more fully addressed in Chapter 2, Ethical Perspectives.

The implication for the effect of these issues and trends on the health care environment is significant. As is common with competition, there is likely to be the development of multiple tiers of service based on ability to pay. Whether quality will be significantly reduced by such developments is difficult to predict. In any case, the health care environment remains in a state of change, which provides both frustrations and opportunities for health care providers.

REGULATION AND LEGISLATION

Health care has for some time been one of the most regulated industries in the nation. Multiple agencies from every level of government provide regulations for the health care institutions. Fifty years of health care policy in the United States have produced a complicated system of health care that has had multiple consequences—good and bad—for American consumers. Legislation that has addressed health care has continued to be revised as needs or desires have changed. Support for health care for the elderly and indigent has received emphasis for many years. The recession of 1981–1982, with its repercussions; the election of President Reagan, with his ideas for private-sector solutions to health care cost problems; and threats to the financial survival of Social Security and Medicare finally resulted in legislation of the prospective payment system, which was investigated in the mid-1970's (Friedman, 1986). This system has resulted in changes in health care delivery and shifting of responsibility for health care. These regulations regarding prospective payment may soon be mandated for physicians and other health care providers, such as nursing homes.

Other regulatory changes are currently having a more positive impact on the health care environment. There are continual changes occurring in the rules and regulations that determine how or if health care planning occurs. Many states have eliminated certificate of need requirements, which controlled the expansion of health services and increased costs for health care. Regulations regarding brain death determination, organ donation/retrieval, and indigent care are heading the list of health care legislation in many states. Indigent care funding, unavailable through previous funding sources, is being addressed in some states through special taxation or collections from health care institutions. Organ donation legislation has included mandated requirements to ask families about organ/tissue gifts with any death of a potential donor.

Medical professional liability or malpractice insurance concerns have also become the center of legislative debate. Costs for malpractice or liability insurance for physicians, hospitals, and many other health care professionals, including nurse specialists, have skyrocketed, if the insurance is even available. States are addressing and Congress will likely produce legislation to limit malpractice awards if costs for health care are to be controlled. Tort reform in many states may receive attention because of changing practice patterns, changing services, and the effect of these changes on health care costs. For example, obstetricians or family practitioners in many rural areas have found the cost of malpractice insurance is so high they cannot deliver enough babies in those areas to pay for the insurance. The options open to them include moving or ceasing obstetrical practice.

Regulatory burdens related to rate control, certificate of need, and planning, as well as others, may be excessive. Regulations related to safety, quality control, licensure, drugs, equipment, and accreditation, among others, have helped to create this high cost of health care. However, it is unlikely that the government agencies will withdraw the regulations. Any changes that occur may be minimal when compared with the extent of regulation. Even more of concern is the rate at which changes occur. Often changes occur before health care institutions are prepared to deal with the changes. Since the regulators and legislators are sensitive to the economic health of the nation, balancing the needs of society with the economic realities must also impact on the health care environment (Anderson and ACHA, 1984).

ECONOMIC AND FINANCIAL CONSIDERATIONS

The impact of prospective payment on the health care environment is one that has threatened the economic viability of many hospitals. Occupancy declined as incentives to reduce length of stay and reduce costs took hold. Pressures on physicians in this arena will continue to influence the health care environment. Hospitals and other health care facilities have tried innovative approaches to improve fiscal positions, with varying degrees of success. Cost shifting within health care institutions has been helpful at times, but with all payer systems predicted for the future, this may be only a short term solution. Other third party payers have already begun to negotiate for discounts as competition among providers increases.

For many years, the medical care components of the Consumer Price Index (CPI) have exceeded the overall CPI. As some regulations attempt to control health care costs, others such as those related to licensure and accreditation have driven those same costs higher. Inflationary pressures on hospitals related to increased labor costs and increased expenditure for services purchased by hospitals also affect the total costs for health care. Creativity in program development and improvements in productivity are methods being used by health care institutions to stabilize the rising costs.

A greater competition for capital is also occurring among health care providers. Uncertainty about the outcome of the prospective payment system on health care institutions has produced a tendency in some financial situations to avoid providing capital to hospitals. Additionally, other health care institutions, such as freestanding surgery centers, urgent care centers, and diagnostic centers, will compete for the capital.

Hospitals will be expanding services and looking at other ventures to improve their financial status. These ventures might include growth in outpatient services from diagnostic to various treatment facilities. Joint ventures between hospitals or between a hospital and a group of physicians are now common and are expected to continue to provide new sources of revenue and perhaps to reduce some of the detrimental competition faced by the groups. Another example of methods by which hospitals are expanding services is the involvement with HMO's and PPO's, which are increasing as health care providers seek other ways to improve referrals and, therefore, revenue.

In spite of the various methods that health care institutions are and will be using to improve their financial position, hospital failures are continuing to surface and will surface into the 1990's. Small hospitals are most likely to succumb, and unless legislation is passed that will better compensate hospitals that have high percentages of Medicare, Medicaid, or indigent populations, they will be hit first. Costs for care of more seriously ill patients continue to rise as the high acuity patients consume resources.

The major concern of health care administrators today is financial viability. Efforts to control expenses have generally been successful, as revenue growth has risen faster than expenses. However, payment inadequacies, competition, and declining utilization have adversely affected some hospitals and may continue to produce problems, especially in smaller hospitals (AHA, 1986). Providers of health care face greater financial risk now and in the future, as other prospective payment limitations, problems with accessibility to capital, and competition combine with low patient census. No longer can simply maximizing revenues be adequate for health care institutions. Increasing efficiencies and reducing costs have gained importance for financial managers. This means improvements in productivity through productivity management (see Chapter 10, Productivity Management), which is the key to financial success for hospitals.

HEALTH CARE PRACTITIONERS

Health care practitioners have been caught up in the health care environment, and the impact on them has been significant. The impact of prospective payment, which reduced revenues, reduced occupancy, and increased competition, also resulted in reductions in the work force of health care institutions. Downsizing, which focuses on strengths and reducing costs, including staffing costs, across the nation's hospitals, has been common. Layoffs, reduced hours of work, and attrition have reduced the work force in hospitals (Glenn, 1984). As hospitals continue to face further census declines, more of these staff reductions may occur. As staff reductions occur, the importance of training, recruiting, and retaining competent and highly productive staffs becomes clear.

Greater involvement by hospital boards has been occurring and will continue to occur into the future. As boards become more involved and liability insurance becomes less available for these groups, compensation for the boards may be considered. Education of trustees and increased involvement in marketing, planning, and finance decisions is noted.

The health care environment has also significantly influenced the practice of physicians. The patients cared for today and tomorrow have changed to an older population and to more females. Physicians have had to adjust already to those changes. Specialty practice has also changed. There are many specialties that now are nearly completely practiced outside the hospital setting. Ophthalmology, dermatology, plastic surgery, otolaryngology, and urology, for example, are primarily ambulatory specialties. As technology increases, other specialties may also be found outside the hospital setting. Certain specialties are well suited for the aging population (cardiology, rheumatology), whereas others may have fewer patients (pediatrics). Fewer patients is the result, too, of the increasing competition among physicians resulting from increases in the number of physicians. Although enrollment in medical schools is tapering off, there still will be a surplus of physicians in 1995 (Kirchner, 1986).

The change in physician relationships has been occurring for some time, as physicians have begun competing with hospitals and demanding greater involvement in decision making. Physicians now practice more in groups, and these groups will continue to grow as physicians attempt to join forces for negotiation ability. HMO's and PPO's will be working more with physicians to negotiate agreements for services as competition among physician groups grows. Capitation and other third party payment plans have already begun to affect physicians as PRO's plan for control of medical care costs. For many physicians, this may mean reductions in pay from the practice of medicine.

Related to the practice concerns facing physicians is another issue—competition among practitioners. As the roles change and the health care economy demands more productivity and less personnel, competition for the work may rise dramatically. Already there are situations in which changes in duties are threatening developed positions. Health care administrators are looking for the most cost effective methods for care delivery. Practitioners are protecting their turf and hanging onto roles. Affected by this competition are nurses, therapists, social workers, physicians, and others.

The oversupply of nurses that occurred recently has reversed, and there is now a shortage of nurses once more. Decline in nursing school enrollment, shifts in employment to non-nursing jobs, and improvements in the overall economy with unemployment being down have resulted in fewer working nurses, so that there is need once more for more nurses than are available. In any case, the emphasis now and in the future may be on selectivity— choosing the *best* qualified person rather than *any* qualified person. The reason for the emphasis is the need to improve productivity through well motivated, well educated, and trained staff members. The entry level into nursing issue is one that has a great impact on this particular discussion. At a time when a shortage of nurses is again occurring (Bezold and Carlson, 1986), the BSN entry level into practice issue may be pushed back again. Because of the importance of selectivity at this time, it is critical that this professional issue receive appropriate attention. Credentialling of these employees may continue to gain importance as well. As acuity rises, the need for better trained, more qualified nurses will also rise. Credentialling has provided a mechanism for some standard by which to ensure that those needs are met.

As the health care environment has changed and continues to change, well qualified managers also are needed. More complex organizations have grown out of the changes occurring now, and these organizations require competent, skilled managers from the department director to the chief executive officer. For the nursing department, the nursing administrator must be well qualified in all aspects of health care management. She has faced multiple changes in the system and has had to be involved in the serious decision making, from financial planning to downsizing to corporate restructuring. Her role as a key individual in the health care institution has become clear as the environment has changed.

TECHNOLOGY

Technology has advanced the practice of medicine so significantly in recent years that it is nearly unrecognizable. Improved technology has affected diagnostics with imaging, laboratory studies, and invasive and non-invasive studies in cardiology and other specialties. Computer assisted diagnostics has expanded the field even further. Artificial red blood cells, chemotherapy, anti-rejection drugs, and implantable devices for medication delivery and defibrillation have opened the field of medicine even further. Artificial hearts and organ transplants continue to arrest disease or replace destroyed tissues. Laser surgery, fiber-optics, and microscopic procedures have expanded the capabilities of medical practice.

Technology in clinical information systems is yet another way in which the health care environment has been and is changing. Computer information systems, not new to hospitals, are expanding to complex integrated networks providing financial, billing, record maintenance, organization, and monitoring services, which are connecting hospitals with physician offices, clinics, and remote care facilities. Computer assisted instruction, documentation, care planning, and even treatment are expanding daily. All these technological changes have been costly but are aimed now at improving efficiency to increase productivity and reduce costs.

STRATEGIES FOR THE FUTURE

What can be done with a health care environment that has on one hand produced magnificent technologies but has on the other hand threatened the very existence of health care institutions? Several strategies may be helpful to prepare for and face the future environment of health care.

As advances in medical technology continue, lengthening life spans and creating ethical dilemmas, health care providers should have developed mechanisms such as bio-ethics committees to help answer the questions regarding access to care and reasonableness of care. The public must also be made aware of and be given incentives to take more responsibility for caring for the elderly or chronically ill to help keep costs down. More emphasis on a family orientation, with societal rewards for maintaining family members needing care, will be important. Sharing in care of the elderly for tax benefits may be the needed incentive. For example, incentives in the form of a tax credit for caring for this type individual could be used. An emphasis on wellness and health promotion should continue, and there should be more emphasis on health education. Encouragement of individuals' involvement in health care decisions is another critical point.

Reforms in malpractice legislation will be necessary to control health care costs. Involvement in the political process will be important for health care providers. Changing regulations will continue to be difficult, but development of communication networks and working relationships with legislators will be helpful in this process. It will also be important for providers to recognize and consider the regulations during decision making.

Hospitals should collaborate more with physicians in joint ventures or other innovative ways to treat patients. Networking and cooperative involvement in strategic planning constitute one mechanism that may be used to accomplish this. Involvement of physicians on hospital governing boards is another. Involvement in HMO's and PPO's as alternative delivery systems will be important as well, to maintain a competitive edge in the health care environment. Strengthening the public image and marketing must be emphasized as full services are offered through affiliated arrangements, and pricing for competition will be of even greater importance.

Strong governing bodies and chief executive officers will be essential strategies for surviving health care institutions of the future. Nursing departments, still composing the greatest share of the labor force in health care, will have increased responsibility in the management of patients to improve productivity and reduce costs for care. This can be expanded even more through involvement of nursing in more external ventures in health care. Credentialling and support for baccalaureate entry level into practice in the future can improve even further the credibility of nursing as a driving force in health care. The nursing administrator will need to ensure excellent medical staff relations, since these relationships will be a top administrative priority.

Research in all aspects of the health care environment will have a very high priority. Use of research to assist in product differentiation will be necessary as competition for services increases. Nursing research will gain in significance, too, as it supports the need for well educated practitioners not only to provide the services but also to help create the market for health services.

Health care institutions will be faced with so many opportunities in the future that minimizing risks will be essential. Successful competition can, however, be engendered by networks and joint ventures of various types. Flexibility in expanding services will be important, as profitable outreach services are developed by hospitals. Strategic planning and enhanced productivity will be critical for the future success of every health care organization.

The nursing administrator of tomorrow will likely be one who understands all the changes that have occurred today. Today's health care environment is fraught with changes—in technology, in human resources, in finances, in regulations, in societal position. There is no clear direction in health care. The health care policy in America is no real policy. Forces of indecisiveness, fiscal ambivalence, infighting, quality versus cost, power shifts, and structure versus financing have left Americans surprised that some logic resulted from the decisions (Friedman, 1986). The opportunities for nursing, however, are tremendous in this changing environment. The focus of services may change toward outpatient services—home health, health education or wellness, diagnostics, rehabilitation—but with that change comes the challenge for nursing. Who better can adapt to the changing focus? Who better can develop innovative approaches to nursing patients in the new settings in which patients will find themselves? The role of nursing has evolved dramatically over the last 50 years. Marketing of nursing expertise and establishing nursing units as revenue centers are ways in which nursing administrators of tomorrow may meet the challenge of maintaining high quality care in a cost efficient manner in the continually changing health care environment.

The development of nursing units as revenue centers is based on specific charges for nursing care. Just as other "revenue departments" have charges for procedures or time utilized in care, charges for nursing care can also be established. Charges have been based on such things as level of care required. This method links the charge to the acuity of the patient and the amount of care needed by each level. For example, a level I patient may need 2 hours of nursing care per day, whereas a level IV patient may need 16 hours per day. The charge associated with care of the level IV patient would likely be much greater than the charge for the level I patient. This type of charge system considers the acuity of the patient and provides an approach to billing that may be more reasonable than simply a room and board charge. This is especially true as patient acuity rises.

Determining the charges for nursing care can be accomplished by first identifying cost. Nursing care hours must include support hours (unit secretaries, monitor technicians, etc.) and indirect care (documentation, preparation for procedures, errands, etc.). Costs for patient supplies, equipment, and office supplies not individually charged to patients must also be included. Once costs are determined, the necessary charge may be established.

As hospitals seek better ways of identifying and increasing revenue, the nursing unit as a revenue center will become more important. Objective mechanisms to determine acuity will be essential, so that patient classification systems will be under scrutiny for their objectivity or lack of it. Computerization in nursing will be gaining even more importance as this trend occurs.

References

AHA (American Hospital Association) (1986). *EconomicQQY Trends 1*(4), 1–11.

Arthur Anderson and Co. and the American College of Hospital Administrators (ACHA) (1984). *Health care in the 1990's: Trends and strategies.*

Bezold, C., and Carlson, R. (1986). Nursing in the 21st Century: An introduction. *Journal of Professional Nursing, 2*(1), 2–9.

Detmer, S. S. (1986). The future of health care delivery systems and settings. *Journal of Professional Nursing, 2*(1), 20–26.

Freedman, S. (1985). Megacorporate health care: A choice for the future. *New England Journal of Medicine, 312*(9), 579–582.

Friedlaender, G. (1986). Toward rational rationing: Defining public rights and responsibilities. *Health Management Quarterly*. First Quarter, 21–23.

Friedman, E. (1986). Fifty years of U.S. health care policy. *Hospitals, 60*(9), 95–104.

Fries, J. F. (1986). The future of disease and treatment. *Journal of Professional Nursing, 2*(1), 10–18.

Glenn, K. (ed.) (1984). DRGs, LOS, and FTEs. *Washington Rep Medical Health/Perspectives.* October 1, 1–4.

Goldsmith, J. (1986). 2036: A health care odyssey. *Hospitals, 60*(9), 68–76.

Kirchner, M. (1986). Which specialties will prosper? *Medical Economics*, March 31, 54–67.

Levenstein, A. (1985). Adjusting to the new environment. *Nursing Management, 16*(10), 74–76.

Management Rounds (1985). Ventures show cooperation with MDs up. *Hospitals, 59*(19), 37–39.

Moore, W. B. (1985). CEOs plan resource shift for 1986. *Hospitals, 59*(24), Dec. 16.

Naisbitt, J. (1982). *Megatrends*. New York: Warner Books.

Neely, C. (1985). Hospital goods and services to go up in '86: Forecast. *Hospitals, 59*(19), 74–78.

Owens, A. (1986). Who will be your patients? *Medical Economics*, March 31, 35–53.

Powills, S. (1985). Hospital industry price wars heat up. *Hospitals, 59*(19), 69–73.

Shimberg, B. (1984). Licensing in the year 2000. *Issues, 5*(2), 1–8.

Teitelman, R. (1984). Taking the cure. *Forbes,* June 4, 82–91.

GAMES AND POLITICAL STRATEGIES

INTRODUCTION

Health care organizations, like other organizations, have long been recognized as political. Organizational structures operate through the distribution of authority and responsibility to various individuals in various positions. Through this authority structure, individuals have opportunities for career development and for expression of their interests and motives (Stone, Berger, Elhart, Firsich, and Jordan, 1976). In the setting of authority and position, power can be exercised, and the exercise of power places many individuals in a position of conflict.

When conflicts occur, game playing follows as a mechanism to achieve goals or objectives. Games are not unique to organizations. Games have been used historically by groups to achieve various purposes. Through manipulation, rewards, and punishments, people have sought to meet their

14

specific goals. Health care organizations are no different than other groups in this respect.

Political savvy, necessary for survival in organizations today, has been identified as a part of good planning in order to benefit fully from one's efforts (Research Institute of America, 1984). Politics in organizations may be thought of as only pulling strings or manipulation to get ahead or get even. However, more importantly, politics can be considered a skill in which resources are fully utilized to accomplish effectively those objectives important to the manager. Political behavior in organizations, then, can be defined as that behavior used to maintain or attain power, status, or prestige in the organization and to influence decisions about resource allocation.

Words such as manipulate, power, play, and games have negative connotations. There is often hesitation or resistance to consider use of game playing or involvement in organizational politics. Avoidance of organizational politics or game playing is merely an attempt to deny reality. It is essential for nursing administrators to embrace organizational game playing with an open mind.

Every organization has its own culture or set of norms and values by which it operates. This culture conveys an identity to the organization, provides stability, guides behavior, and facilitates commitment (Smircich, 1983). It is the organizational culture that permits or inhibits political behavior within an organization.

A number of factors contribute to the necessity of politics in organizations, especially health care organizations. The presence of bureaucracies in these settings and the resultant formation of informal groups within the organization foster the use of political strategy for accomplishment of goals. The development of power bases and the struggles by groups or individuals to achieve, maintain, or increase a power base contribute significantly to political game playing. Trust versus distrust, which may actually grow out of power struggles, plays yet another role in the development of politics within organizations.

Organizational politics can be divided into three categories. One type of organizational politics is that associated with self. The political maneuvering associated with advancement of the individual within the organization includes those strategies that serve to promote individual ideas, to protect the individual from the actions of others, and to maintain the individual in the upwardly mobile group. Another form of organizational politics is that associated with the teams or groups to which an individual belongs. It may involve the subordinates of a manager, members of the peer group, or supervisors. Essentially, this form of politics within an organization encompasses the interpersonal relationships developed in the various groups to which one belongs in the institution and is closely associated with roles and with role conflict. Conflict, including role conflict, is a predecessor of game playing. The third category of organizational politics is the politics associated with growth or with change within an organization. There is obvious overlapping of the categories of politics within organizations. The politics related to self and that associated with growth, for instance, are identified in the power struggles to attain more prestigious positions or control a larger number of departments. Change and growth in an organization often result in restructuring of the organization, with accompanying political ramifications for individuals or groups. Even without the restructuring, change, including growth, sets the stage for game playing by individuals with interest in the changes.

Nursing administration's success within the organization has required more active participation in institutional politics as nursing administration's position in the formal organizational pattern has changed (Longest, 1975). Because of changes in the scope and practice of nursing over the years, nursing administration has become increasingly involved in political games as a matter of survival. Much of what was formerly the responsibility of nursing departments has been assumed by other departments (Physical Therapy, Respiratory Therapy, Cardiovascular Services, etc.). Many departments that formerly reported to nursing may no longer have that association (Central Supply, OR, Emergency Services, etc.). The emerging role of physicians within health care institutions has to some extent diluted the authority of the nursing hierarchy. While these changes may have many positive benefits for the consumer and for nursing, the changes have fostered the need by nursing administrators to re-examine the power bases they have and to resort to political game playing to accomplish goals. Countering some of these changes in which the role of nursing has evolved, leaving behind it many functions such as those described, is the fact that many nursing administrators have assumed responsibility for departments that are non-nursing oriented, such as clinical or ancillary departments. Much of this has been accomplished through political game playing and building of power bases.

The following sections will address the factors that influence politics and game playing within health care institutions and will identify many of the most common political games in those organizations. Each section will address specific strategies for games, and the final section of this chapter will identify strategies for nursing administrators to use in organizational politics.

HEALTH CARE POLITICS

Formal vs. Informal Organizations

Health care institutions have such well established bureaucracies that politics becomes necessary for the organizations to survive. Bureaucracies are characterized by policies and procedures, by a clear chain of command, by impersonal attitudes, and by job assignment according to specialization. Formal organizations expend large amounts of time and energy establishing organizational charts to define the chain of command, position descriptions to define the specialist jobs, and rules and regulations to define the when and how of procedures. There are, however, many interactions among members of organizations that will not fit into the formal organizational structure.

The relationships and communication between members of the organization that do not exist in the formal structure create the informal organization. The informal organization, just as necessary to the institution's existence, results from social interaction between individuals. Unlike the formal organization, which places emphasis on authority, the informal organization emphasizes people relationships. Another differentiating characteristic between the formal and informal organization is the fact that management cannot eliminate the informal organization because management did not create it. The informal organization consists primarily of small groups whose membership exerts significant influence over the behavior of the group members. In exchange for the power the informal group gains, the group members receive rewards that the formal organization does not provide.

The rewards that members of informal organizations receive may vary with the group but generally are categorized into four types. Each informally organized group is distinct and somewhat unique. There is *status* afforded to group members through belonging to a special, perhaps exclusive group. An informal group provides *security* to its members, since the individual is viewed as an equal to his peers. The individual may be better recognized in the small informal group for his participation than within the formal organization. Interpersonal relationships in informally organized groups often produce *relief from stress* found in the monotony and pressures of a formal organization. Finally, *information* through informal channels (the grapevine) is a reward the informal group members receive. Communication within formal organizations frequently is restricted, resulting in individuals who have no sense of belonging. This need to belong is a strong basic human need.

Informal groups, like formal groups, have leaders and may have a complex structure. The leadership of informal groups is developed in an unofficial manner and may never be specifically identified, but it can be observed. Informal organizations, unlike most formal organizations, tend to remain small and to fit the patterns of behavior associated with small groups.

The rewards associated with membership in informal organizations help to maintain the stability of these groups, which is important to the formal organization. Lack of flexibility in formal organizations may hinder action in meeting objectives. For example, if a new program has been developed, but the organization requires concurrence of the board before any marketing efforts are begun, the delay may hurt the new program. The lack of flexibility hinders action in meeting the objective. The informal organization may "informally" leak information about the program to improve the marketing of the program. Spontaneous action by informal groups is permitted and may improve the accomplishment of the overall goals of the organization.

Obtaining cooperation and support of an informal organization or its leadership may be essential to a manager, since the manager's formal authority alone is often not adequate for supervising groups. The informal communication channel, while inaccurate at times, can serve the manager well in obtaining information about employee attitudes and feelings or in ensuring that information is rapidly disbursed to employees.

One major problem associated with the existence of informal organizations is the possibility that the goals and objectives of the formal organization are at cross purposes with those of the informal organization. The individual group member may even desire to meet the objectives of both groups, but may be unable to without significant role conflict. Interaction between individuals and the interdependence of individuals further complicate achievement of goals, since achievement of certain goals or work toward certain goals may jeopardize relationships. Role conflict between these groups increases the necessity for game playing.

Power

Power struggles are the basis of many of the games found within any organization. Use of power was discussed more fully in Chapter 5. Essentially, power derives from three major sources—personal, social/interpersonal, and organizational (Claus and Bailey, 1977). Personal power from a strong self-concept can be found in individuals at any level within an organization. It can be achieved through expertise or perceived expertise. Social power is built on interactions within groups and tends to be stronger than any individual's power. This type of power can be seen in formal and informal organizations. Organizational power, dependent on functional authority bases, is found in formal organizations. Sources of organizational power include the control of resources; access to more powerful supervisors; authority to make decisions, take action, and enforce policy; control of information; and title.

There is competition for the power that exists within organizations. Because power is scarce, shifts in power may occur at any time. True power is derived from assuming responsibility for decisions or actions rather than from command or authority (Claus and Bailey, 1977). Power can be a positive force in affecting the behavior of others. The strength of the positive force is tempered with the reality of limitations, and the energy associated with the power can be transmitted to others to facilitate goal achievement through motivation and behavioral change.

Each of the power bases identified may result in conflict with the others. One individual's or group's personal, social, or organizational power base may be in conflict with another's. In either case, power becomes a factor that, rather than being positive, necessitates game playing to achieve individual or group purposes.

Trust vs. Distrust

There is found within most institutions some level of distrust either between individuals or between groups. A number of factors contribute to the trust/distrust problem, creating still another avenue for game playing. Many of the contributing factors result from the business nature of organizations, which emphasizes the maintenance of hierarchies. Such hierarchies inevitably include some individuals who, through the Peter Principle, have risen to their level of incompetence (Peter and Hull, 1969).

Placement of individuals into positions for which they lack knowledge, skill, and/or adequate preparation is a significant factor in development of distrust. Other managers in similar positions are unable to communicate on a peer level and lack trust in the relationship that develops. Subordinates may find themselves in a position in which they recognize the incompetence yet are unable to cope effectively with it through formal organizational channels.

Assumption of the responsibilities of one group by a second group leads to distrust by one or both groups. One group tends to feel quite threatened and defensive, while the group that assumed new responsibilities might feel the need to be constantly on guard.

When an individual has been in a position for a short period of time, distrust arises in other individuals who feel insecure in developing relationships. The individual who is new to the position will not have developed alliances, and other individuals (both subordinates and peers) will be unable to predict behaviors in relationship to them. The inability to make predictions breeds a lack of trust. This lack of trust results in more motivation for game playing.

HEALTH CARE GAMES

Economic, sociological, and psychological needs of various groups will eventually be expressed in political form as individuals and groups attempt to exert control over decision making (Kovner and Neuhauser, 1983). Every group and individual in the organization must cooperate with others to some degree to ensure the survival of the organization as a whole. The extent to which cooperation is available depends on the needs of the groups or individuals and the degree to which the needs are met by the formal organization.

When a group or individual is unable to have its needs met formally by the organization, political game playing often results. Although the kind of game utilized by a particular group or individual may vary, the games described in the following paragraphs are common to health care institutions.

Male/Female—Doctor/Nurse Games

Two political games, difficult to separate because of sex-role stereotyping, are the male/female and doctor/nurse games. The American culture has produced, through social conditioning, sex-role stereotyping, which typically places females into the nurse role and males into the physician role. Although there are male nurses and female physicians, the political game playing emphasizes the sex-role relationship.

From early childhood, social conditioning has stressed passivity and dependence in females (Burgess, 1979). A lack of cohesiveness and a concern for interdependence of people rather than things are attributed to females as characteristics that influence their power needs and expressions. Females tend to have a diffuse awareness of the wholeness of nature and the link of individual to the whole (Masson, 1981). The same characteristics are often attributed to nurses. Additionally, nurses are described as obedient, having less intelligence, submissive, and lacking political awareness. Studies on the image of nursing by Kalisch and Kalisch verify this view of nurses in the media and further attribute to nurses a lack of career commitment and subservience to physicians (Kalisch and Kalisch, 1982).

Nursing evolved from two sources: religious and secular. In the religious group, devotion through service and sacrifice was required. The secular source brought females without homes or families into the profession of nursing. Subservience was seen as essential to nursing (Spitzer, 1981). From nursing's origin, the characteristics that are synonymous with weakness have been those most valued for nurses. The failure of nurses and women to be assertive and the use of "feminine charms" to influence others have been major obstacles to leadership development. Because of the rejection of the use of confrontation and negotiation by nurses and women, it has been the view of others within health care organizations that nurses attempt to solve problems from a position of weakness rather than a position of strength (Duncan and Partridge, 1980).

Males, through social conditioning, are characterized by aggressive behavior, independence, commitment to career, and political awareness. They have been described as better able to analyze, and to formulate logical relationships. The abilities to identify and solve problems and to formulate logical relationships are also considered masculine characteristics.

Team play, recognized as a primary value in goal achievement, is established in early childhood in males and is the result of a military mentality. There is generally a female ignorance of military protocol and a lack of team concept among females that further differentiates females from males (Spitzer, 1981).

Physicians, from their training in medical school, are taught that completely independent, aggressive thinking may be justified by the physician's responsibility for human life (Trinosky, 1979). For this reason, the mostly male physician group assumes the dominant role and gives orders for care. Further conflict occurs when the mostly female nurse group responds in the

| TABLE 14–1 | | |
| Dimensions of Work | | |
Dimension	Nurses	Physicians
Sense of time	Scheduled, hourly	Course of illness
Assigning of work	Bed or room	Case
View of resources	Scarce	Abundant
Reward	Hourly wage	Fee, salary
Sense of mastery	Weak	Strong

Adapted from Sheard, T. The structure of conflict in nurse-physician relations. *Supervisor Nurse*, August, 1980. Reprinted with permission.

manner so frequently attributed to females—resentful of the physician's authority, yet obedient, passive, and dependent.

Conflict between physicians and nurses may be complicated by the differences between five basic work dimensions of the two groups (Sheard, 1980) (Table 14–1). Nurses, of necessity, maintain an hourly sense of time and follow rather rigid schedules. Both in hours worked and in ordering their patient contact, nurses tend to perform tasks by schedules and, when interrupted, may commit errors in care delivery and develop resentment of the interrupter. Physicians measure their time with the patient not in actual time with the patient (which may be quite brief) but in duration of the illness or treatment for that illness. Their time is rarely scheduled with any strictness, and they fail to be able to fully appreciate the nurse's sense of time.

Physicians carry patient loads and view each patient as a case assignment. The relationship with the patient often begins before hospitalization and generally endures beyond discharge of the patient from the institution. Nurses, however, are often assigned to patients by bed number rather than by patient needs, with changes in assignment occurring on a daily basis. Although primary nursing has reduced much of the problem of continuity, transfer of patients within an institution prevents even the primary nurse from developing a therapeutic and ongoing relationship with patients. Failure to develop a therapeutic relationship with the patient diminishes the dedication of the nurse and may make the nurse less willing to provide much extra effort for the patient.

A third work dimension that differs between nurses and physicians is a sense of resources. Nurses often view resources as scarce or limited. Obtaining necessary supplies, drugs, and equipment is frequently a chore for the nurse. When a physician, who sees the hospital as an abundance of resources, requests an extra procedure or test that increases the workload of the nurse, another conflict surfaces. For the physician, the task is simple. The physician need only write the order, even when the test or procedure may be unnecessary. The reason for ordering the test may be a good one or may result from fear of lawsuits, but the reasoning is rarely shared with the nurse.

The nurse, on the other hand, must carry out the order within a reasonable time frame, including arranging the test, obtaining supplies that are often difficult to obtain, ensuring that the test is performed, obtaining the results, communicating the results with the physician, and receiving more orders. Nurses may become angry when asked to perform tasks they view as unnecessary. When nurses request that the physician discontinue orders that increase the number of tasks they perform, they may only be attempting to reduce the heavy workload. The physician may feel that authority and judgment are being challenged or that the nurse is apathetic.

Physicians are rewarded very differently for their work than nurses. Nurses tend to earn hourly wages, whereas physicians, who work by case assignment, are generally paid a fee for service. Nurses value their work in terms of pay per hour, including overtime and vacation or holidays.

Because of the strong relationship established between patient and physician and the sense of responsibility the physician takes for a patient's recovery, physicians have a strong sense of mastery over their work. Nurses, however, often feel they are unable to master their work because of difficulty they encounter in completion of tasks within the bureaucracy of the institution. Inability to develop or maintain therapeutic relationships because of mode of work assignment contributes to this weak sense of mastery and sense of powerlessness by the nurse.

In their doctor/nurse games, the participants continue to play out the relationships of the males and females in our society (Masson, 1981). Skepticism by physicians for the changing role of the nurse has resulted from a shifting of responsibility from one group toward the other. While the nurse becomes specialized and qualified to offer intelligent suggestions, the physician is threatened by what may be viewed as an attempt to challenge orders. The nurse may have excellent ideas for patient intervention, yet withhold the suggestion because of a lack of confidence or fear the physician would not listen or would be threatened.

Despite attempts to keep nurses powerless and inhibited, the realities of cost control that face the nursing and medical professions today force nursing to move toward a more masculine mode than perhaps desired by either group. This may be exemplified in the increasingly assertive behavior of some nurses to meet the expectations of an administration that encourages them to begin to plan discharges early after admission. However, the physician often views this as a loss of control over the patient's stay. A lack of understanding by each profession for the other's work and rationale for the work fosters the conflicts described. Game playing has become essential in the struggle between the groups, but a number of strategies may be utilized to permit successful competition between physicians and nurses (or males and females).

STRATEGY

The feminist movement has strengthened the power base of many nurses and has encouraged confrontation between the physician/nurse groups (Shiflett and McFarland, 1978). Such confrontation encourages professional growth. Barriers to communication between the groups must be recognized and minimized. Too often, one group makes assumptions about the other group without validation. Such action by either group results in loss of respect, inadequate understanding, and resentment. Adequate and clear communication is essential. Each group should evaluate role expectations with the other group. Respect and appreciation for the contribution of one group by the other will foster understanding and improve communication. Accountability should be an expectation of any responsible position, regardless of sex and profession. Commitment is a personal choice, unrelated necessarily to profession or sex.

The team concept, generally easier for males, provides an approach for professional association in which contributions to goal achievement by physicians, nurses, or others is valued, yet recognition of the various hierarchies within the political structure is necessary to integrate any proposed change. Mutual consideration of the hierarchies and professional associations may at times require delicate role playing for the nursing administrator. As long as physicians and nurses, or males and females, view one another as competitors for some reward, conflicts will continue. The challenge for the nursing administrator is in preserving the balance between those attributes associated with males and those associated with females, and in maximizing the strengths of each to enhance professional contribution to goal achievement. This may be accomplished by the nurse executive through positive reinforcement to the individual (male or female) of the appropriate or desired characteristics, such as compassion, dedication, and rational thinking; and negative reinforcement of those less desirable ones, such as aggression and lack of confidence.

Credentials Game (Technical Guru)

Another kind of political game identified in hospital settings is the one commonly known as the technical guru game. This game is most characterized by the individuals or groups who insist that only they are able to accomplish some specific procedure or task. The procedure is often one that has previously been performed by a different group, but currently requires specialized training in order to be performed accurately.

This game is associated with another one (territoriality), discussed in the next section. Blurring of roles of professionals has resulted in this particular conflict (Ryan, 1981). Over time, roles of various groups have overlapped, with changes occurring necessitated by economics, demands for improved productivity, and changes in expectations. This overlapping of roles and changes in role expectations have fostered the necessity for playing the credentials game to ensure survival.

Individuals subject to this game are the individuals who have specialized training for their positions. The individuals have been taught and believe they are the only individuals qualified to perform certain functions. The individuals function very well in their positions, and usually there is no disagreement that they function well. The game begins evenings, nights, weekends, and holidays. On these days or during these hours, there are other individuals who can perform the same functions.

Conflict arises between groups when one group attempts to convince others that specialized knowledge or training is essential for tasks that can be assumed fairly easily by another group at other, less convenient times. Because each group desires to control decisions that directly affect that group, the group will develop its own mechanism for maximizing its role within the organization. The credentials game is one mechanism that is utilized but that has significant adverse effects. Inconsistent application of requirements for performance, which is seen in this political game, breeds loss of respect and increases group conflict.

STRATEGIES

Strategies that may be utilized successfully with the credentials game are related to maintaining control. Departments and individuals most affected by the game are those that (1) are the most versatile and (2) are already working those less convenient times. To prevent abuse by other departments or individuals, a few basic guidelines are needed. It is important that acceptance of additional responsibilities is associated with appropriate rewards. For example, if one department begins performing a procedure for another, it would be appropriate that revenue for the procedure be assigned to the department performing the procedure. Rewards for acceptance of additional responsibility may include a strong power base. Groups or individuals who desire to have others assume responsibility for some procedure or task should place emphasis not on the required skill for performance but on other factors influencing goal achievement. These other factors might include improved productivity, more consistent performance, and lower costs. Negotiation for changes in responsibility and associated rewards is necessary to ensure that affected departments or individuals are comfortable with the outcome. (See also section on negotiation in this chapter.)

Another strategy that may be utilized would be performance of the function during undesirable situations in exchange for other resources or future support. There must, however, be a clear understanding by both groups of the "debt" that is owed. If there does not appear to be any mutually agreeable way to assume responsibility for the function, it is necessary for managers or administration to lay firm groundwork as to the expertise and abilities, and for both parties to network sufficiently with all other interested and affected groups as to the goals and motives of the two groups or individuals involved.

Territoriality

Territoriality, defined as the acquisition and defense of a specific area by an animal, individual, or group, is another political game commonly observed in health care institutions. Animal and human behavior has been driven to a great extent by territoriality. Dogs mark their territory and guard it vigorously against intrusion. Man has protected his territory since the days of cave men. Many wars have been fought because of territoriality.

Human beings have developed numerous methods for displaying their territories—licensure laws to protect jobs, separate departments within organizations, areas of specialty practice with associated organizations, and fences to surround property (Holl, 1981). In humans, the need for identity and security, characterized by territoriality, is high in Maslow's hierarchy. Territories, such as specialty practice, claimed by a group provide the group with a psychology, recognition, and a certain amount of cohesiveness.

Many nurses have ambivalent feelings of territoriality related to the identification of nursing with different roles (educator, administrator, clinician), different specialities (obstetrics, critical care, orthopedics), and different locations for practice (hospitals, home health agencies, physician offices). Variations in educational preparation and confusion about the place of nursing in the common health care framework may also create ambivalence within nursing groups about territory. The socialization of nurses to the expectations of the organization versus the objective of service to mankind results in further maladaption to the concept of territoriality.

As with many other political games, territoriality may be viewed negatively, but the basic need for security can drive individuals or groups to fight or defend their territory against invasion. Examples of this game are noted in situations in which changes in responsibilities are considered. If one department has responsibility for a procedure that another department requests to perform, even on a limited basis, the first department may be very threatened by a loss of territory. This threat to the first department may evoke numerous defensive tactics, including the technical guru game. Some groups may go to elaborate ends to build up the importance of procedures or to increase the use of a particular space if that particular "territory" is threatened. This feeling of potential loss of territory by a group is enhanced when other threats to security co-exist. For instance, if job layoffs are rumored at the same time a suggestion is made for another group or department to assume responsibility for a particular procedure, the threat to the first group is significantly increased.

STRATEGIES

An understanding of the factors that influence feelings of territoriality in an individual or group is necessary to approach this game. Controlling any of these factors related to insecurity can be positive in resolution of the conflict that often occurs. The timing of the confrontation or approach may be extremely important. Choosing a time at which the individual or group has a feeling of control and an ability to negotiate can be utilized to prevent such feelings of total loss. Maintenance by the individual or group of some control is essential to that individual or group's effective survival. Knowledge of environmental or situational factors related to the individual or group can also be helpful. A reduction of the feeling of a loss of territory by an individual or a group may be essential to satisfactory resolution. This may be accomplished through successful negotiation (see section on negotiation).

Passive-Aggressive Behaviors

Overt aggression is often considered unacceptable behavior for managers at all levels. Anger and hostility, characteristic of aggression, and expression of the anger and hostility through physical or emotional abuse of threats, violence, loud verbal attacks, or profane language are frequently viewed as immature and more harmful to the abuser than the abused in management circles.

An individual or group, however, may use passive-aggressive behavior to undermine the efforts, the success, or even the respect of another individual or group. The person(s) who uses this type of behavior is characteristically very friendly and supportive of the person or persons being undermined. Behind the scenes, however, that person is pointing out weaknesses of the maligned individual or group. An example of this might be recognized in J. Doe and S. Smith. J. Doe has discussed a particular decision with S. Smith. S. Smith has told J. Doe that he agrees the decision was best under the circumstances. Later, S. Smith shares his concern with the mutual boss of the two that the decision had not been thought through clearly and that another alternative would have been much better. Such "concern" is appreciated by the boss, and the decision making ability of J. Doe has been somewhat undermined. This type of passive-agressive behavior has also been called "whistle blowing." This same example applies to a lower level manager who undermines his supervisor's decisions with lack of support to the employees for management decisions.

Passive-aggressive behavior can also be more open than the behind-the-scenes example. When one person is attempting to undermine another, a number of techniques can be utilized. One method is the "I only just remembered the criticism of your department I heard" game. In this version of passive-aggression, the criticism is always recalled in front of the boss. The two individuals may be in conference for hours, but five minutes after the boss arrives, the incident is recalled and mentioned to the person under attack. The attacker does not tattle to the boss but rather makes sure the boss sees the attacker as sharing information with the person under attack. The disadvantage to the person attacked is that he is continually viewed as ineffective because the feedback always appears negative.

Another type of passive-aggression is characterized by the stealing of credit by one person from another. Although one individual may have contributed a small portion of the work on a particular project, he may take equal or full credit in the meeting at which the project is presented. At times this credit stealing is not done through any particular malice, but through an attempt of one individual to receive positive strokes for himself. Unfortunately, this action, whether accomplished with malice or not, is detrimental to the individual who actually did the work.

Playing individuals or groups against each other is a form of passive-aggressive behavior requiring much behind-the-scenes work. Support for those persons by the attacker is usually pretended, but in actuality undermining of each individual occurs. The attacker's primary purpose may be personal gain or merely survival. In either case, the attacker will agree with each of the two persons or groups under attack (A or B) while in their individual presence. Away from one individual (A), the attacker will be critical (either openly or subtly) of the views expressed by A and will instead support the view of the person (B) with whom he is talking. The attacker will even "confidentially" share with person A, in the presence of A, contrived and false criticism or lack of support by person B of person A.

Another act of passive aggression is noted in the failure of a lower level manager to complete his responsibilities in following the advice of the higher level manager. The lower level manager may carry out this attack in several ways. One avenue for the lower level manager to use is through firm promises to his supervisor to complete assigned work necessary for efficient operation of a department. The manager then fails to satisfactorily complete the work. When confronted, the manager openly or subtly blames his supervisor (higher level manager) for his lack of understanding regarding completion of the work. For example, he might say, "No one told me it needed to be done today." This same passive-aggression is identified in the manager who requests advice from his supervisor in handling a disciplinary problem. The supervisor may tell the manager that he may carry out strong disciplinary measures against the employee if the documentation is adequate. The manager then carries out discipline without appropriate documentation. When confronted, the manager again blames his supervisor, saying, "I asked my supervisor if I could carry out the discipline, and he told me I could."

STRATEGIES

In considering the strategies to use in dealing with passive-aggressive behavior, it is very important to answer several key questions (Research Institute of America, 1984): (1) Who is talking? (2) Who is listening? The larger the number of those listening, the larger the problem. (3) Who is telling you? Although you could be hearing the truth, exaggeration to win points is a possibility (Crawshaw, 1982). If a decision is made to take action after the questions are answered, there are several strategies that may be used.

One strategy is publicizing the reasons for decisions—up and down the chain of command. This may help reduce resentment. Confrontation without betraying confidences is another alternative for dealing with an individual who is undermining you or your efforts. If there has been a lack of understanding or miscommunication that has resulted in a grievance, this action is necessary.

In situations in which passive-aggression has led to others stealing undeserved credit, other action may be necessary. Taking an offensive approach may prevent defensiveness after the fact. Keeping your superiors informed of projects you are working on or sharing your ideas with them can prevent theft of the idea or the credit later. Rather than reporting the person who has inappropriately taken credit for your work (which would be defensive), subtle information that can be pieced together by others may be appropriate. For instance, a remark may be made that while you were developing the marketing plan for project X, you found that the market research done by the Corporate Office was supportive of your plan. This action voids accusations that might prove harmful to you, yet permits you to receive credit you deserve.

In the situation in which an employee or lower level manager fails to complete responsibilities and blames the supervisor, strategies may require more thought. Confrontation can still be utilized to clear the air. Any legitimate grievances can be identified and discussed in a mature and professional manner. Motivation of any employee to become accountable for his actions is difficult. Reasonable expectations should be clearly defined, and the potential result of not meeting those expectations should be explained carefully.

Sometimes, particularly with a new manager, a testing period occurs in which an employee, including the lower level manager, attempts to test the endurance of the supervisor. Even between managers this type of game may occur. Confrontation may again be necessary to resolve the conflict between individuals. It becomes important for the individual to clearly identify expectations and to firmly and consistently act when expectations are not met.

Pet The Ego

Related to the physician-nurse and male-female games is a game frequently referred to as "pet the ego." The purpose of the game is maintenance of the favor of an individual by petting his or her ego. Compliments that induce very positive feelings in an individual are sometimes used to soften the individual. Softening may be described as conditioning the individual to respond in a more receptive or a more positive manner. This mechanism serves a multiple purpose. It helps to remove barriers between individuals to improve interaction. Additionally, it can place the individual being "stroked" into a more receptive mood for communication and negotiation. While giving positive feedback is an acceptable mechanism to improve communication, problems related to this game occur when "petting the ego" is essential for any communication. Some individuals in groups have demanded such strokes to the extent that the entire group has been generalized as having the characteristics of being egocentric.

Demands for compliments and positive strokes vary widely in degree. Everyone needs positive feedback to function well. Only when the demand for such compliments is excessive does the game begin. Withholding cooperation and withholding information are two mechanisms by which individuals apply pressure until their ego needs are met. Another controlling technique used to demonstrate self-importance is manipulation of patients or employees. These techniques are used as power tools by individuals to maintain or attain control over some aspect of the organization.

STRATEGIES

Understanding manipulative behavior is a key to effectively playing the "pet the ego" game. This requires prediction of behavior. Effectively applying preliminary influence can affect decision making. For instance, if A demands attention and ego petting to cooperate, one might be wise to approach A early regarding an idea and influence him to consider the idea. Use of legitimate authority may be effective in this (Claus and Bailey, 1977). Convincing A that an idea is good may require his thinking the idea is his own. If the desire is to reach a certain objective, and reaching the objective requires cooperation of A, presenting the idea as originating from A may accomplish what is desired. The alternative is that A get improper credit for the idea. However, if the group understands A's egocentric behavior, it will also understand that the idea was not necessarily his.

Finance/Paper/Budget Game

Within the political framework of health care institutions is found another game referred to as the Paper Shuffle, the Budget Game, or the Finance Game. This game is played at several levels in the institution. Several categories fit into this game.

Allocation of expenses from one department of the hospital to another and cost shifting to maximize reimbursements are examples of one category. Under prospective payment, this category will be utilized much less than previously and may eventually become extinct. Cost shifting and expense allocation are discussed in detail in Chapter 9, Financial Management.

The category related to budgets becomes a political game through one or more mechanisms. With fixed budgets (as opposed to flexible budgets), the lack of flexibility supports the predilection toward game playing. The game playing may include such aspects as padding the budget, or "going in fat," so that budget cuts will not adversely affect the department. When this aspect occurs frequently over time, the finance department is continuously suspicious that all the departmental budgets are padded. This encourages larger cuts to really effect improvements in productivity and further game playing to pad the budget even more. Those who do not play the game may suffer because of the belief that all budgets are padded. There is, therefore, no reward for not playing; there is only punishment.

Changing personnel mix, requesting large numbers of additional personnel, and altering numbers of procedures, with reams of documentation for justification, are other categories of the paper or budget game. In these categories, the desired outcome frequently is to boggle the minds of the administrative group with requests for more and better in hopes that the status quo can be maintained. This is another version of padding.

Inappropriate blame is placed on this game at times, related to lack of understanding of forecasting or budgeting. Appropriate cuts in budgets may lead to inaccurate accusations that departments or administration is playing a paper game. Adjusting personnel or other expenses to reach a bottom line figure is part of good financial management rather than being a part of a game. However, inflexibility in budgeting may result in this game being played inappropriately to meet the bottom line.

STRATEGIES

Flexible budgeting is a method by which game playing may be discouraged (see Chapter Nine). Because budgeted expenses go up when expected workload goes up, departments only need to justify variances not related to workload. Unfortunately, this does not eliminate padding, since some managers may still pad the budget to encourage favorable recognition of their departmental management.

Education of managers related to budgeting, accounting, and forecasting is extremely useful in discouraging budget padding. Education can provide tools for managers to use in justifying their predictions, and related needs, and can prevent a perceived need for games. Mutual respect by department heads and administrators for each other and respect for the institutional objectives are essential in reducing or eliminating the paper game.

Power Game

Influencing many of the games already described is the Power Game. This game is probably played more than any other game in all businesses. Power had been discussed briefly in an earlier section of this chapter. Politics in organizations results at least partially from a need to use the power one possesses. Groups and individuals within organizations desire control of decisions that directly or indirectly affect them. These groups or individuals utilize their power to develop, maintain, and increase a zone of authority within the organization (Kovner and Neuhauser, 1983). Game playing begins as the groups or individuals vie for each other's zone or for those areas belonging to neither.

Several key factors affect the success of the power game between various groups or individuals. When the *responsibilities of a group or individual are considered essential* to the organization, that group or individual is more successful in the power game. In this situation, there may be control over some source of unpredictability (resources, expertise) within the process of production (of products or services). A group or individual may also attain or maintain a power base through the autonomy of a group or through *standards of behavior* for the group. *Commitment* of the group members to the group, to the individual, or to a professional may affect the power each has. *Possession of knowledge or skills* can provide expertise, which also enhances the power base. Individuals in organizations generally attain or maintain their power by virtue of the position held within some group. Groups of individuals may, however, more obviously hold power over other groups than is seen with individuals.

The traditional groups within health care who wield power are physicians, administrators, and trustees. However, the influence within the organization does not necessarily correspond to the position held on the organizational chart. Nursing has been characterized as being placed between the positional authority of administration and the professional authority of the medical staff (Weisman, Alexander, and Morlock, 1981). Such a position produces a role conflict but may not positively influence the power base of nursing.

The unique relationship that exists between the administrative hierarchy and the professional expertise of the physicians results in attempts by these groups to regulate each other's and their own behavior (Hamm, 1980). They may accomplish this through withholding or selectively sharing information. The groups also attempt to control others by teaching and delegation of responsibilities. This has been noted in the relationship of physicians to many of the clinical departments in hospitals. Physicians do maintain a professional monopoly (Alford, 1975). They have nearly complete control over their work setting and continually utilize this powerful position to attain their objectives. This control, however, may conflict with the organization's responsibility to maintain quality and to control costs. Examples of physician power can be noted in the control over hospital accreditation, demand for ancillary services, length of stay, patient admissions, and even patient behavior (Crawshaw, 1982). This control of resources (patients) results in a significant influence within the organization.

Power games, whether between physicians and administration or between groups, imply rules, goals, and players. Rules are implied rather than written down, and the goal may be achievement of specific objectives or the position of power itself. Granting support to another group is a power game in itself, since returning favors is a rule of the game (Peterson, 1979). The returned favor may be tucked away for future use or identified at the beginning. Power games may be very subtle, or quite obvious. They do occur despite any dislike of or resistance to them.

When power games occur and favors are exchanged, it is important that risks be considered on both sides. Some groups or individuals feel that high risks are needed to succeed. Others feel risks should be low if success is to be achieved. Some will risk little if there is a possibility of failure, but others take high risks to avoid failure (Silber, 1981). In communications between powerful groups, the potential for gain versus loss is necessarily considered in decision making.

STRATEGIES

Power games are so widespread that elimination of this type of game is unlikely. Strategies, therefore, are better directed at understanding the behavior, gaining and maintaining appropriate control when possible, and cooperating to ensure survival of the organization as a whole. Administrative accountability and professional accountability are not necessarily at cross purposes. For instance, within the nursing department professional account-ability is directed toward provision of quality care. Administration desires quality care delivered in a cost effective manner and desires to be able to evaluate the outcomes (Clifford, 1981).

To maintain or prevent a loss of control of persons and policies within the organization, several strategies may be useful. Obtaining and sharing accurate information is a countermeasure to the action by the power players of withholding information. Action, then, can be based on facts rather than rumor. Expertise, communicated through performance and documentation, must be perceived by others and demonstrated to attain respect from group members. Promoting ways in which subordinates can identify with the leader helps to prevent their seeking another leader. Communication is a key element in this activity. Effective use of rewards and punishment in a consistent and fair manner may allow the leader to control the work environment and shape the relationship of an individual to the organization. Clear, frequent communication of how, what, and where one's responsibil-ities contribute to the organizational goals makes one less susceptible to power plays.

Understanding manipulative behavior permits the manipulation of cues affecting a decision. It requires prediction of behavior and acting on the prediction. Making the risks of some action seem relatively unimportant in relation to an anticipated reward is an example of manipulation (Claus and Bailey, 1977). Control of the environment can be considered manipulation and may be utilized successfully to alter behavior or response. For example, limiting the number of committee members may cause overwork and dis-courage the committee, slowing down or stopping the committee process.

Strategies to gain some control within an organization are dependent somewhat on where control is desired. For nursing to gain or share control with physician groups, for example, it would be essential for the true physician leaders to be identified. Improvement in communication with the physician group and gaining influence in any policy-making group would also be helpful. However, for influence within the hospital governing board, an understanding of the fiscal operation and the hospital's priorities would be essential. Appreciation of timing of institutional politics would be crucial as well. The nursing administrator may achieve the desired objectives in relation to board activities through use of expertise, logical presentation of factual information, and continual support for the final decisions of the board as a demonstration of abilities to function at or above the desired level. Active participation and assertiveness within the groups' interactions are strategies that would stress the positive effect of an individual or group on others (Niederbaumer, 1979).

Although power games have occurred for some time, there are new and stronger forces in the health care environment. Problems related to power games may be the result of the forces continually acting on health care institutions. Outside forces, such as governmental regulations, prospective payment, and competition; and internal forces, such as the medical staff and hospital departments, are continually affecting the operation of the institution. Physicians are threatened by changes in reimbursement, by certificate of need programs, and by PSRO's (Professional Standards Review Organizations). Competitive pressures are forcing hospital boards to become more active in decision making, thus threatening the power base of the physician group (Kovner and Neuhauser, 1983). Threats to various groups may encourage additional game playing.

Power relations may be weakened significantly in situations in which coalitions have not been well established. Decision making may be adversely affected when support is lacking. Stress related to rapid or numerous changes may mobilize a group's defenses and paralyze decision making as well (Stone et al, 1976). The redistribution of power will undoubtedly continue and is most certainly affected by such factors as stress and support within and without the group. Organization and delegation are required for power to be exercised in this type of environment (Ganong and Ganong, 1976). The presence of stress and the absence of support adversely affect delegation of responsibility. Recognition of these problems is another important strategy for power game players.

Negotiation

Negotiation may be identified by some as yet another game. Others may consider it a means of accomplishing goals. In either case, negotiation is a mechanism to reach goals in a manner that is satisfactory to both parties. The purpose of the negotiation is that both sides can win, although not necessarily equally. Successful negotiation requires an understanding of people and the needs of the persons/groups negotiating.

There are two basic rules in negotiation. The first rule is to always enter negotiations with room to bargain. The second rule is to begin negotiating now with low risk areas to improve skills and to improve confidence (Laser, 1981).

The elements of negotiation include (1) conflicting and non-conflicting goals, (2) variable values, (3) mutual victory, and (4) incomplete information. Both parties in a bargaining session must desire essentially the same objective, but some goal(s) must be different, or dickering would not be necessary. Identification of the conflicting area is necessary early in the process. The original values may be replaced or modified by information gained during negotiation. If values were fixed, bargaining would be unsuccessful. Mutual victory in degrees has already been identified as essential for successful negotiation. Assumption that all information is shared by both sides may result in unsuccessful negotiations. A shift in negotiating power may occur because one side has more information than the other. One piece of information that is concealed intentionally is the hidden or secret agenda, the underlying reason for agreeing to negotiate. An example of a hidden agenda might be a desire to obtain support for another project or program totally separate from the discussion and unrelated to the subject under negotiation. The secret agenda may be identified through conversational slips or through non-verbal cues such as looking away or obvious discomfort. This agenda is better understood as the negotiation process continues.

STRATEGIES

Setting deadlines is important in negotiation, with a cushion built in for safety. If the other side sets the deadline, one should always test it. Nibbling to determine what else may be gained can result in many additional features or advantages later. Even when confronted with a demand to which one could concede easily, one should leave doubt in the mind of the other party. The other party will feel they gain more, while actually little is lost. Concessions are another way to gain little victories, both in the receiving and in the making aspects. Identification of concessions may provide an edge for later negotiation. The first major concession must come from the other party for the success of this party. Any concession one makes must be recognized as such by the other side. Use of trade-offs is another method of negotiation. In either case, one should be sure that concessions are given in order of decreasing value. This implies that the limit is approaching and the other party will be reluctant to demand more.

With negotiation as well as other types of communication, listening plays an important role. Listening permits talking by others to allow the cues to be revealed. Negotiation may be very useful in meeting objectives and may result in gaining other concessions not anticipated previously.

TOMORROW'S STRATEGIES

Politics exists in health care institutions, as in other organizations, to accomplish the recognized objectives of the organization or groups within the organization. Specific strategies have been identified to address each specific game. General strategies related to institutional politics may be viewed in light of nursing theorists and their respective conceptual frameworks (see Chapter Four). Nursing administration usually fits snugly into the overall organizational structure of the institution. In today's environment, nursing administration must be involved in hospital decision making and must effectively interact with other groups in that structure. Adaptation to changes occurring within the health care environment has been essential for nursing administration. The success of the adaptation is and will be determined to a great extent by the strategies utilized.

Keeping informed of occurrences and their significance is a key strategy for nursing administration. A straightforward approach may be all that is necessary. If this is unsuccessful, calling in the favor granted in the past may provide information essential for survival. Assessment of the situational and environmental factors can assist in strengthening defenses or in preparing for necessary action.

Gaining allies can provide support for plans at a later time. Cooperation with others now may reap benefits later. Giving credit to those who deserve it will enhance loyalty in those individuals. Positive feedback is a mechanism that can be advantageous in several ways. It indicates observation and assessment, and it shows a caring attitude.

Planning is another strategy that fits well into the framework of any nursing model. Although assessment can be considered the primary step, planning involves several elements. Identification of the objectives of each project or program is essential in successful planning. Once objectives are identified, selection of alternatives and the pathway to each will be necessary. This may include selling the ideas to key groups, negotiating for a particular alternative, playing power games to accomplish a purpose, or identifying ways to gain important information.

Implementation of the ideas or alternatives involves many of the strategies identified (such as negotiation). Knowledge of the plan, organization, and delegation will help in the implementation process of any plan. Assertiveness and planning are essential in accomplishing the desired goal.

Evaluation of the process and refining the plan based on new information constitute yet another strategy. Flexibility, lacking in many groups in organizations, may assist in goal achievement and successful fulfillment of the role of nursing administrator.

Teamwork, interdepartmental involvement, and an accurate grasp of the goals of the organization are important for successful competition in health care environments. Political astuteness is a major characteristic necessary for power acquisition and success for the nursing administrator of tomorrow.

References

Alford, R. (1975). *Health care politics*. Chicago: The University of Chicago Press.
Burgess, G. (1979). Nurses as women. *Nursing Leadership*, 2(4), 26–28.

Cavanaugh, D. (1985). Gamesmanship: The art of strategizing. *The Journal of Nursing Administration*, 15(4), 38–41.

Claus, K., and Bailey, J. (1977). *Power and influence in health care*. St. Louis: C.V. Mosby Company.

Clifford, J. (1981). Managerial control versus professional autonomy: A paradox. *Journal of Nursing Administration*, 9(9), 19–21.

Crawshaw, R. (1982). Professional growth through politics. *Medical News*, September, 15.

Duncan, J., and Partridge, R. (1980). Peer polo: Overcoming the obstacles to leadership development. *Nursing Leadership*, 3(2), 18–19.

Ganong, J., and Ganong, W. (1976). *Nursing management*. Germantown, MD: Aspen Systems Corporation.

Hamm, S. (1980). The influence of formal and informal organization within a modern hospital. *Supervisor Nurse*, 11(12), 38–42.

Holl, R. (1981). Identities in nursing: A territorial issue. *Supervisor Nurse*, 12(8), 25–29.

Kalisch, P., and Kalisch, B. (1982). Nurses on prime time television. *American Journal of Nursing*, 82(2), 264–270.

Kovner, A., and Neuhauser, D. (1983). *Health service management*, 2nd ed. Ann Arbor, MI: Health Administration Press.

Laser, R. (1981). I win–you win negotiating. *Journal of Nursing Administration*, 11(11–12), 24–27.

Longest, B. (1975). Institutional politics. *Journal of Nursing Administration*, 5(3), 38–41.

Masson, V. (1981). Nursing: Healing in a feminine mode. *Journal of Nursing Administration*. 11(10), 20–24.

Niederbaumer, L. (1979). The director of nursing service: A participant in top management. *Supervisor Nurse*, 10(12), 22–27.

Peter, L., and Hull, R. (1969). *The Peter principle*. Toronto: William Morrow and Company, Inc.

Peterson, G. (1979). Power: A perspective for the nursing administrator. *Journal of Nursing Administration*, 9(7), 7–10.

Research Institute of America (1984). *How to win at organizational politics*. New York: Management Reports, Inc.

Ryan, M. (1981). Professional survival. *Supervisor Nurse*, 12(92), 16–17.

Sheard, T. (1980). The structure of conflict in nurse-physician relations. *Supervisor Nurse*, 11(8), 14–16.

Shiflett, N., and McFarland, D. (1978). Power and the nursing administrator. *Journal of Nursing Administration*, 8(3), 19–23.

Silber, M. (1981). Nurse power: Projecting self and ideas. *Supervisor Nurse*, 12(7), 65–68.

Smircich, L. (1983). Concepts of culture and organizational analysis. *Administrative Science Quarterly*, 28(September), 339–358.

Spitzer, R. (1981). The nurse in the corporate world. *Supervisor Nurse*, 12(4), 21–24.

Stone, S., Berger, M., Elhart, D., Firsich, S., and Jordan, S. (1976). *Management for nurses*. St. Louis: C.V. Mosby Company.

Trinosky, P. (1979). Nurse-doctor dissension still thrives. *Supervisor Nurse*, 10(4), 40–43.

Weisman, C., Alexander, C., and Morlock, L. (1981). Hospital decision making: What is nursing's role? *Journal of Nursing Administration*, 11(9), 31–35.

RISK MANAGEMENT

INTRODUCTION

Risk management programs have gained popularity within health care institutions since the early 1980's for a number of reasons. Although health care providers, as service organizations, were always thought to have a moral obligation to provide a safe environment and high quality patient care, laxity in the health care institutions resulted in less than optimal risk management programs (Salman, 1979). Reaction to the laxity from consumers and third party payers occurred, with a renewed interest in risk management resulting.

As health care has become more accessible, consumer expectations have increased. Particularly within the United States, consumers see health care as a right. Additionally, the level of care expected is not always realistic. There are, therefore, more consumers utilizing the health care system and demanding more from it. Third party payers who are paying the majority of the costs for health care also play a role in the concern for risk management programs.

Other factors that relate to the increased interest in risk management include the rising number of malpractice claims filed within the United States. Malpractice does unfortunately occur, but patient-physician relationships previously based on loyalty and devotion have deteriorated to such a

15

point that consumers may seek remedies for results they did not expect or desire, regardless of whether "malpractice" occurs. Rapid settlement of claims "out of court" without regard for whether liability actually existed also contributes to an increase in lawsuits (Salman, 1979).

So, as health care has become more technologically advanced and has developed more services for consumers, it has increased the risks that may be associated with the new services and technology. Management of those associated risks has gained significance in terms of priorities within health care institutions. The costs of malpractice and negligence claims, regardless of guilt, are extremely high. As more claims are paid, insurance costs continue to climb. Incentives to health care institutions to control expenses must also consider these insurance expenses. It behooves those health care institutions, then, to examine carefully their risk management programs and to ensure that resources are available to establish programs that will manage risks effectively.

This chapter will define risk, risk management, and the elements of a risk management program. It will explain the effect of external environments and internal attitudes on risk management. The elements of a risk management program will be presented and described. The prerequisites of such a program will be included. The integration of risk management and quality assurance will be emphasized. Organizing a program, including the handling of liability problems, will be discussed. The role of the nursing executive in relation to risk management and her strategies for the future will also be addressed.

RISK MANAGEMENT

Risk has been described as the probability or predictability that something will happen. A negative connotation is associated with risk. Management, on the other hand, implies positive results achieved through some activity (Brown, 1979). Schmitt (1983) further defines risk management as the "treatment of loss exposures." A loss exposure, or exposure to loss, is quite common in health care settings. These exposures to loss result from interaction of organizational elements (see Chapter 8) and the unlimited number of circumstances that give rise to potential loss. It is for these reasons that all decisions related to services, programs, facilities, and personnel, as well as direct patient care activities, involve risk management (Schmitt, 1983).

It may be said that risk management is a planning approach to risk problems or loss exposures (Brown, 1979). As such, it is a critical part of strategic planning and must be considered as such. It is important that there be an understanding of what composes a loss exposure or risk problem. Brown (1979) has identified three major elements: the subject of the loss, the value of the loss, and the cause. The subject of the loss includes anything of value and can of course be subjectively determined. The value of the loss is based on financial value and relative value. An example might include the effect of bad publicity on a new health care program. Finally, the cause of the loss may be human, economic, mechanical/electrical, or natural. This, of course, broadens the scope of risk management to include much more than the falls or medication errors previously considered. An earthquake exemplifies a natural cause; a mechanical/electrical cause might include an electrical fire; an economic cause might include changes in reimbursement regulations; and human causes might include errors in judgment. These facts and the trends in health care, economics, and law, have significantly influenced the position of risk management within health care institutions.

The external environment for health care has undergone tremendous change in recent years, and such change will continue to occur. As health care costs have risen, consumers have demanded cost control and third party payers have instituted incentives to reduce costs. Changes in reimbursement and cuts in government supported programs have jeopardized the very existence of many health care institutions. Conflicting demands for high technology, equal access, and comprehensive health care programs versus cost containment have greatly complicated the system under which health care institutions operate. In all of this is seen a basic change in attitudes about health care organizations, from one of awe to a requirement for accountability (Brown, 1979).

Within the institutions, attitudes are also changing. Whereas previously health care workers were dedicated to service regardless of the reward or the demands, the worker of today is often confused by the desire for service versus the desire for appropriate reward. This change in attitude is reflected in changes in public attitude as well. It is important, for example, to consider the current demand for the "service one pays for," when previously there was less "demand" and fewer real expectations. The dynamics of the formal and the informal organizations within health care institutions further influences the role of risk management in health care (see Chapter 14).

Another major factor impacting on risk management in health care is the crisis of liability insurance. Cost of premiums for liability coverage in health care institutions and for health care practitioners has increased at enormous rates. The crisis has had such an impact on obstetricians, for example, that many of this group of practitioners are no longer practicing OB. In many cases, liability coverage is not even available. Coverage for directors and officers, and, in some areas, for ambulance services is almost non-existent at any price. Additionally, it must be noted that these rate increases are not related to the individual institution's claims history. The stated reasons for such increases include removal of charitable or government immunity from many hospitals, a trend toward increased litigation, huge judgments or awards granted by courts, the escalating costs of living, and an increase in the number of attorneys (Brown, 1979). In any case, insurance costs are excessive and continue to rise within the health care industry.

The role of risk management in health care organizations has been and will be influenced by a number of factors that have been identified. As a result, health care institutions have found themselves in a situation in which the practice of risk management must be different than it was previously. No longer can the hospital, for example, assign risk management functions to a middle manager as an additional task. Rather, employment of a full time risk manager may be essential. In fact, many states are requiring such an individual in the health care institution. Education for the risk manager is another necessary change. Instead of an occasional workshop or vendor supplied information, in-depth training courses have become a key ingredient for successful risk managers (Schmitt, 1983).

RISK MANAGEMENT PROBLEMS

Although there are many types of risk management problems in health care, the problems that occur in risk management within health care institutions involve primarily two categories: negligence and malpractice. Liability, defined by some as responsibility, has four principles that apply to these categories and to other forms of litigation. There must be a duty to be performed. There must be a breach of the duty. Damage or harm must have occurred, and the breach of duty must have been the proximate cause of the harm or damages (Creighton, 1981).

Negligence has been defined as the failure to act as a reasonably prudent person would act in similar circumstances (Creighton, 1981). Common acts of negligence within health care institutions include falls, burns, incorrect medication, failure to communicate, property loss, failure to observe or take action, mistaken identity, foreign objects left in patient, and defects in apparatus. In every example, there must be the breach of duty, damage or harm, and proximate cause. The duty that is owed to the patient by persons who render direct health care flows from three basic duties: compliance with statutory duties such as drug laws, proper consent for care, and provision of care relatively equal to that offered by similar providers (Richards and Rathburn, 1983).

Malpractice refers to an unreasonable lack of skill in professional duties, illegal or immoral conduct, or professional misconduct. It includes disregard of rules or principles, carelessness, and acts occurring as a result of a lack of knowledge that the professional should have. As with negligence, there must be a duty, a breach of duty, and an injury that resulted from the breach. The major difference between negligence and malpractice seems to be the involvement of the professional (Creighton, 1981). Any individual may be negligent, but the professional has a specific duty to perform that requires some skill, knowledge, and behavior that meets a standard. Failure to meet the standard in performance of the duty by the professional constitutes malpractice.

Health care institutions may have multiple situations in which negligence and malpractice may occur. Patients, or the consumers of health care, have

TABLE 15-1
Elements of a Risk Management Program

1. Identification	5. Retention
2. Analysis	6. Education
3. Investigation	7. Prevention
4. Transfer	

certain reasonable expectations. It was partially because of these expectations that nurse practice and medical practice acts were created. Licensure laws were designed to protect the public and to ensure that certain expectations were met. The major expectation of the public in health care institutions (and all other public buildings, for that matter) is the safe environment. Patients also have specific rights that they may expect will be upheld. These include a right to privacy and a right to consent for treatment or to refuse treatment. When patient expectations are not met, liability and the potential for litigation are increased. A risk management program should be designed to address the problems in risk management in a variety of ways.

RISK MANAGEMENT PROGRAM

A risk management program must be designed with a purpose in mind—to manage risks. The objectives of such a program may be numerous but should certainly include those identified by Mehr and Hedges (1974): survival, stable earnings, reduced interruption of operations, lower risk management costs, continual growth of the organization, satisfaction of the institution's desire for a positive image or satisfaction of the institution's social responsibility, and peace of mind. Williams and Heins (1981) identify another objective, which is to meet regulations of certain regulatory agencies. These objectives can be met with a well designed program, but such a program must be well organized and operated well.

Elements of Risk Management

A well planned risk management program will have seven essential elements that define the responsibilities or expectations of the program. These are outlined in Table 15–1 and include identification, analysis, investigation, transfer, retention, education, and prevention. Each element is important and is an essential part of the entire program. Failure to include these essential elements in a risk management program may prove fatal for the success of the program.

Risk *identification* is the first step in successful risk management. Identification of various risks in terms of the potential loss confronting the health care institution and the likelihood of occurrence and severity composes risk identification (Williams and Heins, 1981). The identification process should be a deliberate rather than an accidental process. It should be continuous and systematic, and it should look at all potential losses to the institution. Potential losses are, of course, related to assets, which may be categorized into physical assets and intangible assets.

Physical assets of a health care institution may include property, buildings, equipment, machinery, furniture, art work, supplies, vehicles, cash, securities, animals, radioactive property, promotional displays, aircraft, or watercraft. Intangible assets refer to such assets as markets, consultants, location, availability of resources, credit lines, insurance, personnel (especially "key" personnel), foundations, and reputation. It is easy to see from this incomplete list of assets that losses could be extremely detrimental in a number of ways.

Exposure to loss of assets, then, becomes even more important. Identification of potential losses begins with a recognition of the type of loss. Exposures may be direct, indirect, or third party liabilities (Pfoffle and Nicosia, 1977). Direct exposures may be uncontrollable, including lightning, power surges, volcanos, earthquakes, sound waves, war, flood, snow, hurricanes, or falling trees. Controllable or predictable direct exposures to loss have more concern for the health care institution because of their nature. For example, equipment malfunction, spillage, fire, corrosion, employee negligence, strikes, or structural defects are within the control (to some extent, more or less) of the institution. Other controllable direct exposures to loss include embezzlement, theft, or inventory shortage.

Indirect exposures to loss of health care institutions are less concrete at times but definitely impact on the organization. Increased costs for replacement of equipment, loss of key individuals, changes in demand for programs or services, errors in managerial decision making affecting the market or the product/service, and economic fluctuations are examples of indirect exposures. Third party liabilities as exposures to loss are those compensatory or punitive damages potentially paid to third parties. Employer's liabilities such as worker's compensation, malpractice liability, negligence of employees, easements, and vehicle liability are examples of this type of exposure.

Once risks or potential risks have been identified, the severity of the potential loss must be measured. This is often referred to as risk *analysis*. Potential frequency of the loss, and its probability, are important aspects of this step, since judgments related to insurance coverage may depend on these measurements. For example, if the probability of hurricane damage is extremely low, payment of high insurance premiums for protection against such loss would probably not be considered.

Analysis of risks is accomplished so that appropriate action may be determined. In determining the extent of a potential loss, data are gathered that may come from external or internal sources and that affect the decisions related to the management of the identified risks. Sources of information include reports, medical records, quality assurance (QA) studies, protocols, outside organizations, standards, and consultants. The process for risk analysis begins with data collection from these and other sources; examination of the data to determine loss experience, especially cause and effect; estimation of costs of such losses; and the total impact of the loss.

Investigation of risks can occur during the analysis phase before loss occurs. However, this step is generally utilized after an incident that resulted in loss. Investigation is accomplished to determine cause and effect and to place responsibility when possible. Investigation requires skill and specific knowledge about risks and liability. Investigation of incidents and losses is important because of the difficulty in determining liability. Investigation may identify the duty, the breach or potential for breach of duty, the damage or harm that occurred or may occur, and the association of the breach of duty to the damage. Investigation may also be used to determine trends or patterns.

Several steps are basic to the process of investigation. Data collection is the first step and is necessary to separate opinion from fact. Obtaining reports, interviews, or physical type of evidence is a part of this data collection. Diagrams, photographs, and sketches are also tools for data collection. Determination of cause and responsibility is the next step. Defining these aspects should be viewed in terms of a potential course of action needed to direct, to the extent possible, the outcome of the incident as well as future occurrences. Finally, a thorough report, including the who, what, when, where, and how of the incident, should be completed. It is unfortunate that many health care institutions either have not formalized or do not practice these investigative techniques. Because of increasing emphasis on risk management in health care, the need for thorough investigation has become critical in the management process.

Tools for management of risk also include handling the risk once it's been identified and validated. This is generally accomplished through one of two measures—risk transfer or risk retention. Risk *transfer* is a method by which the risk is transferred to another person or group. There are several ways risks may be transferred. The most common method is purchase of insurance, in which the insurance carrier assumes responsibility for the risk in terms of financial obligation. It should be very clear that a transfer such as this, called a "risk financing transfer," does not excuse the transferor from liability. It simply shifts the financing of losses related to the risk.

There are two other ways to transfer risks. These are risk control measures that have not been as common in health care organizations previously as they are currently or will be in the future as health care institutions diversify into multiple business arenas. One such transfer technique involves transferring the property or activity responsible for the risk to another person or group. In health care, this may be exemplified by joint ventures in which all or part of the activities or programs are performed by another group who assumes liability for the activities. Selling a building to another individual or group will also shift the risk associated with ownership of the building. Associated with this transfer of risk is the transfer of risk without actual transfer of the property or activity. This is often accomplished through release forms that release from responsibility an individual or organization. In these situations, a person may be giving up his rights to hold the organization responsible. One example of this might be the release from responsibility signed by the patient who leaves a hospital against medical advice.

If risks cannot be transferred, they must be retained. *Retention* of risks is sometimes the only option an organization or business has, but retention may also be the chosen management tool. For example, if the costs for transfer are excessive, such as with liability insurance, a hospital may decide to self-insure. One specific type of example in which this could occur is insurance for emergency vehicles. If claims history has been low and there are no known factors to indicate this will change significantly, the health care institution may decide to self-insure its comprehensive coverage since the cost of coverage otherwise would be excessive.

Retention of risks may not be planned but may nevertheless occur because an organization has not realized that the loss exposure exists or has not realized the magnitude of potential loss. This, of course, is poor management of risks. There are other risks that should wisely be retained because the potential for loss is minimal and/or the costs for transfer are excessive. These risks include losses related to personal property of minimal value. This may be compared with the deductible amounts on personal property (homeowner's) insurance or automobile insurance.

Another consideration in risk retention is tax advantage. Insurance premiums are a deductible business expense, whereas the deduction of actual loss is complicated by irregularity of losses and by limitations in deductions related to property value determination (which involves depreciation versus actual cost to replace). Consideration must be given to these factors as well as others identified before decisions are made regarding risk transfer versus retention.

Education about risks is another essential element in a risk management program. For a risk management program to be effective, every employee must be involved. Employees must understand the significance of hazards and associated liabilities. In health care, this means all those liabilities associated with negligence and/or malpractice. Each manager in the health care setting must also be knowledgeable about risk management and must practice those principles necessary to manage risks effectively. For example, a manager must be knowledgeable about competent practices and take appropriate action to ensure that each employee is competent in the performance of duties. Failure to do this indicates the manager lacks understanding of risk management.

Education in risk management can be general in only a very limited manner. It is, therefore, important that specific targeting of groups for risk management be accomplished. Employee needs may then be identified and met, but, more importantly, education about risks related to the specific group's activities/functions can be discussed. This comprehensive type of program can be the key to an effective risk management program.

TABLE 15–2	
Prerequisites for Risk Management Program	
Preventive activities	Education
Corrective activities	Administrative activities
Documentation	

Prevention of loss begins with this type of educational program. Through the educational process, the staff of the institution will develop a constant awareness of potential risks, which in turn will help to prevent loss. Prevention of loss in health care is dependent on a number of variables that can help to abate potential risk situations. Patient relations is one of those variables.

Improved relationships between patients and the institution can be determined by courtesy, adequate information or mutual understanding, and open communication. Resolution of patient complaints is a part of the courtesy expected by patients. Information needed or desired by the patient is critical in his judgment of the institution in relation to his concerns. An established mechanism for dealing with complaints should be developed in every risk management program to ensure satisfaction by the patient. Many times, this is the only action a patient requires in otherwise potentially litigious situations. The importance of handling patient complaints in preventing loss cannot be overemphasized. Attention to complaints and concerns may provide the needed safeguard from those who feel no one is interested in them.

Identification of loss exposure (risks) and planning for risk transfer where appropriate are other factors in a program of prevention. Only through identification of risks can the associated losses be controlled or prevented. Planning ahead for management of those potential risks is the other part of the prevention objective.

Finally, prevention of risks can be achieved to a great extent by ensuring quality service to the consumer or patient. That quality service is important and must be included in an overall program of positive patient relations and staff education.

Prerequisites of Program

In the development of a risk management program, several prerequisites should be met. These prerequisites may already exist or may need to be established in order for the program of risk management to be effective. There are five categories (Table 15–2) into which the required activities generally fall: preventive, corrective, documentary, educational, and administrative (Brown, 1979). These correlate very well with the essential elements of a risk management program.

PREVENTIVE ACTIVITIES

Preventive activities that serve as a prerequisite for risk management begin with quality service. In health care quality service, of course, means that the patient receives care that meets acceptable standards and is delivered appropriately. As was previously mentioned, excellent care must be combined with good relationships if patient satisfaction is desired. The use of patient representatives to speak or act on behalf of the patient is an approach recommended by many organizations. The patient advocate is certainly needed in many situations. It is interesting to note that nurses for many years were "the" patient advocate. Patient advocacy, however, cannot exist in adversarial relationships, which unfortunately sometimes exist between nurses and patients. Nurses, however, may be ideally suited to this role, especially in the cost conscious environment that exists in health care. Advocacy roles are certainly best when direct contact can exist. However, a substitute that may be considered as an option is a 24 hour phone service for patient complaints (Brown, 1979). Another consideration in developing the patient advocacy role is the potential conflict between patient advocate and staff. Selection of the advocate as an objective, open-minded individual is quite important to maintain the cooperative, supportive relationship needed between advocate and staff.

Satisfying patient needs/desires is the key that is critical in preventive activities. Approaches to this include hotel services concepts, patient attitude surveys, and more diverse services. Additionally, nursing continues to change its approach to patients to involve the patient and family more in the care and to move nurses back to the patient's bedside. Many of the technological improvements in computerization, for example, are aimed at reducing indirect tasks such as writing care plans or charting and increasing direct care time. In a world in which sicker patients are the most common, this can have a significant impact.

Preventive measures for risk management must also include measures to improve personnel relations. Satisfied employees provide better services to patients to prevent patient dissatisfaction. Medical staff relations and public relations are other areas that require consideration. A positive image of the health care institution to the public and the medical staff is necessary. This may involve marketing (see Chapter 11) and certainly must involve physician participation at all levels of activity within the organization. Physicians control a great deal of the activity within health care organizations, including much of the patient's opinion. Support from and involvement of the medical staff in decisions related to the institution may be critical in the preventive activities of that institution.

Provision of safe, secure physical environments is another preventive activity. Joint Commission on Accreditation of Hospitals (JCAH), the Department of Health and Human Services (HHS), and state health agencies or boards, as well as numerous other regulatory agencies, play roles in ensuring that these health care institutions meet stringent standards for safety. From equipment maintenance to fire safety to infection control, health care organizations practice safety measures daily.

CORRECTIVE ACTIVITIES

In spite of preventive measures taken to avoid risks or loss exposure, risks will nevertheless exist. The situations that produce risk may be identified and analyzed as was previously described. Ongoing monitoring for such risks is an excellent tool for the risk manager. Such monitoring is necessary to identify potential problems so that corrective action may be implemented as needed.

Action initiated may take several forms, based on the consequences of the problem and the potential solutions to the identified problems. Where problems are identified, some form of action (as opposed to none) is usually necessary. While action may be deferred, it should be noted that failure to take action to correct identified problems may later be construed as negligent action, further increasing the risk of loss for the institution.

DOCUMENTARY ACTIVITIES

Documentation, often the most important of the prerequisites, is also frequently the most difficult to obtain in the desired format and at the desired level of detail. In health care, the persons most in contact with patients or clients are those persons who are giving direct care to the patients. Completion of paperwork is "part of the job," but the addition of incident reports or anecdotal reports about incidents is often met with resistance. In fact, even the documentation of the care patients receive, minutes of meetings, and personnel counseling records are at times difficult to obtain as desired. It must be emphasized that this documentation as well as many other records is essential in good risk management. Brown (1979) identified a number of records that he considers critical: medical records; personnel records, policies, and procedures; quality assurance reports; financial records; minutes of all committee meetings; contracts; deeds; correspondence; bylaws; and regulatory reports. Loss control reports and risk management records are also important and will likely be even more important in the future.

The place of documentation in a risk management program can be continually seen in nearly every malpractice suit or employee hearing. Repeatedly, it may be seen that documentation or lack of it can determine the outcome of a case. Particularly in light of the time lapse that routinely occurs from an occurrence to an action filed, documentation may provide credibility to the plaintiff's allegations or to the defense. Documentation serves to provide not only information relative to incidents but also information that may reveal trends, monitor quality, and/or identify problems.

It is also important that documentation be non-judgmental and state facts rather than opinions. Accusatory remarks in incident reports make such documents legally sensitive. Incident reports, for example, should be neutral, since they are often discoverable documents (i.e., able to be used as evidence). Follow-up investigation, on the other hand, is easier to protect from discovery, since it is clearly related to preparation for litigation and falls under the attorney/client privileged information (Richards and Rathburn, 1983).

EDUCATIONAL ACTIVITIES

Education has perhaps the most influence on the development of a good risk management program. Education, as a prerequisite, is understood when evaluated in light of its potential in identification, analysis, and prevention of loss. Education has been recognized by accrediting and licensing agencies as an essential element in attaining and maintaining quality practices in health care.

Education is usually divided into two primary categories—staff education and patient education. Staff education as a risk management tool prepares the staff for the steps in the risk management program. More importantly, staff education is often directed toward effective methods for task completion or toward explaining the theory that supports specific duties. Education provides orientation to responsibilities and specific standards required of staff members. Education may produce behavior modification or reinforce attitudes that can positively affect relationships.

Patient education is yet another tool for risk management in that it helps patients by improving their satisfaction. Understanding better what may be expected reduces anxiety, which too often leads to dissatisfaction. Patient education may assist patients in learning skills necessary for follow-up care or in understanding what kind of changes in their condition should produce concern. Compliance with treatment and positive attitudes are additional outcomes from good patient education programs. These are excellent prerequisites for good management of risks.

ADMINISTRATIVE ACTIVITIES

Involvement and support by administration are necessary ingredients in risk management. By providing a framework for risk management operation, administration may develop and implement organizational goals that guide the efforts of the organization, ensuring quality, consistency, and purpose (Brown, 1979). Administrative activities that serve as the prerequisite for the risk management program include development of a meaningful philosophy, open communication, well-organized structure, sound judgment, and strategic planning.

All levels of management have a role in the administrative activities identified. Support of the risk management program is essential for success. Development and implementation of objectives are important responsibilities of the managers in achieving the framework into which the other employees of the organization fit. Providing a sensible organizational structure and good communication will improve relationships and outcomes.

Decision making, which is so important at all management levels, is, of course, a function of the activities previously described—judgment, communication, structure, planning, and certainly philosophy. Once decisions are made, action becomes necessary. Evaluation or analysis of all action, preferably before it occurs, in relation to risk or loss potential is another administrative function. Obviously, excessive time cannot be spent in performing this task. However, once principles or philosophies are established and policies are developed to guide actions, management of risks becomes less of a burden.

Proactive thinking and planning, then, become important in risk management. Strategic thinking, as it is called in Chapter 8, is critical in the success of such a program. Reaction to problems, on the other hand, may result in failure or loss unnecessarily. A supportive and proactive attitude for the administrators and managers is just as important as it is for other staff members in the development of a good risk management program.

QUALITY ASSURANCE/RISK MANAGEMENT PROGRAM

There has been a trend developing in the health care industry toward formalizing a relationship between risk management and quality assurance. Because of the similarities that exist in the purposes of these activities, the trend is one that is understandable and logical. Both risk management and quality assurance must have continuous and ongoing monitoring that will identify problem areas that may result in a loss of some type. In risk management, the loss covers a variety of forms, whereas quality assurance is generally tied to the patient. For example, both medication errors and an inaccurate malfunctioning time clock should fall under the category of loss. However, only the medication error would be patient related. Both risk management and quality assurance look for trends or patterns of noncompliance, either with safety practices or with goals, objectives, policies, procedures, and standards. Quality assurance and risk management also have as a major purpose prevention of future losses.

Even with the identified similarities, it must be recognized that there are a number of areas within quality assurance and risk management that do not overlap. Orlikoff and Lanham (1981) identify five of these areas (Table 15–3). The focus of risk management is on the protection of the various assets (tangible and intangible) of the organization, whereas quality assurance must focus on the quality of patient care. Whereas risk management has concern with the legally acceptable level of care, quality assurance must seek the optimal level of care. Quality assurance activities are directed only

| TABLE 15–3 | | |
| Differences Between Risk Management and Quality Assurance | | |
Area	Risk Management	Quality Assurance
Motivation and focus	Protection of assets of institution	Quality of patient care
Level of care	Acceptable from legal perspective	Optimal
Direction	Toward all persons, events, and surroundings in health care setting	Toward patient care
Specialization	Loss prevention and risk financing activities	Quality of care measured against standards
Role	More of focus in loss prevention activities	Improve quality care through activities

Based on Orlikoff, J. E., and Lanham, G. B. (1981). Why risk management and quality assurance should be integrated. *Hospitals, 55*(11), 54–55.

toward patient care activities and outcomes, but risk management deals with all events or persons in the health care setting. Risk management specializes in loss prevention and risk financing activities, with a focus on loss prevention. Quality assurance, on the other hand, measures the quality of care against standards and seeks to improve that quality.

Consolidation of risk management and quality assurance programs can be advantageous to the organization in several ways. In the health care environments facing institutions today and in the future, such integration can reduce budgetary expenses. Even more importantly, however, is the effect of such action on the overall focus of both programs. Risk management may see beyond "acceptable levels" to the impact of improved quality on potential loss. For example, improved quality of care can significantly impact on attitudes of patients in a positive way and reduce the risk of litigation that is unwarranted. Whether a patient wins or loses a lawsuit, litigation is costly to the institution because of attorney fees, investigation, employee time, etc. Quality assurance, in the other direction, may be able to better understand the need for cost control and the "best quality for the most reasonable cost" when it is integrated with risk management.

Perhaps the major reason for consolidating risk management and quality assurance programs is to provide effective planning for these programs. Reacting to problems has been the general thrust of risk management in the past, yet the mechanisms needed to monitor and provide data beneficial to risk management have been in effect in most health care institutions for some time. Coordination of risk management and quality assurance programs can improve the effectiveness of both programs by enhancing communication and by providing a mechanism for review of quality assurance to ensure adequate risk detection and control. A good example of how this can work in the hospital setting is medication variance reporting. Monitoring medication variances is a quality assurance tool to identify potential problem areas or trends. Risk management and quality assurance programs may find the data useful in different ways. Risk management reviews the data in terms of potential loss for the institution. The same data, when reviewed by quality assurance personnel, reveal problems that threaten the level of quality care the patient receives and can often pinpoint serious problems requiring action. Action taken can eliminate the threat to the patient, shift the responsibility from one person or group to another without eliminating the threat, or reduce the loss potential with or without affecting the quality issue.

ORGANIZATION OF A RISK MANAGEMENT PROGRAM

The organization of a risk management program in the health care institution may take one of several paths; but several considerations are important in the initial stages of development. As was exemplified in the previous section on quality assurance and risk management, the risk management program should be coordinated with existing programs such as safety, security, and quality assurance. Although risk management programs generally are designed to advise and support other departments, it is important that all hospital departments be included in the scope of activities. Involvement of the medical records department is especially important, since this department may be called upon to locate records on a frequent basis. Commitment of resources, including human, material, and financial, is essential, and the result should be that the program will be able to justify its existence from the service and fiscal points of view (Brown, 1979). Measurement of results may include reduction in litigation, complaints, reported losses, dollars spent in settlement, etc.

All activities in the health care institution are involved with risk management. Organization of a risk management program should provide the mechanisms by which input from and feedback to each department can be accomplished. Attitudes are, of course, important as the program is developed. Department managers must understand that the risk management program has the responsibility of reviewing policy, procedures, and activities and of making recommendations for changes that will prevent or reduce potential loss. If there is inadequate support for a risk management program, this responsibility cannot be fulfilled.

The structure of the risk management program may vary from institution to institution, but basically it requires formation of a representative committee. Related committees may include quality assurance and safety committees. Depending on the size of the institution, other overlapping committees may also include disaster planning, infection control, education, and environmental control committees. Each of these committees may provide important data for risk management, but will usually need to function separately from the risk management committee.

The risk management program must also have a manager whose expertise must primarily be in management. Although many states have already implemented legislation to require full time risk managers in health care institutions such as hospitals, in other states the decision for the time commitment required of the risk manager in a particular institution must be based on the current and anticipated needs and problems in the areas of risk prevention and loss control. Certainly, consideration must also be given to the environment relative to potential litigation. One approach that may be helpful is initiating a part time position with planning toward full time as the need arises. This may be accomplished by expanding an existing position. One major danger in developing this position is overloading the individual by inadequately planning for changes in responsibility.

Experience and education for the risk manager are important. As was previously discussed, education for this role has been limited in the past, but more and more training programs are being offered. Experience that would be helpful for the risk manager includes knowledge of or training in the areas of insurance, safety, nursing, claims management, quality assurance, education, research, finance, personnel management, and investigation. Because of the close contact with all departments and the sensitive nature of many of the activities, the risk manager must have good interpersonal relation skills as well.

Responsibilities of the risk manager may vary from place to place, so long as the identified elements of a risk management program may be accomplished (see Table 15–1). The risk management program will have specific policies and procedures that define how risks are identified, how incidents are reported, and what action may be taken. Additionally, all policies and procedures may need to be reviewed by the risk manager to ensure that risk detection and loss prevention goals are addressed as necessary. The risk manager should also review all reported incidents, initiate adequate investigation, and follow-up as appropriate. Review of insurance coverage in all areas should be a part of the risk manager's responsibilities.

Besides analyzing the role of the risk manager in the program, it is also wise to review the expectations from other employees with respect to the program (Brown, 1979). Department heads are generally responsible for development and enforcement of safety policies within their department, for identifying and correcting problems or potential problems, for staff education in safety practices, and for appropriate equipment maintenance and repair. All employees have responsibilities for following safety practices and rules, for participating in drills as requested, and for reporting injuries or unsafe conditions or practices to the appropriate supervisor. Even the medical staff of the institution is expected to cooperate with a risk management program through credentialing, participation in committee activities, documentation, quality assurance activities, and education. Hospital attorneys primarily are responsible for representing the hospital in litigation proceedings. However, attorneys may also advise the governing body, administration, and medical staff in relation to legal implications of contracts, policies, bylaws, rules and regulations, committee activities, or operational activities. Occasionally, consultants are also utilized in risk management to assist in establishing services or programs that will fit with risk management objectives, including self-insurance functions.

TOMORROW'S STRATEGIES

In all of the discussion about organization of the risk management program, the role of the nursing administrator has not been specifically addressed, for one major reason. The nursing administrator has no specific separate role in such a program. However, both today and tomorrow, the nursing administrator may serve as a major catalyst for the development and support of such a program. As a labor intensive department, nursing generally has the largest percentage of employees of all hospital departments. As such, it has the greatest impact on potential risk or loss. As the only department with 24 hour continual contact with patients, nursing has, unfortunately, tremendous potential for liability. The nursing administrator, then, must first recognize this and then must identify the mechanisms by which she may work with the risk manager to control liability and reduce risks.

Risk management is aimed at eliminating harm and reducing costs associated with harm (Brown, 1979). Cooperation between risk management and nursing is essential in accomplishing those objectives. With the somewhat hostile external environment that hospitals and other health care institutions are facing, including demands by consumers and increasing liability hazards, the difficulty of a risk management program is more pronounced. The internal environment, including interdepartment competition, program development, and staffing problems, has also become more complicated, which creates even more problems. Without a cooperative and well developed relationship between nursing and risk management, the program cannot succeed.

The nursing administrator can support the risk management program by first recognizing its benefit and usefulness to the nursing department and the institution as a whole. Good communication between the risk manager and nursing administrator is essential to ensure that adequate monitoring of nursing activities is done (quality assurance; QA), that identified problems or trends are recognized and adequately addressed, that documentation is appropriate, and that continuing education is ongoing. Integration of the nursing quality assurance program into the hospital risk management program is a proactive stance that would be beneficial to the department of nursing and the risk management program. This may be accomplished through coordinated planning of QA monitors, appropriate reporting, and follow-up. Utilization of data from either program by the other could provide the necessary input for sound decisions about alternatives in problem resolution. Mechanisms that will serve to accomplish goals of both programs include documentation and education. Education, especially, must be supported by both the risk manager and the nursing administrator to maintain and improve nursing practice and to assist the nursing staff in dealing with ever present risk management problems. Coordination of the two programs is important. An example of this type of coordination may be seen in patient falls. This is an obvious risk management problem, since falls lead to fractures, which may mean litigation. This is also a QA monitor, since falls mean complications and impact on quality of care. Monitoring falls and recognizing trends, associated factors, and causes can be dually performed. Action may be initiated jointly, and follow-up studies the combined efforts of both departments.

The major focus for the nursing administrator in the management of risks will continue to be documentation. No other activity can substitute for written evidence of action, behavior, intervention, or response. Given the delays in litigation, accurate and thorough documentation is essential. Mechanisms that improve documentation should be investigated and implemented by the nursing administrator. Computer programs available currently will expand to support this need even more.

The nursing administrator can also support risk management in the elements identified in Table 15–1: risk identification, analysis, investigation, transfer, retention, education, and prevention. Especially in the situation in which the risk manager is not a nurse, the nursing administrator can interpret policy and procedure and can assist the risk manager in the decision making processes necessary to achieve the specific elements described.

A risk management program is an essential part of current health care institutions. Risk management is—must be—a team concept. The nursing administrator can contribute much to the program through participation on the risk management team. Through the activities and functions described, the risk management program can make a significant difference in the control of liability. The nursing administrator needs to be a part of that difference.

References

Brown, B. L. (1979). *Risk management for hospitals: A practical approach*. Germantown, MD: Aspen Systems Corporation.
Creighton, H. (1981). *Law every nurse should know*, 4th ed. Philadelphia: W. B. Saunders Company.
Mehr, R., and Hedges, B. (1974). *Risk management: Concepts and applications*. Homewood, IL: Richard D. Irwin, Inc.
Orlikoff, J. E., and Lanham, G. B. (1981). Why risk management and quality assurance should be integrated. *Hospitals*, 55(11), 54–55.
Pfoffle, A. E., and Nicosia, S. (1977). *Risk analysis guide to insurance and employee benefits*. New York: Amacom, a Division of American Management Association.
Richards, E. P., and Rathburn, K. C. (1983). *Medical risk management: Preventive legal strategies for health care providers*. Rockville, MD: Aspen Systems Corporation.

Salman, S. L. (1979). A systems approach can assure high quality care and low costs. *Hospitals*, March 16, 79–82.

Schmitt, J. (1983). Risk management—It's more than just insurance. *Hospital Financial Management*, March, 10–22.

Williams, C., Head, G., Horn, R., and Glendenning, G. (1981). *Principles of risk management and insurance*, 2nd ed. Malvern, PA: American Institute for Property and Liability Underwriters.

Williams, C. A., and Heins, R. M. (1981). *Risk management and insurance*, 4th ed. New York: McGraw-Hill Book Company.

NURSING
ADMINISTRATION

V

The first four sections of this book have provided the framework for Section V, Nursing Administration. Each section has identified specific building blocks and has discussed the materials necessary for the foundation. Section V pulls together these building blocks to produce the synergistic practice of nursing administration, which is administration, nursing, and human relations management. Both chapters in Section V are devoted to a major portion of the nursing administrator's responsibility.

Human Relations Management, Chapter 16, will include sections on recruitment, placement, and retention. Direction of careers with counseling, evaluation, and disciplinary action will be discussed. Labor relations, including employee benefits, responsibilities, and accountabilities, will also be addressed. Primarily, the nurse executive must manage resources (human, material, and financial) to achieve specific goals (optimal care of patients). Whether hiring, educating, directing, consulting, or controlling, the nurse administrator fits into this role. Adequate preparation for the role certainly includes the foundations identified and the development of each aspect of the desired role.

Chapter 17, Patient Care Management, will look at care delivery, quality assurance, standards of care, staffing, and education. Specific emphasis will be placed on patient acuity systems, discharge planning, continuity of care, mode of care delivery, and certification. Staff and patient education program development will also be included.

HUMAN RELATIONS MANAGEMENT

INTRODUCTION

This chapter addresses the most significant resource of any organization—its people. Despite the significance of this chapter, it cannot stand independent of the other chapters because a leader and manager's attitudes, philosophies, knowledge, and skills are inherently tied to her personnel management. The attitude of this chapter is to accentuate the positive approach to people management. However, the darker side, such as labor union activity and chemically dependent personnel, does exist and therefore must also be addressed.

The supply of professional nurses will be restricted because of such factors as the BSN requirement for professional practice and the growth of alternative health care delivery systems. Higher patient acuity, more technologically complex care, and alternative delivery modes will demand a more flexible professional nurse who can practice efficiently and effectively

16

in a variety of settings. Therefore, personnel management will become even more critical.

RECRUITMENT

Although the big recruitment budgets and aggressive nurse recruiters were once considered things of the past, recurring shortages of nurses have necessitated their resurgence. Historically, the sheer numbers of nurses required to operate a health care organization were the focal point of most recruitment. Rapid expansion of services and capacity of physical plants demanded large head counts. Currently, the nurse leader and manager is faced with the situation of selected vacancies. Economic pressures mandate a short orientation period, yet one that effectively produces a highly pro- ductive nurse in that short period of time. This need implies the obvious advantages of recruiting nurses already experienced in the area in which the particular vacancy exists. Experienced nurses can only be obtained from two sources. A limited number are currently not in the labor force, either not working or in school. It may be possible to identify these nurses and recruit them on an individual basis. The other source of experienced nurses is found in other health care organizations. Actively recruiting nurses from other organizations is not considered a "nice" thing to do among administrators. It is acceptable if the nurse is unhappy or dissatisfied and seeks out another organization. But going after another hospital's ICU or nursery nurse does not improve that organization's community image. As a result, organizations will advertise their selected vacancies and hope the right nurse will read the advertisement. The aggressive organization will contact these nurses through an associate and offer incentives to switch employment. Both recruiting strategies can be effective, but there is a difference in time and cost. Competition among health care organizations has already increased tremen- dously, and a little less good will might not significantly impact on the existing relationships. A recruitment strategy that may not appear to be as devious could involve recruitment at a meeting of the local group of specialty nurses. This type of recruitment is more directly targeted at the group in demand than a newspaper ad, and is somewhat more tasteful than a bounty hunt.

Recruitment of new graduates will also continue. However, the lack of quantity needs will result in a shifting to an emphasis on quality. This quality emphasis should reinforce the move toward the baccalaureate degree as the entry level into practice. Nursing administrators of patient care services should target specific schools that are interested in working with them to deliver the type of practitioner the organization needs. Schools will be more interested in working with health care organizations that are willing to guarantee the placement of their graduates. Declining enrollments can be offset when the school can ensure its graduates of a place of employment.

The maldistribution of available nurses still exists. Rural areas still have many more vacancies than urban areas. The closing and downsizing of urban health care organizations create opportunities for rural areas to maximize their recruitment efforts.

Inherent in any recruitment discussion is the understanding that the patient care service area in need of nurses must market itself in the recruitment effort. All nurses are much more selective in their choices of employment than in the past. There are fewer differences in benefit packages than there once were. There is greater concern over seniority and job security, making nurses less eager to change employers. Nurses have a better understanding of what they are looking for in a practice setting. Therefore, it is necessary for the recruiter to communicate clearly the advantages and disadvantages of the area in need. Where competition is fierce for one subspecialty group of nurses, the marketing program must emphasize the unique aspects of employment with that particular organization.

Nurses have not been and still are not good at selling themselves. The nursing shortage of the early 1980's helped to overcome some of this shyness. However, in the late 1980's and early 1990's, the successful marketing strategy for nurses will emphasize the proper fit between the professional nurse and the job that needs to be done.

The mechanics of recruitment should be based on a master strategy that addresses the major components identified thus far. General recruitment should focus on two components. The first component deals with the relationship of the organization with one or more schools of nursing. The second component deals with community profile. Responsibility for these two components can be delegated to some extent to the human resource department or shared through a recruitment committee. A recruitment committee composed of both nursing and human resources personnel provides flexibility and also the necessary resources for a third component that recruitment should address—that of specialty needs. A group of experienced people, such as the committee, is responsible for the master plan and materials for recruitment to ensure that the organization will not be unprepared for a new service initiated at a competitive organization. Likewise, this group provides the general expertise for recruitment, but can draw specialty nurses into the group as needed to recruit for special vacancies as they occur.

The master strategy and ongoing responsibility of this recruitment committee and group include several aspects. This group reviews all advertising to ensure that it is accurate, is timely, and communicates the desired impression. Handouts and other printed material are reviewed at least annually to keep them fresh and current. Meetings with executive level administrators should occur as needed, involving either the group or the chairperson, so that recruitment activities are consistent with the movement of the organization as a whole. Finally, the annual development of a recruitment budget is the responsibility of this group.

Although there are fewer recruitment dollars available than in the past, the job they have to accomplish is of smaller magnitude and focus. It is, however, inappropriate to say that there is no need for a recruitment budget because turnover has been reduced and fewer vacancies exist. Recruitment will always be necessary to some extent. As the nursing shortage reappears and increases, the organization that has sharpened its recruitment skills and maintained a profile in the community will have a definitive advantage over other institutions.

RETENTION

The concept of retention involves more than reducing the rate of turnover to some preordained level. In actuality, turnover is not the terrible indicator it is usually made out to be. A certain amount of turnover is inevitable, and it varies based on the locale. Normal turnover is due to spouse transfer, pregnancy, illness, and retirement. Desirable turnover also involves the elimination of undesirable employees. There are some behaviorists who would argue that every firing or termination is a failure on the part of management and the organization. This type of attitude is unrealistic and places unnecessary guilt on these parties. Attempts should be made to place individuals in the job that is correct for them. However, sometimes there just is not a job that they can do or someone makes a human mistake in hiring. Turnover also allows for the infusion of fresh ideas into a system. When there are no new inputs into a product, the output never changes. Lack of turnover can also lead to a condition known as group think. Group thinking involves a similar thought process, shared values, and goals. With group thinking, alternatives are not positively sanctioned.

Retention begins with the initial contact made by the prospective nurse with the organization. First impressions, including the ease of entry into the system, can do a great deal to form a good opinion. Difficulty in accessing a system in order to find out about a position and its benefits indicates to the potential employee that there is a complex bureaucracy and that communication is not valued. Although due processing of applications is necessary in order to adequately protect the institution, an applicant should not have to work through several different people in order to find out the precise expectations of a position. The manager directly responsible for the vacant position is usually the person best able to hire for that position. Therefore, it is only common sense to establish that relationship as quickly as possible.

Interview

There are three main purposes of an interview. Ideally, these purposes are shared by both the employer and the potential employee. Unfortunately, however, that is not always the case. Employees who have previously been unsuccessful in positions are sometimes so anxious to relocate, they will seek any job they can obtain. Other employees, usually new graduates, are truly not able to discern the information they need in order to make an informed decision. As a result, in both of these situations, the employer is ultimately responsible for the outcome of the interview. Even if the prospective nurse is not hired, she can leave the relationship feeling good about both herself and the institution. This will occur if the three purposes of the interview are accomplished.

The main objective of the interview is to find the right person for the duties of the position. This is much more difficult than it sounds, as any experienced nurse administrator can attest. Every position is unique, even if the title is staff nurse and there are 365 staff nurse positions. That is because each position has a unique relationship to the other positions with which it interfaces, and each operates within a unique environment. In order to hire the best individual for the position, two other objectives have to be accomplished during the interview.

One essential objective is for the employer to accurately describe and effectively communicate the expectations of the job, and the atmosphere and conditions in which the job is performed. This objective is essential in order for the applicant to make an informed decision about her abilities to meet the expectations, as well as about the desirability of the work environment. The manager directly responsible for the position is usually the person most qualified to discuss the expectations of the job and the work environment. It may be helpful, however, to include a staff member's perspective of the job sometime during the interview process.

Finally, in order for the right person to be hired for the job, the third objective is the applicant's accurate communication to the employer concerning her strengths, weaknesses, and career goals. It is only when there is a close fit between what the employer is communicating and what the applicant is communicating that the best person is found for the position. When this occurs, retention of the employee has begun on a firm foundation.

In order for the three objectives of an interview to be accomplished, several details need to occur. The setting is important. The interview should proceed through several settings. Initially, privacy and comfort are important in establishing rapport and ensuring there are no distractions or interruptions to communication. At some point, introduction to the actual work environment is indicated. Depending on the organizational level of the position, it may be appropriate to include interviews with other key individuals. These individuals should expect the applicant, be familiar with the applicant's resume and know what their responsibilities are during their interview time. Following this active part of the interview, there should be another private time. This provides an opportunity for questions, clarification of issues, review of main points and significant benefits, summary, and closure. When this process is complete, the employer and applicant know where they are, who is responsible for the next step, and when the next step is to occur.

Interviews that accomplish the three stated objectives are primarily the result of a skilled and experienced interviewer. Although the applicant's ability to communicate and her accurate appraisal of her own abilities do contribute to the effectiveness of the interview, the fact remains that the majority of applicants are anxious and uncomfortable in this unusual role. Becoming a skilled and experienced interviewer should not be left to chance in the development of any nurse administrator. Planned experiences to observe different types of interviews as well as being observed interviewing are two strategies to acquire skill and experience. During these experiences, the nurse administrator can learn techniques of putting people at ease. These include meeting the applicant at the door with a handshake, showing her where she is to sit, and offering her coffee or a cold drink. The sitting arrangement can also communicate messages to the applicant. If there is a desk between the interviewer and the applicant, it implies distance and impersonalization. Sitting together at a table creates fewer barriers, as does sitting in comfortable chairs with no table between the participants. It is helpful to open the interview with non–job-related questions or comments, either about the individual, such as a compliment, or about the institution. It is then helpful to outline the process of the interview so that the applicant knows what to expect and can mentally prepare himself for the flow of events. For example, the employer might say:

Mrs. Jones, I usually interview potential employees by first finding out about you as a professional, such as your strengths and weaknesses; what is important to you in a position. What are your career goals. Then, I try and tell you about us as an organization. Where are we going, what our strengths and weaknesses are. Then, I will cover the specific job in some detail, including salary, orientation, and benefits. Following that, we'll visit the patient care area, where you will meet several coworkers. Then we'll come back here and tie up any loose ends. This will take us about 90 minutes. If this is agreeable to you, let's get started.

In discussing the applicant's strengths and weaknesses, it is helpful to be familiar with the employment history. Gaps in dates need to be explained, as do short tenure or drops in successive salaries or position. Strengths and weaknesses can be identified by discussing responsibilities that the applicant felt confident performing or types of patients he or she enjoyed. Identifying situations in which the applicant felt anxious and angry can also provide insight. These types of questions encourage applicants to talk about themselves, whereas short answer questions put the burden of the conversation on the employer. If you suspect an undesirable situation, such as a previous termination, it is difficult not to ask a leading question or present an opinion and ask for confirmation. Nevertheless, it is better to avoid doing this. More information will be gained in the long run if these types of questions and opinions are avoided because the applicant will not be put on the defensive.

Once the process of the interview has been outlined, return to the first section and begin with one question at a time. As the applicant is led through her professional career, impressions, signals, and further questions are forming in the interviewer's mind. The interviewer should make short, inconspicuous notes as necessary, but should concentrate on listening.

When the time comes in the interview for the employer to inform the applicant about the job and the work environment, two strategies can be very effective. First moving from big to little, the employer can put the individual job in perspective to the total organization. The applicant then develops a sense of how she can contribute to the total operation. It is not necessary to bore the applicant with complex organizational charts. Herein lies the second strategy. In order to communicate, it is necessary to use language understood by the applicant. Abbreviations unique to the organization are a mystery to the applicant and can be demeaning. It is best to describe the total organization using common terms and simple explanations. Detail is not essential or necessary. Beginning with the total organization, one can break down the responsibilities for goods and services to the main area where the particular job is located. In this manner, career mobility, in terms of lateral or upward mobility, can be better illustrated. If career mobility is just alluded to, the applicant is without reference points in this particular organization to determine actual possibilities. Lines of authority and responsibility immediately surrounding the position should be reviewed in some detail. Likewise, specific job responsibilities and evaluation criteria, process, and frequency are specifically covered. During this period, the applicant is receiving a great deal of information and as a result may not have many questions. A visit to the work environment followed by a summary time allows the applicant to internalize some of the information and raise questions.

Job Placement

Assuming that the right individual has been hired for the position, retention continues through the process of job placement. For the purposes of this chapter, job placement refers to the socialization of the individual into the organization and the role prescribed by occupying a given position. There must be a commitment in the philosophy of the organization, by the nurse administrator and by the individuals involved in the role set to this socialization process. Obviously, one of the major components of job placement is orientation. However thorough and comprehensive an orientation program may be, it frequently is regarded as the responsibility of a few key individuals. The concept being presented here concerns the recognition of all members of the role set, including superiors, peers, and subordinates, in helping one another to reach their maximum potential within their respective jobs. Clearly defined expectations and open communication are the best ways to ensure that the socialization is accomplished in a positive way. Job placement implies the knowledge of not just what one job entails, but also how it relates to every other job. When an employee is confident about boundaries, relationships, and expectations, she is free to concentrate on the duties of the job. This security frees her from unnecessary anxiety and confusion, which drains employees of motivation, enthusiasm, and energy.

As employees perform well in their jobs, they gain confidence. This is reflected in their evaluations.

EVALUATION

Evaluation of an employee's performance has four objectives:

- To provide an opportunity for reflection and feedback on work performance and the work environment for a given period of time between an employee and supervisor
- To acknowledge and encourage appropriate and above standard performance
- To identify and remove distractors, dissatisfiers, and obstacles, as well as ineffective behaviors
- To identify areas of growth for the employee and organization (Rowland and Rowland, 1984)

Given these objectives, it seems paradoxical that for many managers and employees evaluations are regarded with dread and anxiety. These negative attitudes are the result of many years of experience by both supervisor and employee with unfair, subjective, cumbersome, and erratic evaluation processes, criteria, and outcomes that begin as early as elementary school. Building on these less than desirable experiences, the evolution of performance appraisal has resulted in the development, adoption, revision, and changes in as many different types of appraisal systems as there are employees. In an effort to find the perfect evaluation tool and method, organizations have changed their policies sometimes as often as every three years. This is extremely frustrating to both employees and supervisors.

Another major problem with employee evaluations is the lack of training of supervisors in coaching and evaluation of employees. Traditionally, in nursing, the best clinical nurses were frequently promoted. It was then assumed that since they knew "good" nursing practice, they were qualified to evaluate their staff. Knowledge of nursing practice is essential, but it is not the only requirement for effective performance appraisal. It is also necessary to be able to break down the performance into discrete behaviors. In doing so, only those unacceptable behaviors can be eliminated. Acceptable behaviors can be reinforced. The ability to communicate this information in such a way as to motivate the employee is an essential component of the evaluation process. Being able to identify employee potential and knowing how to develop that potential constitute one of the most difficult aspects of employee appraisal, for several reasons. Depending on the background of the supervisor, he may not be knowledgeable about jobs beyond or above his immediate area. If the supervisor is not developing his own potential and is not acquiring new knowledge and skills, his perspective is very limited for both himself and his employees. Another reason for difficulty is that developing the potential in others can be perceived as very threatening by some supervisors. The supervisor may be concerned that the employee may be interested in obtaining the supervisor's job or competing with the supervisor for a promotion. It takes a mature supervisor to go beyond this type of paranoia.

Another type of problem experienced by the supervisor who excels at employee motivation and development is the constant rebuilding that has to occur. If the supervisor is known for the wealth of employees in his department, the department experiences frequent loss of employees to lateral and upward promotions. On one hand, this is very rewarding to the supervisor, but at the same time it can be a draining experience. This supervisor may then be tempted to hold back his employees in order to reduce turnover and provide the department with some stability.

As the preceding discussion illustrates, the employee evaluation process is embodied with many types of pitfalls, which are all but impossible to avoid.

There are some basic principles that can help to minimize the difficulties associated with employee performance appraisal:

- Objectives of appraisals are identified to all parties.
- Results of appraisals are clearly understood.
- The appraisal process and tool are developed with input from all levels of employees affected by the job responsibilities.
- The supervisor has received education and training in the use of the appraisal process and tool.
- The appraisal process is valued by the organization.
- The appraisal process occurs consistently.

Although some of these statements may seem somewhat obvious, it is amazing to discover how varied the actual practice of employee evaluation or performance appraisal is among institutions.

The actual types of evaluations or performance tools also vary considerably between and among institutions. Within institutions, tools may vary between classifications of personnel. Many organizations, dissatisfied with standardized forms, have gone to considerable time and expense to develop their own tools for every type of position. At the other extreme, a standard form is used for every employee of some institutions.

Methods of performance appraisals are numerous. There is the rating scale. A rating scale can either be a continuous scale or be composed of discrete scales. These types of scales allow for numerical tabulation of scores. Problems associated with scales involve the interpretation of the total score. Total scores are usually interpreted as being unacceptable, acceptable, average, expected, above average, or exceptional. The main problem involves people's dissatisfaction with being average or acceptable. These middle ratings are associated with the mark of "C." The majority of people feel put down with this classification, because a "B" is actually what is considered acceptable. Some organizations have attempted to avoid these labels and simply attach salary or merit increases to groups of points, or to disassociate wage changes from the process entirely. A variation of the scale is the weighted scale. Specific behaviors are weighted as a result of their degree of significant impact on ultimate job performance. Many people feel this is more accurate than having all behaviors contributing equally to job performance.

Employee comparison methods are not frequently used in health care because they create more problems than they solve unless the comparison is against a standard and not a personal comparison. One form of comparison is a ranking method, and another is the forced distribution. The forced distribution requires that employees be ranked according to a normal bell curve. In practice, the normal bell curve is not necessarily a desirable standard nor does it actually exist. Other forms of evaluations include documenting critical incidences, which unfortunately often emphasizes negative incidences; essay, which is very subjective; and joint appraisal, which may involve more than one supervisor or peer review (Rowland and Rowland, 1984).

Smith and Elbert (1980) advocated a behaviorally anchored rating scale (BARS) that involves specific behaviors anchored to a scale ranging from ineffective to effective performance. The development of this system is one of its major strong points. Although it is a time-consuming process, the system results from input from supervisors and employees, which makes it more acceptable to both groups. These authors also advocated a combination of the behaviorally anchored rating scale with specific objectives. Since many organizations operate under management by objectives (MBO), this is a possible alternative. Many organizations are also introducing incentive-associated appraisal programs in which an employee is compensated according to the increase in production and profit associated with his job performance. Although these incentive programs have largely been introduced among middle and upper management, there are examples of department-wide incentive programs within health care. Examples include monetary rewards based on a specific percentage of the amount of money saved in a department by the employee's idea. It is anticipated that more of these programs will be introduced in order to encourage productivity and maximize cost effective behaviors. Because of these trends, a combination of BARS and MBO appraisal methods may be very appropriate.

Whatever evaluation or performance appraisal a manager is either blessed or cursed with, he has two strategies with which to work. The first strategy is a long-term commitment not to be content with the status quo. Working within the system for change is part of the manager's responsibility. These changes may involve a complete overhaul of the evaluation process and tool. Changes of this magnitude take a long time and involve the marshalling and commitment of many resources. It is not a short-term goal. In situations in which the evaluation process is basically sound, it then becomes the manager's responsibility to ensure that the process remains current and relevant.

The second strategy concerns the manager's or supervisor's ability to use the process appropriately and to maximize its potential to achieve the objectives identified at the beginning of this section. This is determined to a large extent by the manager's knowledge, skills, and attitude. The process must be regarded as a positive, valued experience. The manager or supervisor must also be prepared to complete the evaluation process. No matter what type of performance appraisal is used by an organization, some form of input by the employee is of extreme value and important to the successful outcome of the process. Many supervisors solicit this input at the time of the evaluation, either verbally or in writing. Others prefer to get this input prior to completing the evaluation. In this manner, items of significance and concern to the employee are readily identified, and there is assurance that they will not be overlooked during the actual evaluation. Some employees resent providing input. These employees may feel they are doing the supervisor's job for them because in some instances, the supervisor has simply used the employee's self-evaluation. This is inappropriate and does not remove the supervisor's responsibility for completing a thorough evaluation of the employee's performance.

The evaluation is scheduled for a time and place that ensures privacy and adequate time. As part of the performance appraisal, the manager communicates how well the employee is performing his job responsibilities, which behaviors are appropriate, and which behaviors are not effectively contributing to good performance. It is during this time that there is mutual discussion on those things that are interfering with appropriate behaviors, how best to remove these obstacles, and who is responsible for removing them. An evaluation of the supervisor's performance is not appropriate at this time. Supervisors or managers desiring feedback on how their performance is affecting their employees' performance or wanting to improve upward communication should request this feedback at another time. It is inappropriate to use this time for those purposes. Information of this nature obtained during evaluation times will undoubtedly be distorted and shaded, owing to the natural anxieties of the employee concerned about repercussions.

Institutions are now gearing their performance appraisals to address behaviors that directly affect productivity. As a result, the impact of changing behaviors should be more measurable through changes in productivity. Likewise, strategies agreed upon by both supervisor and subordinate may be chosen only to the extent that they affect productivity. For example, a supervisor inquires of an employee what kind of additional information would help him perform his job better. The employee should like to learn more about a new procedure that is being done at the hospital, but not in the employee's patient service area. The employee's rationale is that he would be able to answer questions about the procedure if asked by his patients. Although this request is not without some validity, it does not directly impact on the employee's productivity. Using this as a standard, the supervisor can objectively make a decision concerning the request. Of course, the supervisor may not choose to flatly deny the request, but rather choose the method to provide the employee with the information he desires at minimal or no cost to the institution. Likewise, requests to attend inservice or continuing education programs can now be evaluated in terms of their impact on productivity. As staff members become cognizant of this relationship, they will become more adept at demonstrating a direct relationship between the two.

CAREER COUNSELING

Career counseling, job placement, and performance appraisal or evaluations are all part of the larger picture of productivity and motivation of human resources. The importance of an individual's contribution to an organization as well as the importance of the employee as an individual is expressed by the manner in which these components are carried out. Initially, an employee is placed in the right position. Because he/she has the right knowledge, skills, and motivation to do the job, he/she performs well and is accordingly recognized. But as most theories of motivation suggest, an individual must experience some form of personal growth in order for him or her to remain motivated and happy.

Personal growth is an extremely individual experience. Therein lies the challenge for the nurse manager, who must identify what constitutes personal growth for individual employees. Frequently, the employees may have insight into their personal growth. However, there are many employees who do not possess this insight. Instead, they only know they are dissatisfied or, even worse, they are without desire. These two last types of employees can present the greatest challenge for the manager. For these two types, initial discussions about career goals are totally unproductive, because the employees have no comprehension of the concepts involved. These individuals must be brought along more slowly than the employees who have insight into their personal growth. Nevertheless, all types of employees can recognize the genuine concern for them by their supervisor.

Career counseling can begin with the initial interview, in which the applicant is made aware of the manager's interest in assisting the applicant to realize her greatest potential. It continues with the completion of an orientation designed to ensure success in the position. Career counseling then takes both an informal and formal direction. Informal career counseling occurs spontaneously when the manager observes the employee in various roles and behaviors. Feedback and validation regarding the employee's performance and reaction can be helpful to clarify strengths, weaknesses, and new interests for both the supervisor and the employee. Formal career counseling should occur at least once a year, not necessarily during the time of the employee's performance appraisal. During a private conference, career goals should be discussed. These career goals can be short term, such as acquiring a new skill within the patient service area. Likewise, career goals can be long term and project over the next five years or more.

Career counseling is more than just an identification of goals. It also involves at least two other steps. One is to identify specific actions on how to achieve the goals. Then the responsibility and timetable must also be identified. The manager can specify how the institution can assist the employee in reaching the goal. Or, if there is no specific assistance such as tuition assistance, the manager can identify obstacles that he may be able to remove or prevent from occurring. Likewise, having a shared common knowledge of the employee's career goals goes a long way in explaining the behavior of the employee. It also enables the manager to be more cognizant of alternatives and opportunities that fit with the employee's career goals. If the employee's career goal includes acquiring a master's degree in another state, for example, the manager can plan for the turnover of the employee in a much more objective manner. When an employee and a manager both understand that the goals of the institution are not incompatible with the goals of the individual, a more harmonious and effective relationship exists. When the employee understands that the organization truly wants the employee to do well and grow, he/she will be motivated to be productive for himself/herself and the institution.

There are several other essential components of any career counseling program that also certainly count as part of the institution's benefit package. These components include a definitive career mobility program, both lateral and upward within the department and organization, and a well-developed management training program. A career mobility program includes any number of methods to promote growth among employees. It is based on the philosophy that a happy, growing employee is ultimately good for the organization, both intrinsically and in very tangible, productive ways. It also recognizes that growth does not automatically mean vertical growth. Some employees are not management material and grow best through lateral growth opportunities. In the late 1970's and early 1980's, many hospitals developed career mobility programs consisting of at least two parts. Variations of the concepts of career counseling and job placement may be necessary because of an institution's size and limited resources. The important thing to remember is that the plan must be available to all employees, not just a selected few. The plan can include different opportunities, depending on the individual and the capabilities of the institution. For some hospitals, tuition reimbursement or sponsoring collegiate courses on hospital premises may be the best way to promote growth for their employees. Not all employees may choose this type of option. Therefore, it is important to design a career mobility program that has a menu of alternatives from which to choose. For example, a career mobility track may be in a clinical area, research, education, or management. The manager and employee can determine which method is the best for the employee and proceed from there.

Kaye (1982) identified at least six career options that nurse managers should be cognizant of when counseling employees on their career development. Career development is no longer confined to only one career path. It is now anticipated that many people may perform in two or more unrelated or related careers during their life span. One reason for this is the rapid technological growth, which creates new jobs previously unknown. Secondly, the longer life span of people, with improved nutritional and health status, makes them more active and productive for a longer period of time. The idea of a person having more than one career is still fairly unorthodox. As a result, the majority of individuals have not allowed themselves the opportunity to brainstorm about a wide variety of alternative careers. At best, individuals and counselors will usually examine parallel or expanded careers. These remain definitive and sound options for many people, but the opportunity to consider multiple options simultaneously can and should be encouraged by the nurse manager. These multiple options encourage flexibility and help the employee to be more open to changes as they occur. As a result, the employee feels more in control of his destiny because he has more choices and is not strictly at the mercies of the bureaucracy.

Vertical mobility has traditionally been emphasized as the best and only way to go. The last decade has tarnished the shine on this option. Vertical mobility is getting harder because there are fewer upper level positions and more qualified individuals to fill them. The disadvantages of increased responsibility are now better known, and the effects of stress and strain are not always considered worth the benefits.

Lateral mobility is a career option that has become much more attractive in the last decade. Nursing has especially benefited from the development of lateral career mobility programs. Excellent clinicians are no longer promoted away from the bedside unless they desire to develop a new level of skill and knowledge for management. With lateral mobility, a clinician can receive recognition and status for her expertise. Additionally, lateral mobility can involve movement across function boundaries. For example, if an excellent medical nurse wants to develop into an excellent cardiac nurse, most of her skill and knowledge transfer over to the new subspecialty. Because lateral mobility is encouraged and valued, the medical nurse is not held back in order to retain her expertise for patients with medical problems. Likewise, a head nurse may aspire to become a department head over a non-nursing department. The head nurse should receive equal consideration as any other qualified applicant.

Downward mobility within an organization has traditionally held a negative connotation. However, Kaye (1982) illustrated downward mobility as a deliberate strategy for future career opportunities. Some employees desire to change fields completely, or in order to make vertical moves, require additional formal education. In order to acquire this education, it may be necessary to free time and energies required of a current position. For example, a head nurse may assume a part time staff nurse position while attending school full time. Likewise, a unit secretary may take a lower level technician's job in the cardiovascular lab in order to gain clinical and technical experience. Downward mobility can also occur where organizations provide for employees who attempt a new position but for a variety of reasons are unsuccessful. Allowing such an employee to return to a level or position comparable with the previous position without emphasizing failure encourages the employee to try again and reinforces the concern the organization has for the employee as an individual.

Another career choice can involve participation in exploratory research, new ventures, and consultative or special projects. These opportunities are especially well suited for the tenured experienced employee who would enjoy the change of pace and challenge of such a project. At the same time, these employees are mature enough to know how to approach these types of situations. For example, suppose a hospital is planning to computerize its nursing stations. One year will be spent in research and development and the second year in training and implementation. Several experienced, mature unit clerks are recruited to participate in this project for its duration. Their job security is maintained, yet this type of mobility is enriching for both employee and the institution.

Job enrichment opportunities are another form of career counseling. Hackman and Suttle (1977) suggested that job enrichment can occur through either changing the individual or changing the job. The number of skills or variety within the skills used to perform the job can be changed. Allowing the employee to be involved in a task or project from the beginning to the end can make the job more rewarding. Primary nursing is a variation of this concept. Assisting the employee to understand the importance of his job in relationship to the entire organization can also make a job more rewarding. An employee who has never worked outside one small area could perceive his job differently if given the opportunity to rotate through other related departments.

A final alternative to be considered by the nurse manager involves assisting the employee to relocate outside of the immediate institution. This may mean remaining within a larger system or moving outside the system entirely. Ideally, a manager and institution are interested in keeping employees within the institution. However, this is not always realistically feasible. The need to consider alternative career options outside the institution can occur as a result of retirement or downsizing. However, this is also a possibility when the career goals of the individual cannot be actualized within the organization. Regardless of the reason, a positive attitude toward this option is necessary. In being realistic and objective concerning the institution, the manager leaves the employee with a positive attitude toward the institution. Additionally, the economic resources of the institution are not being spent on an unproductive employee. It can also be an opportunity to seed another organization within a system with expertise or leadership that the other institution sorely needs.

The second component of a career mobility program is the existence of an effective management development program. Theory of leadership and management was presented in Chapter 5. Depending on the theoretical and philosophical orientation of the institution, the management development program should be structured accordingly. Socialization to a new role in management will be more successful it if proceeds along a definitive path.

Managers and leaders need specific knowledge and skills in order to accomplish their job responsibilities. Prepackaged or commercial management development programs have their strong points in presenting basic management concepts and principles. However, it is still necessary to develop a specific segment that covers philosophies, objectives, and policies of that particular institution. All newly promoted managers need orientation periods, regardless of their prior position. The management development program should be structured in such a manner that ongoing continuing education and educational experiences are made available periodically. In this manner, the manager is expanding his knowledge and skills. As a result, the manager is better able to perform his current job and is also preparing for the next opportunity in the development of his career. Mentoring can also play a significant part in the development of effective managers. Mentoring relationships should not be confined to the patient care area or nursing service department. Mentors are available outside of nursing and as such provide experiences from an entirely different and often beneficial perspective.

HUMAN RESOURCE PROBLEMS

Managing people inevitably means having to deal with their problems and the problems they create for the organization. This is undoubtedly why human resource management is considered simultaneously the greatest challenge and the greatest source of frustration for managers and leaders. Included in this section are discussions concerning the concept of constructive criticism, the process of disciplining employees, and alternatives for dealing with troubled and impaired employees.

Constructive Criticism

The concept of constructive criticism is composed of the essence of the two concepts construction and criticism molded together to form one concept. Construction means to build or put together or change form. In order to build something, it is necessary to have resources such as tools and supplies. Construction is considered a positive process. Criticism means to examine for the purpose of evaluating, giving feedback, or judging someone or something. In order to evaluate or judge something, it is necessary to value that something. As a result of this value, standards or expectations are developed by societies, or in this situation, by departments and institutions. A message is prepared that contains information on how the item being evaluated compares with the standard. The message contains information such as strengths and weaknesses in relation to the standard. It also includes information on how to alter the weaknesses. The message can be non-verbal,

verbal, or written. Up to this point, constructive criticism is composed of an item or person of value, a standard, a message, and someone to deliver the message. The individual delivering the message, usually the manager or supervisor, is generally considered to be the person who has knowledge, expertise, or interest in the employee being evaluated. The message will not be valued by the receiver if the sender has no merit. Constructive criticism occurs within an environment that is conducive to effective two-way communication. Frequently, this means a quiet, private, uninterrupted place where the involved individuals can concentrate on the messages. Group constructive criticism, such as that found within quality assurance programs, can also be effective. However, group constructive criticism involving specific individuals is rarely successful. Alternative methods of delivering the message to an individual other than by or in a group ensure the greatest likelihood of success.

Constructive criticism can occur at several different times, all of which can be appropriately used by the nurse manager. Constructive criticism can occur during the development or training phase of an employee. When constructive criticism occurs during this time, there will usually be an impact on the outcome or product. In other circumstances, constructive criticism may be withheld until the outcome or product is finished. A third time for constructive criticism to occur is during periodic monitoring, such as in the form of annual evaluations.

As the term implies, constructive criticism should be done in a positive manner. In order to do this, the supervisors or managers must be secure and comfortable with themselves, non-threatened, and genuinely interested in the employee. It is obviously also advantageous for the employee to have an open mind and be interested and willing to receive the message.

Employee Behavior Modification

Any time an evaluation or performance appraisal is to occur, constructive criticism is an inherent part of the process. It is, however, not the only process that has to occur. There is usually an evaluation form to be completed. This serves as a guide for the nurse manager, but it is not sufficient in itself. First, the nurse manager must perform an analysis of the employee's performance. Identifying performance as satisfactory or unsatisfactory can be done globally without too much difficulty. Pinpointing the specific behavior(s) that adversely affect the performance is a much more difficult and time-consuming task. It is critical, however, to the ultimate correction of the behavior. A great deal of time and effort can be wasted if this initial task is not carried out, because not emphasizing the specific behavior will not correct it. Identification of the specific behavior is also necessary if the supervisor is going to be able to evaluate whether the performance has changed or not. Fournies (1978) also makes a valuable point when he raises the question of whether or not correcting the behavior is worth the supervisor's time. It is not unusual to find nursing administrators and managers getting hung up on isolated, irritating behaviors or behaviors that really do not impact on job performance. The behavior's impact on job performance determines the importance of the behavior. If the behavior is not important, the nurse manager should not waste time discussing it or attempting to change it.

The most common reason for unsatisfactory performance is that the employee thinks he is performing satisfactorily. In other words, the employee does not know that there is a problem, frequently because there is a lack of feedback. This feedback should not come at the time of the performance appraisal. Feedback should occur as frequently as necessary to establish the necessary level of performance before the performance is evaluated.

Another reason why an employee's performance or behavior is unsatisfactory is because he/she does not know what he/she is supposed to do or how he/she is to do it. Simplistically, this should be taken care of during the employee's orientation. It is amazing, however, the number of times that employees indicate that expectations of them are unclear or that insufficient training has occurred. If the desired level of performance is the outcome or product, this should be made clear to the employee. For example, if all physicians' orders are to be correctly implemented, the unit secretary needs to understand that this is the basis of satisfactory performance. The manner in which the unit secretary accomplishes the outcome should not be evaluated. If, however, the level of performance desired is the orderly transcription and integration of orders, the process is also significant, and this must be communicated to the employee. The knowledge and ability of the employee in acquiring the desired behavior should be adequately tested before release from orientation (Fournies, 1978). Individuals responsible for the employee acquiring the behavior need to be given the resources to perform this job correctly. Whether the staff educator or clinical preceptor, this person must know how to teach in addition to possessing the behavior to be passed on to the new employee.

Obstacles may exist that prevent the employee from performing the desired behavior. These obstacles can be identified when the nurse manager analyzes the factors that may be influencing work performance. Some obstacles may be beyond the employee's control. It is then the nurse manager's responsibility to remove them.

Fournies (1978) also suggested that the nurse manager examine the consequences of the desired level of performance or behavior. If the consequences are perceived as negative, the desired behavior is less likely to occur. Considered as classic behavior modification, this analysis can assist the manager in identifying strategies to improve the likelihood of the desired behavior occurring. If, for example, the efficient unit secretary is rewarded with more work to do from less efficient secretaries, she may not maintain the desired level of performance. Likewise, if all the troublesome employees are transferred to one particularly effective head nurse, that head nurse may discontinue being an effective problem solver. Two strategies for the nurse manager are elimination of the negative consequence and the provision of a positive consequence at the same time that is better than the negative consequence. Similarly, if positive consequences follow lack of achievement of the desired behavior, the nurse manager can address these consequences by removing the positive consequence and replacing it with a negative consequence.

As a result of this performance analysis, the nurse manager has a great deal of information on how to approach the problem. At this point, the manager can accumulate the other elements necessary to perform the evaluation. The nurse manager must be in control of her emotions. Frustrating employees can be very difficult to deal with. In order for the evaluation to be successful, the manager must remain in control of the situation in order to direct it through all the necessary steps. It is necessary to have all the facts and objective data to document and specifically describe the behavior under discussion. The nurse manager should also determine what is the minimum change in the employee's behavior that is acceptable and at what point these changes are to occur.

In presenting an evaluation, the concept of constructive criticism should be brought into play. As a result, both parties are open-minded and not defensive. It is then necessary for the nurse manager to obtain an agreement from the employee that a problem does exist. For unless the employee agrees that the behavior is not what it should be, there can be no change in the behavior. Fournies (1978, p. 137) stated two reasons that convince an employee that a problem exists:

1. The subordinate perceives the results or outcomes of what he or she is doing wrong or failing to do right, or

2. The subordinate perceives the consequences to himself if there is no change.

Based on these reasons, the nurse manager can identify to or with the employee the effect his performance is having on those dependent on his performance in the work setting. Secondly, the effect of his performance on the employee himself can also be identified. Once a behavior is identified as a problem, both parties can begin to work together to solve the problem. This is done by using the decision making process described in Chapter 5. Alternative solutions are specifically directed at changing the outcome of the behavior, and therefore have to involve changing the behavior.

After a thorough discussion of the various alternatives that are available, both the manager and employee agree on the action or behavior change that is going to occur and when that action or change is to occur. It will then be essential for the nurse manager to follow up on the employee's performance to ensure that the agreed upon change has occurred. This follow up should occur immediately at the time agreed on for the change to occur. This prompt form of feedback can be very effective because it indicates an obvious degree of interest and commitment by the manager. Follow up can also occur periodically depending on the nature of the behavior. Regardless of the occurrence or frequency of the follow up, the important thing to remember is recognition of the achievement of the desired behavior as well as any incremental improvement in the behavior.

Not all employees can completely turn over a new leaf in one night. An employee does not usually come to the job performing badly (he/she would not have been hired or gotten through orientation in the first place), but rather develops unacceptable patterns of behavior. It is the manager's responsibility to recognize these unacceptable behaviors early and counsel the employee regarding them. Most institutions have policies regarding the discipline procedure. This procedure usually begins with a verbal warning, followed by a series of written warnings and probation prior to termination. If the employee's behavior has deteriorated to the termination stage, immediate and complete change or improvement is expected. Short of that, however, it may be more realistic to work with the employee on gradual improvement, depending, of course, on the seriousness of the behavior. This can also be true in situations in which a manager has inherited an employee whose behavior has gone unchallenged. In almost all situations, it is necessary for some form of documentation of the counseling and/or evaluation to occur. Obviously, the more objective, specific, and complete the documentation, the better for all parties involved. This type of documentation does not occur automatically. Emphasis must again be placed on the planned development of these skills in the nurse manager. Secondly, the presence of a formal and operational grievance procedure process within the institution is necessary. Grievance policy and procedures ensure the process of two-way communication and thus a protection of the employee's rights. A nurse manager should not ignore the presence of this system, nor should its indiscriminate use be encouraged. The vast majority of employees who are familiar with this process will never feel the need to exercise it as an option. The remaining few need it as an option because it can effectively handle real problems between employee and employer.

Impaired Personnel

There have always been impaired employees, but the limelight has not been focused on them. The changing emphasis in human resource management as well as increasing societal interest in substance abuse has contributed to the attention on this subject. This heightened awareness is also the result of studies that have demonstrated the presence of alcoholism in approximately 15% of the nursing population. Other studies have indicated that nurses are twice as likely as the general population to become drug dependent. In the past few years, the majority of nursing licensure suspensions and revocations by state licensing boards have been due to substance abuse (Naegle, 1985). In these situations, the nursing administrator and manager is faced with difficult obligations and responsibilities that often overlap and conflict. Undoubtedly, there is the responsibility to protect patients and consumers. But it is also a professional responsibility to maintain and restore the members of the profession. The worst thing that can occur is for the nurse manager or administrator to ignore the problem, whether it be the knowledge of a specific individual or the presence of the issue within the institution. The reality and presence of impaired employees do exist in every institution. The termination or encouraged turnover of an impaired employee only spreads the problem to another institution. Unfortunately, there are still nursing administrators who choose to deal with the presence of the impaired employee in this manner. The administrator may fear being sued by the employee or fear that news of the problem may affect the institution's image. Both of these concerns are valid and do unfortunately occur. However, there can also be repercussions associated with passing the employee on to another institution or ignoring the problem. Legal action can be taken against institutions who knowingly let an impaired employee continue to work, even in another institution. Secondly, the cost to the patients may be fatal because of erroneous decisions made by the impaired employee. Inefficient and non-productive impaired employees are also very costly for institutions.

Unfortunately, the majority of nurse administrators and managers as well as staff members are unfamiliar and uncomfortable with recognizing and dealing with the impaired employee. State laws, both nursing and controlled substance acts, can influence the methods used to deal with impaired employees. Since 1982, the American Nurses Association has been actively involved in this issue. As a result, the majority of state nurses' associations have attempted to examine and address this issue in some manner. Thus, the state nurses' associations are excellent sources of guidance (Naegle, 1985).

Identification of an impaired employee can occur in several ways. In some instances, visible signs may provide clues. The personal appearance of the employee may begin to deteriorate. Work performance may become unacceptable or inconsistent. Tardiness or absenteeism may be other signs of impairment. Subversive solicitation of prescriptions from the medical staff may occur. Theft of supplies or other employees' valuables may occur. When an impaired employee is suspected, the other employees in the department may assume "enabling roles" (O'Connor and Robinson, 1985). In this role, the staff may consciously or unconsciously take up the slack or cover for the impaired employee. Another type of impaired employee may be at the other extreme from the description just given. Some impaired employees give no physical indication of their problems. They may be perfectly groomed, never miss a day of work, and be well liked and respected by fellow employees. Sometimes the only clue may be chronic health complaints. In these situations, the staff may be totally unaware of the problem. Discovery occurs when a staff member stumbles across what appears to be an isolated discrepancy in drug dosage or administration. Upon closer examination, the discrepancy extends to regular occurrences that are ultimately traced back to the model employee. Occasionally, a staff member will inadvertently observe an impaired employee in an act such as slipping a syringe into his pocket or drinking in the locker room. It is these perceptive and responsible employees who will then initiate action with their supervisor to get the impaired employee the assistance needed.

Ideally, the institution will have developed policies, procedures, and programs to deal with the impaired employee. These usually have resulted from previous haphazard attempts to deal with these types of problems. As awareness and experience have increased, resources have become more available. Most institutions choose to work closely with the professional licensing boards, as well as with the law enforcement agencies. Law enforcement agencies have enough other problems that they generally are very cooperative in allowing the licensing agencies to enforce the major action taken. However, in situations in which the employee is unwilling to participate in rehabilitation, denies criminal activity, or is involved in selling illegal substances, criminal proceedings may be pursued. It is essential for the manager, the institution, the law enforcement agency, and the licensing boards to be in concert about actions to be taken.

The objectives of all action taken are ultimately directed at protecting the public or patients as well as on the behalf of the employee. Fowler (1986) referred to the principle of non-maleficence or "first, (or, above all) do no harm" as being applicable to protecting both the patient and the employee. There should be a resource person available within the institution who is familiar with the policies, procedures, and available programs. These policies include any provisions for rehiring impaired employees who have completed a rehabilitation program. For example, many institutions have policies that place an impaired employee on a leave of absence and reinstate the employee who has successfully completed a rehabilitation program. Some states have developed "diversion programs" aimed at diverting the professional into treatment programs. The nurse manager is usually very involved in the identification and confrontation of the impaired employee. The nurse manager may not be as involved in the professional counseling of the impaired employee; however, the manager should be kept well informed of the progress of the situation. It will be the nurse manager's responsibility to assist the remaining staff members to work through the situation because there will be mixed reactions to it. Reactions can range from disbelief to anger, guilt, or relief. It may be necessary to have special sessions with remaining staff members to discuss the situation. These sessions have to be handled very delicately in order not to violate the rights of the impaired employee.

Proactively, nurse managers are in an important position that enables them to create the type of environment that supports and encourages nurses to take care of themselves (Cronin-Stubbs and Schaffner, 1985). Managers who promote communication and trust between and among staff and supervision can better identify and deal with stressors on staff. Sensitivity to staff members' feelings and perceptive awareness of personal problems can lead to the initiation of a dialogue to help the employees cope. Knowledge of alternatives and resources can be very helpful in assisting employees to better handle their personal and professional lives. All of these strategies are acknowledged skills within the effective nurse manager's repertoire.

LABOR RELATIONS

In the early 1980's, there were some well-publicized situations of successful anti-labor activities by the federal government and private industry. As a result of this selective publicity, it may seem unnecessary to be overly concerned with labor relations in regard to unions, contracts and strikes. Since the end of the recession in the early 1980's, it may be easy to adopt the attitude that employees are too grateful to be working to be concerned with labor activities. Likewise, the tremendous change in human resource management brought about as a result of increased attention and emphasis on the individual employee may appear to preclude the need for labor activities. Despite these occurrences, the labor activities are expected to continue and possibly accelerate in the next decade. This acceleration in labor activity is expected to occur as the result of at least two main trends. The health care industry affects a major portion of our economy. Changes in health care are resulting in cost containment activities that include downsizing and layoffs. These activities increase employees' anxieties regarding job security. Employees frequently are under the erroneous impression that a union can protect their job and hence may view them as more desirable. Secondly, unions are a result of the industrial period. As our society has moved away from heavy industry and into the information age, the number of employees in industry and therefore unions has declined. Unions are simply organized groups of people. Unions need people in order to exist. Therefore, it is essential for unions to gain new members through the unionization of previously non-unionized people. Health care is extremely labor intensive. Because of the large number of employees in health care, unions are especially attracted to attempt activity in this area (Henry, 1985). Because of these two main trends, labor activity will continue to be a relevant issue for nurse administrators and nurse managers.

The first line nurse manager is the individual who represents the employer, or "them," to employees. As such, the manager is the critical element in all labor relations. In order to deal effectively with the issue of labor relations, it is essential that the nurse manager have knowledge about the legalities concerning labor relations, the regulations that govern conduct, and the human resource management principles that significantly impact on labor relations.

The National Labor Relations Act guarantees employees the right to either participate or not participate in union activities. The NLR act further prohibits employers from taking any action that interferes with these rights of employees. The National Labor Relations Board (NLRB) is charged with the enforcing of the NLR act.

A union can achieve recognition in three ways. A union can be certified by the NLRB after winning an election. This is the most common way that unions are recognized. Secondly, an employer can voluntarily agree to recognize a union. Finally, the NLRB may order an employer to recognize a union. This third situation has occurred following flagrant abuse of employees by the employer (Henry, 1985).

Union certification resulting from an election usually occurs after the completion of several steps. The first step is the submission of a petition by the union to the NLRB for the election. This petition must indicate that at least 30% of the employees involved in the unit of concern are interested in holding an election. This group or unit is usually referred to as the bargaining unit. This interest is usually expressed through the collection of cards signed by employees indicating their interest. The institution is then served with the petition, which is official notification of interest in holding a union recognition election. In reality, the institution is already well aware of the interest and activities of employees. A hearing is then usually scheduled. This NLRB hearing is to determine the scope of the bargaining unit; whether or not the employer is under the jurisdiction of the NLRB, because some employers are exempt; if the petitioning unit is an official union; and if there are any reasons to delay or not hold the election.

Depending on the outcome of the hearing, the election may or may not be held. The election results are determined by the majority of the employees eligible to vote. Therefore, it is important that all eligible employees vote, even if they are not supporting the union. Following the election, either the union or the employer may appeal the election outcome. The election may be set aside and another election held for any number of violations. These violations can include unfair labor practices or changes in working conditions that occurred immediately prior to the election. Unfair labor practices include activities that could be construed to interfere, restrain, or coerce employees (Henry, 1985; Rowland and Rowland, 1984).

Nurse managers should understand that it is usually poor relations between employer and employees that open the door for union activities. As such, this again emphasizes the need for well developed managers with skills in human resource management principles. The principles of good communication, consistency, and trust are the best defense against union activities. This includes a willingness to discuss the subject of unions by a well informed manager. Campaigning occurs after the petition has been recognized but before the election. The nurse manager can openly discuss the advantages of remaining non-union in terms such as the current wages and benefits. The objective disadvantages of union membership can also be identified. These include union dues, loss of income during possible strikes, the disadvantages of a picket line, and the increased barriers to communication between supervisor and employee. The nurse manager can also provide correct information to the employee about a union and the election. He can also state that no union can force an employer to pay or provide more benefits than the employer is able. There are several things a nurse manager cannot do or say. These include promising increased pay or benefits, inquiring of employees on how they will vote, forging or altering union or institutional documents, or questioning prospective employees about union activities (Rowland and Rowland, 1984; Henry, 1985).

Following the certification of a union, a strike becomes a strategy available to the union to force the employer to conform to the union's demand. A strike is the refusal of the employees to continue work unless demands are met by the employer. During some contract negotiations, a no-strike clause is included in an attempt to remove this option. This clause may be accepted if the employer will agree to a mandatory arbitration clause. A strike usually includes picketing of the employer. Picketing, but not work stoppage, can also occur during the campaigning that occurs prior to the election. When faced with a strike, most institutions develop a plan that includes the decision of whether or not to continue operating, and if so, at what capacity. Positive publicity for the institution during this time is very critical. Strategies developed by management attempt to ensure that the strike will be unsuccessful. Successful strikes result from widespread support and participation of employees. Therefore, activities that detract from the attractiveness of strike participation should be identified. At the same time, these activities cannot be construed as coercion. The literature repeatedly emphasizes that the best defense against a strike is a good offense.

Metzger, Ferentino and Kruger (1984) emphasized that striking nurses are a breed apart from other health care employees involved in labor activities. The majority of labor activities have historically centered around economic and security issues. Nurses have been concerned about other issues that have made collective bargaining much more difficult and complex. Nurses' strikes have revolved around problems with communication with nursing administration, hospital administration, and physicians. Lack of respect, lack of control over practice, understaffing, and schedule inflexibility have been other issues. These issues have been found repeatedly in studies of nurse turnover and job satisfaction. These issues don't go away by themselves. Nurses have also used the strike as a legal instrument to redistribute power within the health care organization and to implement standards of patient care. The issues surrounding strikes by nurses are complex and are shrouded in ambivalent and highly charged emotions. The understanding that labor activities and therefore strikes are realities of tomorrow behooves the nurse manager to emphasize proactive strategies. There are institutions that are using these proactive strategies. In a study of over 15,000 RN's between January 1979, and April 1982, non-union nurses were found to be significantly more satisfied than union nurses with their jobs, administration, supervisors, evaluations, job mobility, salaries, benefits, and physical working conditions. There was no significant difference between union and non-union nurses in their satisfaction with communication, personnel policies, job security, peer relationships, and resource utilization (Metzger, Ferentino, and Kruger, 1984). Perhaps the institutions where the non-union nurses were employed could collaborate with the magnet hospitals in disseminating their successful strategies.

A strike is not the only alternative open to unions during contract negotiations. The use of a panel or individual to identify the facts concerning the issues is one alternative. The body charged with the fact-finding responsibility may only report the facts, or they may have been given authority to report the facts with recommendations on how to proceed or recommendations on the issues themselves. Another alternative is conventional interest arbitration. In this situation, an individual or panel of arbitrators are given the authority to make a decision that is final and binding to both the union and the employer. A third alternative is final offer arbitration. In this situation, the arbitrator chooses between the final offers of the two groups. Finally, in mediation-arbitration, the individual or panel functions first as a mediator between union and employer. If mediation proves unsuccessful, the mediators then become arbitrators in order for a decision to be reached (Metzger, Ferentino, and Kruger, 1984).

In an effort to move away from the confrontation model promoted by the industrial age of labor relations, another more constructive model is being advocated. A more constructive approach to employee dissatisfaction is seen in the development by employers of employee complaint programs. These employee complaint programs are separate and distinct from formal grievance procedures. Employee complaint programs could contribute to the lack of need for union activities. These programs are developed in order to identify organizational problems at both the individual and system level. Not only do these programs identify problems, they are also intended to resolve the complaint. In this process, needed organizational changes can be identified. As a result, the cause of the complaint is removed and the number of parallel complaints decreases. Employees should be more satisfied, their work life should improve, and ultimately organizational performance should be enhanced (Ziegenfuss, 1985). Although employee complaint programs are viewed by some managers as a way for disgruntled employees to go over the manager's head, such programs represent a strategy to identify problems in communication and relationships.

COMPENSATION AND BENEFITS

All institutions have the means to provide compensation and benefits to their employees. Not all institutions, however, have stated objectives and planned programs to achieve these objectives. Instead, salaries and benefits have often evolved haphazardly and disjointedly in reaction to internal and external pressures. Although the responsibility for the development of the compensation process and benefits programs is usually that of the human resource department, the nurse administrator and nurse manager have to be very familiar with them. There should be five goals for compensation and benefits programs that are developed by institutions. These goals address the objectives of the retirement program, life and health insurance benefits, disability benefits, medical care reimbursement, and compensation. In each of these major areas, it is necessary to identify the needs of the employees, the extent to which these needs are being met through other programs such as Social Security or Workmen's Compensation, and finally, the amount or level of benefit the institution will provide (Rowland and Rowland, 1984). Compensation or salary programs are based on the institution's philosophy about salaries. Most institutions have predetermined how competitive their salary structure will be, based on several factors. These factors include the presence of unions, other market forces such as competition and availability, as well as the use of cost of living increases. All salary programs are designed to attract qualified individuals, retain them, and at the same time not waste the financial resources of the institution.

Both the compensation and benefit programs are affected by several forces. There are an increasing number of laws and regulations from local, state, and federal agencies that must be adhered to by the programs. Fluctuations in the economy, including inflation, require flexibility and changes to occur within these programs. There is also an increasing awareness among employees about internal and external equity, such as the women's issue of equal worth. The magnitude of compensation decisions, because they can represent manipulation of up to 50% of an institution's operating budget, has major ramifications for everyone. Alternating surplus and shortages of qualified individuals can also adversely affect the development of fair and equitable programs (American Society for Hospital Personnel Administration, 1984).

There are three major statutes that affect all programs. The Fair Labor Standards Act, or the Wage and Hour Law, amended twice since its enactment in 1938, covers minimum wage and overtime provisions of a salary program. Included in this coverage are the definitions of exempt and non-exempt employees from overtime. Many employees define these categories as salaried versus hourly status. The Equal Employment Opportunity Commission has established the criteria for minimum job qualifications. Included in these as part of Title VII of the Civil Rights Act is the prevention of discrimination of any individual for a job based on color, religion, sex, national origin, or age. The Equal Pay Act stipulates that there can be no differentiation in pay for equal work on the basis of sex. This federal act has been involved in the comparable worth issue surrounding women's compensation for certain jobs. Institutions that have large contracts with the federal government are required by Executive Order 11246 to have affirmative action programs. There are also the Age Discrimination in Employment Act, the Vocational Rehabilitation Act, and the Vietnam Era Veterans Readjustment Assistance Act (American Society for Hospital Personnel Administration, 1984).

Usually, benefits have included such things as life insurance; Social Security; pension plans; shift differentials; and paid time off for illness, holidays, and vacation. These benefits are sometimes related to the amount of the base salary, in that as base salary increases, so does non-cash compensation. In the past few years, however, there has been an increasing move toward more flexibility and variety in compensation and benefit programs. Institutions have developed a menu of available benefits such as dental and eye care to greater depth of coverage. Employees earn credits based on their job level and seniority. The employees can then select those items on the benefit menu that are best suited to their needs and for which they have enough credits. In this manner, families that are adequately covered under another program at a spouse's place of employment do not lose benefits because of the similar plan. Additionally, the institutions are using these benefits to encourage the use of the institution by the employee whenever possible. An example includes the development of preferred provider organizations, in which discounts are given to employees when the institution for which they work is used. Although these types of benefit programs are more complex and difficult to administer, the majority of employees are more satisfied with their ability to make their own decision regarding which benefits are the most meaningful to them.

A major activity within some institutions' compensation and benefit programs has been directed at the issues that significantly impact on the majority of their employees who are female. As a result, more flexible schedules have been developed with competitive compensation and benefits in order to attract the part time nurse. The high incidence of absenteeism among nursing personnel is due in many cases to child care problems and child illness. A study by Miller and Norton (1986) of nursing unit personnel indicated increased conflict and stress related to child care, child illness, scheduling, and job responsibilities. This study reinforced the need for institutions to give more than lip service to the support of employees performing their jobs and to develop programs that can truly decrease stress and impact on productivity. These programs need to be more than child care assistance, although that would be a major breakthrough for many institutions. On-site child care, after school care, and evening and night care must be made feasible alternatives. Sick child programs are another benefit for employees when children are too ill to attend school but are not significantly ill. The large numbers of single parents without adequate support systems may result in abused, neglected children and impaired employees. Whether institutions consider the larger benefits to society or just self-interest for their own growth and profit, benefits specifically aimed at their women employees and their dependents are quickly becoming essential programs.

TOMORROW'S STRATEGIES

Skinner (1982) identified that there have in fact been massive efforts to improve the management of people. Despite these efforts, which have included sensitivity training, employee attitude surveys, and expanded fringe benefits, there has been no substantial gain in productivity, employee satisfaction, or perceived change in the image of managers in their relationship with employees. The poor results are believed to be due to several factors. The majority of administrators do not recognize the true difficulty of managing large numbers of people, which results in unrealistic expectations. There remains insufficient leadership within administration and in human resource management. Organizations are becoming more diverse and complex. As a result, it is even more difficult to merge or relate the goals of the organization to the goals of the individual employee.

Other societal forces affecting the managing of human resources include demographic changes. The number of individuals in the various age groups is shifting. Older individuals are in the work force longer. There are more individuals competing for limited upper level positions. The low birth rates of the 1960's are leading to a shortage of applicants at the entry level and less skilled positions. The work force in health care is already 65% female, and the percentage is increasing. There is an increase in the employees' desire to participate in decisions affecting their work. As mentioned earlier, there will be increased union pressures on health care institutions (Neudeck, 1985). There are several strategies that have been and will be effective for the nurse administrator and manager to use in dealing with human resources.

The nurse administrator should pay attention to public issues and concerns because they do impact on employees. The media are very effective at marketing pain, panic, and pleasure, and employees are swayed by these issues. Getting on top of these issues and addressing them can go a long way to dispelling rumors and quelling fears and insecurities. Among these issues, the women's issues are of significant emphasis. Along these lines, further exploration into flexible work schedules and incentive programs for nursing units is indicated. Ongoing evaluation of the existing compensation and benefit programs will be necessary in order to adapt to changing employee profiles. Employee development programs that include career counseling can assist employees to prepare for a changing world. The development of skilled managers should be a top priority because it is only in this way that a climate of trust and commitment with individual employees can be achieved (Neudeck, 1985).

References

American Society for Hospital Personnel Administration of the American Hospital Association (1984). *Fair Shakes: The healthcare compensation handbook*. Chicago: Pluribus Press.

Baldwin, L.J., Ramos, N.B., and Baldwin, L.E. (1985). Developing an alternative disciplinary process for the troubled nurse. *Nursing Administration Quarterly, 9*(2), 77–87.

Battle, E.H., Bragg, S., Delaney, J., Gilbert, S., and Roesler, D. (1985). Developing a rating interviewing guide. *The Journal of Nursing Administration, 15*(10), 39–45.

Cronin-Stubbs, D., and Schaffner, J.W. (1985). Professional impairment: Strategies for managing the troubled nurse. *Nursing Administration Quarterly, 9*(3), 44–54.

Filoromo, T., and Ziff, D. (1980). *Nurse recruitment: Strategies for success.* Rockville, MD: Aspen Systems Corp.

Fournies, F.F. (1978). *Coaching for improved work performance.* New York: Van Nostrand Reinhold Co.

Fowler, M.D. (1986). Doctoring or nursing under the influence. *Heart & Lung, 15* (2), 205–207.

Ganong, J.M., and Ganong, W.L. (1984). *Performance appraisal for productivity: The nurse managers' handbook.* Rockville, MD: Aspen Systems Corp.

Hackman, J.R., and Suttle, J.L. (1977). *Improving life at work: Behavioral science approaches to organizational change.* Santa Monica, CA.: Goodyear Publishing.

Henry, K.H. (1985). Health care union organizing: Guidelines for supervisory conduct. *The Health Care Supervisor, 4*(1), 14–26.

Kaye, B.L. (1982). Six paths for development. *Nursing Management, 13*(5), 18–22.

Kjervik, D.K. (1984). Progressive discipline in nursing: Arbitrators' decisions. *The Journal of Nursing Administration, 14*(4), 34–37.

Lachman, V.D. (1984). Increasing productivity through performance evaluation. *The Journal of Nursing Administration, 14*(12), 7–14.

Lancaster, J. (1985). Creating a climate for excellence. *The Journal of Nursing Administration, 15*(1), 16–19.

McConnell, C.R. (1986). The evolution of employee relations: A new look at criticism and discipline. *The Health Care Supervisor, 4*(2), 80–88.

Metzger, N., Ferentino, J.M., and Kruger, K.F. (1984). *When health care employees strike: A guide for planning and action.* Rockville, MD: Aspen Systems Corp.

Miller, D.S., and Norton, V.M. (1986). Absenteeism: Nursing service's albatross. *The Journal of Nursing Administration, 16*(3), 38–42.

Naegle, M.A. (1985). Creative management of impaired nursing practice. *Nursing Administration Quarterly, 9*(3), 16–26.

Neudeck, M.M. (1985). Trends affecting hospitals' human resources. *Hospital & Health Service's Administration, 30*(3), 82–93.

O'Connor, P., and Robinson, R.S. (1985). Managing impaired nurses. *Nursing Administration Quarterly, 9*(2), 1–9.

On the scene: The troubled nurse at the University of Cincinnati Hospital (1985). *Nursing Administration Quarterly, 9*(2), 31–68.

Petersen, D.J., Rezler, J., and Reed, K.A. (1981). *Arbitration in healthcare.* Rockville, MD: Aspen Systems Corp.

Rowland, H.S., and Rowland, B.L. (1984). *Hospital Administration Handbook,* Rockville, MD: Aspen Systems Corp.

Simendinger, E.A., and Moore, T.F. (1985). *Organizational burnout in health care facilities: Strategies for prevention and change.* Rockville, MD: Aspen Systems Corp.

Skinner, W. (1982). Big hat, no cattle: Managing human resources (part one). *The Journal of Nursing Administration, 12*(7–8), 27–29.

Skinner, W. (1982). Big hat, no cattle: Managing human resources (part two). *The Journal of Nursing Administration, 12*(9), 32–35.

Smith, H.L., and Elbert, N.F. (1980). An integrated approach to performance evaluation in the health care field. *Health Care Management Review, 5*(1), 59–68.

Vogt, J.F., Cox, J.L., Velthouse, B.A., and Thames, B.H. (1983). *Retaining professional nurses: A planned process.* St. Louis: C.V. Mosby.

Ziegenfuss, Jr., J.T. (1985). *Patient/client/employee complaint programs: An organizational systems model.* Springfield, IL: Charles C. Thomas.

PATIENT CARE MANAGEMENT

INTRODUCTION

Nursing administrators have responsibility for several major functions, which include financial or fiscal management, personnel management, risk management, and patient care management. It is the patient care management responsibility that offers perhaps the greatest challenge to the nursing administrator. There are several factors that influence this aspect of the nursing administrator's job. Patient care management is often considered "clinical" rather than "administrative" or "management." The nursing administrator may have been removed from the clinical setting for such a period of time that feelings of insecurity or concern about clinical aspects occur within the nursing administrator. In staff members, this removal from what they consider "real" nursing may produce a lack of credibility for the

17

nurse administrator. These perceptions, whether real or imagined, add to the challenge facing the nursing administrator in the area of patient care management. Numerous changes have occurred in recent years in the manner or mode of care delivery, which then influence the role of the nurse administrator in patient care management. Changes have also occurred in the role of nurses and nurse managers. Patient acuity, quality assurance, emphasis on productivity, and discharge planning have also changed. Each of these has had an impact on the management of patient care.

The nursing care process will be reviewed briefly in this chapter and the importance of care planning will be emphasized. This chapter will also discuss the various settings in which nursing care is provided. The modes of care delivery, patient acuity and classification systems will be addressed. Standards of care and quality assurance will be discussed as well. The effect of improved productivity on patient care management will also be described. The impact of computerization will be addressed and its role in patient care management reviewed. Education for both staff and patients has a significant role in patient care management. Each of these will be addressed in some detail with discussion including certification and costs for education.

DELIVERY OF PATIENT CARE

Since the time of Florence Nightingale, nursing care has been planned and provided to assist patients to overcome illness or injury and to become well once more. The nursing process is a systematic approach developed to ensure that the care of patients is planned and implemented appropriately. The nursing process is a problem solving approach that has five basic components—assessment, diagnosis, planning, implementation, and evaluation.

Although the manner in which the problem is identified and the focus of the problem has changed somewhat, the *assessment* step of the nursing process is initiated in the same way as in the past. Data collection about the patient must be the first step. A patient history and physical assessment are the major ways in which the data are collected. The patient history may be obtained through a general interview that is very informal or may be taken in a formal manner utilizing a specific format and form. One responsibility of the nursing administrator in relation to this aspect of the nursing process is to ensure that accurate data are collected and that some level of consistency is present in the department. Because of this type of responsibility, the use of a specific form for the patient history is recommended. A format for physical assessment may provide the same consistent approach desired in data collection. These formats serve to support the standards of care expected of staff in relation to patient assessment. Once data are collected, problems or potential problems can be identified and objectives for the patient can be developed. During the process of assessment, the nurse must not only collect the data but must also ensure that the data are valid and must analyze the data in order to make a decision about needed nursing care. This decision making is often called nursing *diagnosis*.

Nursing diagnosis is differentiated from a medical diagnosis made by a physician. Nursing diagnosis is a judgment about health problems (potential or existing) that nurses are qualified to treat. It focuses on a patient's response to a health problem, whereas medical diagnoses focus on the disease process (Gordon, 1982). Nursing diagnoses are very useful to nurses in focusing on nursing rather than on medical problems. Nurses have had difficulty over the years in establishing nursing practice as differentiated from medical practice. Nursing diagnoses help to organize, define and develop what is nursing knowledge and practice (Baer, 1984). Although there are disadvantages to the use of nursing diagnoses, a major advantage is in directing nurses to think in terms of nursing. Through the framework of nursing diagnoses, nursing interventions can be specific for diagnoses and rationales can be specifically indicated for patient care. Evaluation of nursing practice as well as research about nursing can be facilitated with the approach of nursing diagnosis.

In actual practice, nursing diagnosis is still problematic, however. Although many schools of nursing teach nursing diagnosis in basic curricula, there are many practicing nurses who are far from comfortable with the process. There are many patient problems, too, that do not fit one of the diagnoses that have been approved by the National Conference on Classification of Nursing Diagnoses (Gebbie and Lavin, 1975; Gebbie, 1976; Kim and Moritz, 1982), yet nursing care may be carried out to resolve the patient's problem. Forcing thinking into predeveloped categories can be criticized in multiple ways, and the terminology of nursing diagnosis is often addressed as impractical or intellectual in nature. In actual practice, nurses may feel they waste time intellectualizing about the right wording or category when their valuable time could be spent caring for the patient. Regardless of whether nursing diagnosis is perfect or not, it does fill a need in nursing practice, that of directing the thinking toward the patient and his responses to real or perceived problems. Nursing administrators may be able to affect positively the nursing practice of their staff through assisting that staff to learn about and use nursing diagnoses.

Once a problem or need has been identified for a specific patient, expected outcomes or goals for the patient may be developed. This is part of the second step in the nursing process—*planning*. Planning is accomplished for several purposes. Prioritization of problems is one of these purposes. Primarily, though, planning is done to identify nursing actions or interventions that will help the patient reach the specified goal or the outcome desired. The outcome of the planning is the written care plan.

Nursing care plans have been the subject of controversy for many years. Despite the advantages of written care plans, stressed from basic nursing courses into the practice setting, and despite the standards and regulations of the various accrediting and licensing agencies, the nursing care plan in practical application has been one of the toughest items the nursing admin-istrator has ever attempted to "successfully" implement. Every hospital, of course, has nursing care plans, but getting the nursing staff to complete these care plans and keep them up to date for their patients is a continuous battle for nurse managers. Nurses have difficulty giving a high priority to written care plans. There are a number of factors that influence the thinking of nursing staffs relative to these care plans.

The nurse manager and nursing administrator must identify and address these factors if care plans are to be valued by the staff. The various factors may be present or absent in a particular institution, and the degree to which they are present may vary as well. The factors that influence completion of care plans include attitudes of nursing management, understanding of the process, and valuing by the nursing staff.

The attitudes of nursing management about care plans, although seem-ingly clear, may really be confusing or contradictory. For example, if the head nurse or nurse manager never pays attention to care plans except just before JCAH or state licensure visits, the nursing staff will feel they are important only at those times. On the other hand, if nursing management, including unit managers, supervisors, and even the nursing administrator, obviously believe and show they believe that the care plan has value, the attitude of the staff may also change. To support the attitude, the nursing management group may find ways to enhance motivation for care plans. Such steps as making the care plan a part of the chart, ongoing quality monitors for completed care plans, and recognition or credit for the work required are examples of ways the nurse manager or administrator may help improve the motivation toward written care plans.

Understanding the process for writing care plans seems to be simple. However, the variations in terminology and lack of education in the past about what nursing really is have contributed to the problems facing nurse managers today. Previous use of medical diagnoses, even in some nursing schools, has complicated the issue of care planning. The difficulties the profession has faced in defining its practice are a part of this issue. If a nursing care plan is supposed to address nursing, but nurses are unclear about what is or is not nursing, the dilemma can be seen. Nurses not only perform nursing activities but also carry out medical orders and coordinate allied health services. This can and does create some confusion about exactly what nursing care plans should include. Nursing diagnoses, developed to clarify this type of question, have provided assistance in some ways but have not provided all the answers. For instance, as has been noted, some of the terminology of nursing diagnoses is such that nurses avoid using it. Development of standard care plans was one attempt to assist nurses in the process of planning care using accepted terminology for nursing. However, lack of individualization resulted, and standard care plans lost popularity.

Finally, the valuing of care plans by the nursing staff influences whether written care plans are done. Staff members must believe that the care plan will help more than other methods in communicating the information about the patient's care. They must also see the other ways in which the care plan has value. When nursing management supports and rewards care planning in various ways, the value of the plan to the staff nurse will increase. An excellent way to support the value of the care plan is through its involvement in patient classification or acuity determination. Used as a tool to provide information relative to staffing needs, the care plan's value is in providing additional staff as justified by nursing care requirements noted through the care plan. Rewards for completing the care plan then become clearer, although increasing the complexity of the care plan may occur in order to justify additional staff. This will obviously require monitoring by the nursing administrator.

Implementation of the care plan is the next component of the nursing process. Actual implementation of planned care may be by the nurse, other members of the health care team, or the patient and his family. Interventions to be implemented during this step may vary greatly from patient to patient or from day to day. Interventions or actions are the key to this particular phase of the process. The nurse generally feels more comfortable with this phase because it requires technical and intellectual skills with which she is more comfortable. The implementation phase begins when actions are initiated and concludes with documentation of the actions and the response of the patient to the actions. In the past, interventions were planned without much consideration for resources available. As the economic climate continues to change, it will be more important for health care providers to not only be cognizant of but also to plan for the limited resources that may be available. For example, planning for outpatient follow-up that the patient cannot afford and that will not be provided without charge is not an intervention that is reasonable. The success of interventions in meeting the predetermined goal for the patient is measured by the response of the patient and how well he reaches the expected outcome.

The last major component of the nursing process is *evaluation*. The measurement mentioned in the last paragraph is evaluation. As nursing care is planned, it should be kept in mind that one will need to measure the success toward the specified objectives. Evaluation helps the nursing staff determine whether actions specified in the plan helped to resolve the identified problems. If not, reassessment and planning must continue. It is easy to see that this evaluation should occur fairly frequently to provide optimal opportunities for objectives or goals to be met. Evaluation also serves another purpose in that it helps to identify any new problems that may have surfaced since the care plan was developed initially.

Settings for Patient Care

Where patient care is being delivered has changed dramatically over the years as the type of care required changed and as improvement in care delivery occurred. From earlier times, when patient care was provided in the home, to the days when the majority of care was hospital based, many changes have occurred that influence the setting for health care delivery.

Hospitals and nursing homes still provide a great deal of patient care, but as outpatient procedures become more common, fewer patients stay in the hospital than before. Ambulatory surgery centers have sprung up across the nation with support from third party payers. Additionally, third party payment has provided incentives for shorter lengths of stay, which means that patients are discharged sooner. Often this may result in needed nursing care outside the hospital setting.

Home health services have gained wider acceptance and greater use since hospital lengths of stay declined. Services offered by home health agencies have also changed, and the impact on nursing has been significant. Different skills and knowledge are being required of the home health nurse. IV therapy, IV antibiotics, ventilator care, and chemotherapy are among the services offered by some agencies (see also Chapter 13, Health Care Environment).

Before the patient is ready for discharge and home care, if needed, he must have his care planned, implemented, and evaluated. This may be accomplished by a variety of means. The mode of care delivery varies from hospital to hospital and is dependent upon the goals and objectives of the department and the institution.

Modes of Care Delivery

Nursing care delivery systems, like the settings for delivery, have evolved through the years as goals have changed and as nursing administrators have sought to improve continually the delivery of care to patients. Rowland and Rowland (1985) have identified four basic modes of care delivery: case, functional, team, and primary nursing. Variations on these models may be found, depending on the institution. Each system has a different emphasis on the patient and the personnel providing the care to the patient.

Case nursing, better known in the past as private duty nursing, is certainly the oldest method. Except in some ICU settings, case nursing is unusual today, because of its lack of cost effectiveness and efficiency in the one patient/one nurse relationship. Obvious advantages to this type of care delivery include accountability and continuity.

Functional nursing is a division of nursing by tasks. The nurse manager assigns a group of tasks to staff members. These tasks are related to patient care but not to a specific patient. There is no accountability for care planning, since assessment, planning, etc. is assigned by the task. There is no continuity. Staff members document those actions done by them, or a nurse may be assigned to perform the charting. Shift to shift report is done between charge nurses. Although each nurse is responsible for her own actions, no one nurse is responsible to even identify responsibility for problems that occur with patients. Care delivery with functional nursing is fragmented and lacks comprehensiveness. Patients and families are often confused about whom to communicate with for concerns or problems. Because of minimal involvement with specific patients, nurse dissatisfaction is a common problem with functional nursing. Although functional nursing has been praised as cost effective, other methods of care delivery have been shown to be just as cost effective and certainly more professionally satisfying.

Another method of care delivery that is still quite popular is *team nursing*. In team nursing, there is a team leader who makes assignments of tasks. The team leader has responsibility for care planning. Implementation may be accomplished by team members or the team leader, depending on the ability of each staff member. Care may be fragmented or fairly complete, depending again on the qualifications of the staff member. If, for example, the team member is a RN, the care may be quite complete. However, if the team member is a nursing assistant, several team members may have to perform certain tasks for the patient. Shift to shift report is most commonly by the team leader to the oncoming shift. Accountability is limited with team nursing to the team leader, since it is difficult to determine responsibility at times. Because of the team effort and coordination with team nursing, patient care can be quite comprehensive. As with functional nursing, team nursing can cause confusion for patients who need to communicate concerns or problems and who have no specific individual to whom they may express their concerns. Team nursing's major advantage over functional nursing seems to be in the team effort and care planning aspects.

Primary nursing has been identified as the most satisfying mode of care delivery because of the improved quality of care, continuity, and accountability associated with it. In this form of care delivery, the nurse manager assigns specific patients to professional nurses who are responsible for care delivery and planning for the duration of those patients' stay. Shift to shift report is accomplished by the primary nurse to the associate nurse. The primary and associate nurses implement the care for the patient for their eight hour shift, while the primary nurse has additional planning responsibilities and responsibilities for coordination of other nurses' activities for a specific group of patients. Nursing care under this system is comprehensive, with a patient focus. Communication is enhanced by primary nursing, with resulting improved patient/nurse rapport, trust, and understanding. Continuity of care is enhanced, patient recovery is improved, and job satisfaction is better. The major concern associated with primary nursing is related to costs and staffing. However, numerous studies have shown that because the professional nurse is more productive, costs for primary nursing need not be prohibitive. Nursing care hours per patient per day need not increase because of a shift to primary nursing. Planning by the nursing administrator can prepare for primary nursing if it is desired and can gradually accomplish the changeover as vacant positions are upgraded. If, for example, nursing care hours are too low for the patient acuity being experienced, the nurse administrator should make the change in nursing care hours before the change to primary nursing to differentiate the problem of low HPPD (hours per patient day) from the delivery system.

Modular nursing is another popular type of nursing in which an RN and another staff member (often a nursing assistant or nurse aide) form a team to provide care for the assigned patients. This method may be very efficient in getting specific tasks done, but it lacks the accountability and continuity found in primary nursing. Communication during the shift may be adequate, but communication from day to day is very difficult.

Total patient care, a method that is a modification of primary nursing, provides assignment of patients usually over several days to a nurse who is responsible for total care of the patient for the assigned shift. This method lacks the full continuity and much of the accountability of primary nursing, but it provides better continuity than most other methods.

With each system or mode of care delivery, there are advantages and disadvantages. The nursing administrator's task in mode of care delivery will be in deciding which mode is best. In order to make the decision, the nursing administrator will need to review carefully the basic principles that apply to each system to determine which system best meets the needs of the institution. Each system may be modified in multiple ways to meet the described needs. (See Table 17–1 for a summary of modes of care delivery.) Regardless of the care delivery system that is used, one tool that is helpful in planning for the care is a patient classification tool to assist in determining patient acuity.

Patient Classification for Acuity

One outcome of the changes in reimbursement in the health care system has been an increase in patient acuity. This can be understood when consideration is given to what happens when length of stay is shortened. The days that are eliminated are on the discharge end of the stay when the patient is least ill. Pre-admission certification has had an effect as well, through pre-approval for admissions. This means that patients must be sick enough to be admitted. This has resulted, in some cases, in a hesitation to admit patients. By the time the patient is admitted in these cases, he may be sicker. The overall effect has been that hospitalized patients are more acutely ill.

More than ever before, it behooves the nursing administrator to have a good hold on acuity of patients, particularly in light of the downsizing occurring in so many health care institutions. Patient classification systems, originally developed to determine the nursing needs of individual patients in order to properly allocate nursing staff, have expanded into nursing workload measurement systems that not only identify nursing needs for specific patients but also can actually determine the staffing needs by unit and shift to provide the care needed by the patients. This tool becomes an

TABLE 17–1
Modes of Care Delivery

Elements	Primary	Modular	Total Care	Team	Functional
Definition	Delivery and planning is responsibility of assigned nurse for the duration of patient's stay.	Care delivery and planning is responsibility of team—RN and one other staff member—for a module of patients for one shift.	Care delivery and planning is responsibility of one nurse for assigned shift, usually over several days.	Care is assigned by team leader and provided by one or more team members.	Care delivery is assigned by specific tasks to multiple staff members.
Accountability Planning Care Providing Care	Primary nurse is accountable for care planning and coordination of nursing care; primary or associate nurse is accountable for care delivery during assigned shift.	RN is accountable for care planning and providing care during assigned shift. Accountability difficult, since assignments are by shift and may change.	Assigned nurse has responsibility for some care planning and providing care during assigned shift. Accountability for care planning for delivery is difficult, since assignments are by shift and may change frequently.	Team leader is accountable for care planning. Various staff members are responsible for providing care, but accountability is difficult to identify.	No one is accountable for care planning except perhaps nurse manager. Multiple staff members responsible for portion of care—medication, treatments, bath, etc. Accountability is difficult to identify.
Continuity	Maximal continuity because of patient-centered approach and specific assignment of patients for duration of stay.	Some continuity possible, but approach is more nursing oriented and assignments may change daily.	Some continuity possible because of patient-centered approach but lacks assignment of patient for entire length of stay.	Some continuity when team functions well, but approach is nursing-centered and patient involvement in planning may not occur.	No continuity because of task-centered approach.
Assignment	On admission, patients assigned primary nurse for duration of stay.	Daily assignments of group of patients to team of RN and another staff member (usually nurse aide)..	Assignment daily (usually several days) of patients for total care during assigned shift.	Assignment by team leader of patients to team members. Team member may be assigned all or part of care during assigned shift.	Assignment by task.

Nursing Process	Primary nurse responsible for care planning, assessment, and evaluation. Associate nurses responsible for assessment, implementation.	Nurses share responsibility for all aspects of nursing process.	Nurse responsible for all aspects of nursing process in assigned shift. Shared responsibility between various assigned nurses.	Team leader responsible for care planning. Assessment, implementation, and evaluation responsibility shared by all nurses caring for patient.	No one responsible for care planning. Various staff members share responsibility for implementation, assessment and evaluation by assigned task.
Documentation	Primary and associate nurses document care for assigned patients.	Each nurse responsible for documentation of care provided.	Each nurse providing care documents those aspects that she performs.	Team leader usually does all documentation.	Documentation of specific tasks may occur, or staff member may be assigned charting.
Communication Nurse/Patient Nurse/Ancillary Services Shift/Shift Nurse/Manager	Enhanced nurse/patient/family communication. Nurse is clearly identified. All communications regarding particular patient can be directed at primary nurse, etc. Shift to shift report is primary nurse to associate nurse, etc.	Fairly good by shift, though some difficulty because of lack of continuity. Shift to shift report may be between staff nurses or charge nurses.	Fairly good by shift, and better if assignments are for several days. Shift to shift report between nurses caring for patients.	Communication often difficult, since no clearly defined accountable nurse. Shift to shift report between team leader and staff.	Communication very difficult. No clearly defined nurse, even by shift. Shift to shift report between charge nurses.
Discharge Planning	Primary nurse coordinates and plans for discharge.	No specific nurse has responsibility for discharge planning (shared responsibility).	No specific nurse has responsibility for discharge planning (shared responsibility).	Team leader has responsibility for all patients cared for by team.	No nurse has responsibility, except perhaps charge nurse.

TABLE 17–2
Evaluation of Patient Classification Systems

Is Flexible
Fits Institutional Philosophy
Addresses Subspecialty Needs
Is Objective
Is Quantifiable
Recognizes Individuality of Patients
Reflects Workload
Reflects Direct and Indirect Care Requirements
Reflects Unit Specific Variables
Is Valid and Reliable
Provides for Periodic Revision
Is Capable of Manual and Computer Operationalization
Is Easily Implemented

extremely important one for the nursing administrator, who must justify her staffing needs with census reductions being so prevalent.

In considering how patient classification should be accomplished, there are multiple factors to be considered. A number of packaged classification tools are commercially available. However, because of the importance of patient classification in its impact on allocation of staff and budget planning, understanding the various systems is crucial to the successful use of a system in a particular setting. Benefits that have been derived from patient classification systems include daily allocation of staff, budget planning, development of facilities for more effective provision of nursing care, determination of patient charges, and even the development of criteria for quality measurement (Giovannetti, 1979). In order to select or develop the right patient classification tool, the nursing administrator should examine some basic criteria recommended by the Management Information Systems Project task force (St. Germain and Meijers, 1984). These criteria may serve as guidelines in evaluating classification systems (either pre-packaged or self-developed systems). See Table 17–2 for a summary of guidelines to evaluate total systems for classification (classification tool, methodology, definitions, etc.).

A patient classification system must be flexible enough to be modified for specific units or institutions. Philosophies and goals vary from institution to institution, and these should be considered when a tool is to be used for classifying patients. Standards from JCAH or specialty organizations should be able to be incorporated into a tool. Specific requirements of subspecialties should be able to be addressed. An example of a subspecialty in which specific requirements might be necessary would be an orthopedic unit. Caring for patients in traction on an orthopedic unit becomes almost second nature and certainly would require less time than caring for patients on a unit that usually has only general surgery patients. Such flexibility may be obtained through alteration of definitions or through descriptive statements when appropriate.

The patient classification system should provide a mechanism for objective and reliable selection of indicators of nursing workload. Directions must therefore be very clear, and definitions must be able to be easily understood. Subjectivity has been one of the greatest problems in classification, so this criterion is very important.

Each of the components of a classification system should have a quantifiable value that addresses the workload associated with the delivery of care to the patient. It is not an easy task to develop a measure of nursing workload. These factors are related to objectivity and may include frequency, time required, or how many resources are utilized. (See Chapter 10, Productivity Management.)

Individuality of patients must be recognized by the classification tool. The system should be able to differentiate between patients who have the same medical or nursing diagnosis but require different interventions. For example, two patients with a medical diagnosis of myocardial infarction may have significantly varying needs because of age, complications, family or work situation, or previous experiences. Similarly, two patients with the nursing diagnosis of alteration in comfort may require totally different interventions because of the cause of pain, age, associated nursing diagnoses, or contributing circumstances. An example of a simple patient classification tool is included in Table 17–3. This tool is only part of the total patient classification system.

The classification system should also carefully reflect workload as opposed to severity of illness only, since its major purpose is allocation of nursing resources. As has been discussed, the workload is not always reflected by the medical diagnosis. An example of this may be a patient who is very confused and disoriented related to organic brain syndrome. While this may require increased nursing care to prevent injury, the diagnosis is not usually considered a serious illness.

In developing or evaluating a patient classification system, the time required to deliver care should be reflected. The system should also reflect the specific hospital or unit factors. Unit geography, level of personnel, support systems, availability and type of supplies and equipment, mode of care delivery, and even patient mix should be considered. An example of how this may be applied is in IV therapy. If a hospital has available and utilizes IV controllers and pumps, a different amount of time may be needed for that procedure than in a hospital where such IV equipment is not available.

A good patient classification system should be a credible one in which accurate and consistent data are obtained. If a system is reliable, the classification would reveal the same result when done repeatedly or when done by two different individuals. If the system has validity, it will measure what it is supposed to measure. Monitoring of the system is important to ensure that "padding," or identification of non-existent patient needs, by the nurse is minimized. With a valid, reliable system, such monitoring can prevent this manipulation of the system to obtain more staff.

The system should address total nursing workload, including direct and indirect care requirements. Development of care plans and conferences with

---

386 NURSING ADMINISTRATION

TABLE 17–3
Sample Tool for Patient Classification

Unit _____   Shift _____   Date _____

Room Number											
Bath	Bed Bath	3									
	Partial	1									
	Self	0									
Feeding	Tube fdg. Multiple	4									
	Tube fdg. Continuous	2									
	Feed Patient	2									
Activity	Up in Chair	2									
	Ambulate	4									
	ROM	4									
Vital Signs	q 1 hr. or more	4									
	q 2 hr.	2									
	q 4 hr.	1									
Medications	IV meds. × 2 or more	4									
	Continuous IV meds. or × 1	2									
	Multiple p.o. meds.	2									
Tubes	Chest Tubes	2									
	Foley cath.	2									
	N/G Tube	2									
	T-Tube or other	2									
Monitoring	Non-invasive (apnea, EKG)	4									
	Invasive × 1	4									
	Invasive Mult.	8									
Special Procedures	Dsg. Change × 1	3									
	Mult. dsg. change	5									
	Assist MD with Procedure	5									
	Special Therapy	5									

Unit __2W__ Date __2/29__ Day of Week __Monday__ Observer __M. Smith__

TIME	7:00–7:15							7:15–7:30							7:30–7:45							7:45–8:00					
Activity	RN A	RN B	LPN A	LPN B	US	HN		RN A	RN B	LPN A	LPN B	US	HN		RN A	RN B	LPN A	LPN B	US	HN		RN A	RN B	LPN A	LPN B	US	HN
Adm. Meds																											
IV Therapy																											
Bath																											
AM Care/ Pt. Hygiene																											
Vital Signs																											
Treatments																											
Rounds with MD																											
Documentation																											
Transcribe Orders																											
Meetings																											
Break																											
Cleaning Duties																											
Etc.																											

FIGURE 17–1. Work sample form.

families are not direct patient care but should be included, since they impact on the care significantly. Time spent accompanying patients for procedures is a part of this care. Similarly, documentation is equally important. This inclusion of indirect care may be accomplished in several ways, depending on the system. During system development, indirect care studies may be done that verify the average time spent in indirect care. This time may be built into the system, similar to the manner in which time study and test frequency study assist in developing point assignments for direct care. Work sampling is another name for this type of study. (Figure 17–1 is an example of a work sample form that may be used.) Distribution of the workload from day to day or shift to shift should also be addressed by the system, since there is certainly variation.

Periodic revision of the system should be possible, since nursing care is continually changing and more efficient ways to deliver care are being found. Validity of the system may be dependent on this mechanism. It should also be noted that quality assurance monitoring of care delivered can be incorporated into the revisions to provide quality monitoring updates as well. For example, quality monitors may be developed for specific types of respiratory care provided for post-operative patients. Inclusion of this type of care in the acuity system can also provide a mechanism to monitor quality.

Patient classification systems should address the workload of caregivers—those directly involved in the care of patients. Operational support and management personnel should not be included unless added in separately as indirect time over and above the "per patient" time. These types of data—workload requirements for patients as well as other data retrieved—can be used to prepare budgets and to control staffing at all levels. Hours per patient day (HPPD), shift and staff mix requirements dependent on patient acuity, productivity measures, and trends in acuity can be obtained from good systems. Staff mix, for example, may be determined by the implementation team or a panel of experts and may be based on experience or education required for a desired level of care or classification of patient. The team members may decide, for instance, that a Level I patient who will receive 2.8 hours of care per day should have all his care provided by an RN since the nurse contact is so limited, or they may decide that 50% of the care should be by an RN. Similar determination for other classifications would occur. That figure is then used in determining staff mix requirements for patients. Nurse/patient ratios, equitable workload assignments, admission or discharge criteria, and even patient room assignments can be determined from use of the information (Billings, 1983).

One other consideration in developing or evaluating a patient classification system is how it will be operationalized. A system that requires significant staff time is an added burden. A system should require little time from staff members in recording classifying data or in determining staffing needs. It is important to have a system that can be handled manually, even if computerization is available.

Simplicity of design and ease of implementation are two of the basic requirements of a patient classification system (Johnson, 1984). Even when these requirements are met and the identified criteria are given appropriate consideration, problems may occur, which the nursing administrator may prepare for and address as necessary. Huckabay and Skonieczny (1981) identified 16 such problems. Resistance to change and difficulty in motivating staff go hand in hand and are not unique to patient classification. Feelings of stress among the staff or administrative personnel are also associated with change. Difficulty in motivating the hospital administrator, the nursing administrative personnel, and the inservice instructors may also be related to change but may also reflect a lack of understanding about the purpose and use of the system.

The difficulty in selecting a system can be easily understood when one reviews the criteria that should be used to evaluate a system. Lack of reliability, which is important to the credibility of the system, can be a factor in staff complaints, which also creates the difficulty in getting staff members to classify patients each shift. Cheating or padding is not unusual, especially when there is inadequate monitoring of the system. Difficulty in conducting a research study to test the system is another problem faced by the nurse administrator, who may become frustrated as she tries to implement the system.

Two other problems identified by Huckabay and Skonieczny were recruitment and budgetary problems. These were related to the nursing shortage problems when additional staff needs were identified by the patient classification system. This type of frustration may lead to a feeling of loss of control of the situation. These feelings are important, but it must be recognized that good planning may in fact reduce or eliminate the majority of the identified problems. Patient classification for acuity is very important for the nursing administrator who wishes to have a patient care delivery system that provides quality care to her patients.

Quality Assurance

Delivery of quality patient care for a reasonable cost is the ultimate goal of most health care institutions. Such emphasis has been placed on quality assurance that JCAH standards continue to be revised to reflect the importance of quality care, and departments of quality assurance already exist or are being developed in all health care institutions. Although quality assurance is important for all departments, only quality assurance (QA) for nursing will be discussed.

Quality assurance is a process by which standards of care are developed and care to patients is measured or evaluated in relation to those standards. Criteria are used to determine whether the standards are being met. It is important to differentiate between quality care and quality control. Quality control may refer to specifics of a procedure or policy without any effect on the outcome, content, or process of nursing care. An example of quality control might be a requirement that the temperature be charted on the graphic sheet. While it might be agreed that such graphing is helpful to the physician and nursing staff and therefore is related to quality care, actually the standard is to perform the procedure (measuring the temperature), to document the temperature where it may be noted by others (may or may not be the graphic), to call abnormalities to the attention of the physician, and to institute appropriate interventions (quality of care issues) rather than to chart on the graphic.

Quality assurance requires several steps that are essential to the process. The first step is development of standards of care. Standards of care may take several forms. Nursing organizations such as the American Nurses Association and the specialty nursing organizations including AACN, NAACOG, AORN, and others have developed standards that are frequently the basis for standards of nursing practice. Policies and procedures within the health care institution may serve to direct the process toward the standards of practice, and the criteria developed for quality monitoring are utilized to monitor standards of practice.

Once standards are developed, there must be an assessment or evaluation to determine whether there is compliance with the standards. This is data collection and is perhaps the most time consuming step. There are a number of ways in which this may be accomplished. Nursing care may be assessed in terms of outcome, content, or process, depending on whether outcome, content, or process standards are used. The outcome of care is certainly important. The outcome referred to is the end result in relation to the patient or client. An important question in the evaluation might be how the nursing care affected the patient's outcome. Included in outcome might be effect on knowledge, function or performance of activities, life and well being, comfort, satisfaction, and compliance. A negative outcome is obviously not desired. In evaluating outcomes against standards, one must identify not only problems but causes of problems as well.

Evaluation of nursing care content basically is an evaluation of what kind of care was given. Again, using standards of practice, the care that was provided would be reviewed. For example, a patient who has had abdominal surgery would need certain observation, certain procedures carried out, and certain types of teaching accomplished. Evaluation of that content is a type of quality assurance monitoring.

Nursing care may also be evaluated in relation to process, or how the care is accomplished. Steps in a particular procedure may be important in relation to quality, and that process may be reviewed to ensure that quality is achieved. Included under this type of evaluation of care might be interactions with the patient or family, involvement of the patient in his own care, skill utilized in performing procedures, continuity of care, and use of available resources as appropriate as well as the technique or procedure itself.

As resources have begun to dwindle and efficiency has become more important in health care settings, quality assurance monitors may also look at these items, especially as they relate to the other aspects of care being evaluated (Aduddell and Weeks, 1984). For example, length of stay of patients in an ICU or number of days on telemetry or even the number of a type of laboratory test might be monitored to determine whether there is a decrease in any of these. This would be especially significant if average numbers by pay class could be determined and any trends were noted. Consumer demands for cost effective care must always be considered in relation to the demands for excellent care. All of this must be considered in light of how that consumer measures the quality of care he receives. The standards he uses are not always the same as those of his nurse, since he usually evaluates service rather than quality of care.

The next step in the QA process is determination of compliance with the standard. Before the level of compliance has been determined, the nursing manager must decide the level that is acceptable to her. This may vary from standard to standard. For example, if medication errors are reviewed, the standard is no errors to be made. Realistically, however, as long as humans give medications, errors will be made. The nurse manager may feel that the proper action is only to review each error and counsel staff members involved, without other action being necessary.

The action plan to resolve the problem identified by the evaluation is the next step. In each case, the action should be directed at the identified or presumed cause of non-compliance. Corrective action is an essential step in the QA process, since the purpose of QA is to improve quality. Once the action plan is developed, action must occur. Follow-up to ensure that the action had its planned effect is the next step. It may be the final step if improvement is significant and meets acceptable levels of compliance. However, if the problem is not corrected, a different action plan with reevaluation and additional follow-up becomes necessary.

A QUALITY ASSURANCE PROGRAM

In the development of a quality assurance program, one of the resources is the JCAH standards for quality assurance (JCAH, 1986). These standards address the monitoring of the quality and appropriateness of care. Of special note is the requirement that nursing judgment and competencies be monitored. Understanding the requirement for nursing judgment and competencies is very helpful in program development, since questions that might be raised about the particular monitors can be related at least in part to these items.

One essential JCAH requirement of a QA program is that there be a planned and systematic process identified by which the monitoring for the quality and appropriateness of care can be accomplished. A calendar such as that in Figure 17–2 may be established by unit and can be used to plan various monitors. Monitoring for quality should be regular and planned, but there is no specific requirement for monthly or any specific number of monitoring screens. A plan for monitoring quality must also be specific for the nursing care being provided. In other words, the process, content, or outcome of obstetrical nursing care would be appropriate monitors for an OB unit but would not be appropriate for a medical unit.

Implementation of the QA program for a department involves developing a plan for review or monitoring, identifying or determining criteria or standards, collection of data, analysis of the data, identification of problems, development of action plans, and follow-up. Committees may be formed to implement the program, and any number of resources may be used to obtain data. Utilization of data already being collected is one such resource. For example, patient falls are documented by incident reports. Incident reports then become a data source for a monitor of patient falls. Worksheets of all types may be developed to assist in data collection. An example of a worksheet for data collection about IV therapy is found in Figure 17–3. This type of worksheet makes data collection very simple. Data may be collected by direct observation of care or by review of charts.

Once data are collected, analysis of the data for compliance is done, and results are noted. Previously, percentages were common in the results portion of the documentation. While percentages are acceptable, it is preferable that real numbers also be included so that determinations may be made of significance of any identified problems. For example, 50% of 4 patients has a different significance than 50% of 100 patients. Analysis of

MONTH Monitor	JAN Plan	JAN Done	FEB Plan	FEB Done	MAR Plan	MAR Done	APR Plan	APR Done	MAY Plan	MAY Done	JUNE Plan	JUNE Done	JULY Plan	JULY Done	AUG Plan	AUG Done	SEPT Plan	SEPT Done	OCT Plan	OCT Done	NOV Plan	NOV Done	DEC Plan	DEC Done
Nursing Care Plans			X	X					X	X					X						X			
Medication Errors	X	X	X	X	X	X	X	X	X	X	X	X	X		X		X		X		X		X	
Abnormal Temps	X	P	X	F	F		X	F	X	X	X		X				X				X			
Patient Falls	X	X	X	P	X	F	X	F	X	X	X		X		X		X		X		X		X	

FIGURE 17–2. Quality monitor calendar.

Unit _____ Date _____

Patient Number	IV Site Location Noted		Dsg Change qd		IV Tubing Change q 48 hrs		Site Change q 72 hrs		Site Condition Noted		Comments
	Yes	No	Yes	No	Yes	No	Yes	No	Yes	No	

FIGURE 17–3. IV therapy worksheet—QA

results also begins the process of planning action by evaluating the reasons for non-compliance. During the analysis of results, there may be identified needs for education, for policy or procedure development, or for changes in structure or organization, or for changes in forms or equipment. Practices may be examined to determine effectiveness. The results of the analysis may be used to modify policy or procedure, to improve documentation practices, to provide support for staffing changes, to provide support for needed equipment, or to develop education programs. The nursing administrator may additionally use the results found in the QA programs to identify strengths or deficiencies within nursing as a basis for planning and goal development.

A quality assurance program can be very successful if the nurse manager values the program and works with her staff to monitor those areas of care that reflect quality. Use of the data in a meaningful way to effect needed change can have positive effects throughout the department. Motivation of personnel to participate in patient care evaluation may be the toughest part of the manager's job, but if she is able to get the staff motivated, the benefits will certainly make the effort worthwhile (see heading "Motivation" in Chapter 5, Foundations of Leadership).

Productivity

Nursing care must certainly be of high quality, but because of economic pressures, high productivity within the nursing department has become essential as well. Nursing administrators are being asked to improve productivity without increasing costs or sacrificing quality. In fact, at times they are being asked to improve quality, improve productivity, *and* cut costs. Effective planning and control within the nursing department provide much potential for the nursing administrator to achieve this objective (Kirk and Dunaye, 1986). Measurement of actual versus budgeted hours of care is a tool that may be used in this control or management of productivity. Patient classification for acuity, cost efficient scheduling, and flexible budgeting are other techniques that may be helpful in controlling productivity. Chapter 10 (Productivity Management) addresses productivity in detail.

Productivity measurement has become essential as prospective payment has reduced lengths of stay and increased the demand for cost control. As resources are more limited, controls of productivity become more necessary. Added benefits to such controls come from use of the collected data to plan budgets or to justify staffing needs, particularly in relation to acuity. Maintaining productivity and high quality care provides a challenge for any nurse manager. Delivery of patient care must be accomplished while maintaining both of these if the nursing departments are to survive.

Staffing

Staffing is the process of placing the appropriate number and mix of personnel in a particular unit to provide the desired outcome of high quality and productivity. That outcome in a nursing unit is a desired level of care as determined by the needs of the patients in that unit. Several factors may influence the staffing of a particular unit. The number and acuity of patients are two such factors. Obviously, more patients or patients who are sicker may require more nursing care. The mode of care delivery will also influence staffing. Primary nursing requires a different mix of personnel than does functional nursing. How much flexibility is permitted from unit to unit may also affect staffing decisions. The philosophy of the institution and nursing department may affect the staffing. If psychosocial needs receive a high priority, the staffing mix may need to reflect that priority. Use of clinical specialists is another area in which the philosophy of the institution and department may play a role in the decision. Financial stability of an institution or budgetary constraints may also significantly affect the staffing decisions made in a particular department or institution. If there are not financial resources available to support an all RN staff, all the desire in the world for top notch quality care may not make the wish realistic.

There are still other factors that may have some influence on staffing needs. Educational preparation of staff and experience level may determine to some extent the needs for staff. A unit can usually operate more efficiently with better educated and/or more experienced staff. If a unit has a high number of new graduates who are new to the institution and inexperienced in nursing, more staff may be required to perform the same amount of work. Increased time for orientation is one aspect of this problem. Turnover of staff is also tied to this, since total time for orientation increases as turnover increases. Presence of nursing students may also influence the perceived staffing needs of a unit. If nursing students care for patients two days a week, staff members may perceive that their workload on those days may be reduced. In fact, although many schools of nursing have agreements regarding students being "used as staff," there may be a need for fewer staff when students are present on a nursing unit. The extent of responsibilities that nursing assumes continually or at specific times is also related to staffing needs. For example, if the nursing staff members are responsible for patient transport, errands, dietary tasks, respiratory therapy, etc., more staff may be needed than when these duties are retained by other departments. Standards of care as determined by the institution may impact on staffing. If standards require that a procedure be performed by two nurses, for example, staffing to provide that service would be necessary. In fact, the type and spectrum of services available will necessarily affect the staffing needs of the institution. It cannot be anticipated that services will be expanded unless staff is available to provide the services. Although expanding or adding services does not always result in increased staffing needs, this should receive consideration. Finally, unionization may impact on staffing, since contract requirements may demand specific staffing levels. Each factor identified may have a varying influence on staffing. Each nursing administrator should give consideration to the various factors as she develops a staffing plan to match staffing needs to quality standards and productivity standards.

Human resource management, a major responsibility of every nursing administrator, does not just happen. Like other areas of responsibility, this task requires planning and coordinating. Consideration should be given to several key points as the staffing plan is developed. Tools are needed by which staffing needs may be determined. These tools, as previously identified, include patient classification for acuity and to measure workload. The amount and kind of nursing care can be objectively determined by many such systems. A second part of the tool or a second associated tool is needed to convert the needed care into staffing requirements by shift and category. Many pre-packaged classification or staffing tools assist in this conversion. However, since no two institutions are alike in terms of patient population or needs, it is important for the nursing administrator to carefully examine the data from her own institution to ensure that the tool selected is suitable to determine the staffing requirements. For example, if a classification tool does not consider the tremendous time requirement for counseling family members on an oncology unit, it might indicate a need for fewer staff members than is actually the true need or desire.

Flexibility is one characteristic needed in every staffing plan, since nursing units, probably more than other departments, have difficulty predicting needs consistently. Interruptions in routine, admissions, discharges, transfers, changes in patient condition, and visitors are examples of occurrences that are often difficult to predict but that impact on staffing needs at times. Lack of flexibility in addressing these occurrences can result in significant levels of frustration among staff members.

Once tools have been made available to assist in determining staffing levels, the process of staffing may occur. A staffing program will provide an overall system to project staff needed and to provide that staff at the time it is needed. Such a program may be complex, depending on needs and availability, and must consider a number of factors. As has been suggested, needs may be determined by various tools or methods that look at care requirements and/or acuity. Staff may be viewed in its general perspective of availability for hire or more specifically for ability to work a particular day or shift. Compounding the issues related to staffing may be personnel policies that predetermine paid time off, off days, call in procedure, hours of work, and consecutive days worked. It is, therefore, important that any staffing program be developed in coordination with human resource departments to ensure compliance with those policies. Staffing policies of the nursing department that will be applied are another aspect of the staffing program. These are often associated with personnel policies but may also determine work assignment, floating or pulling policies, and shift rotation.

Actual calculation of required personnel must be based on all these factors. Adjustment for special areas is often included in the calculation, as is provision of supervision or unit management. The major purpose of the staffing program is certainly provision of adequate staff to provide the indicated level of care. However, the program should also determine basic staffing patterns by unit, core versus flexible staffing provision, coordination of staffing needs to include personnel policy requirements, and a mechanism to monitor staffing to ensure that desired quality standards are met.

There are several ways to operationalize a staffing program. A simple method that may be used is conversion of hours of direct care per patient day as determined by patient classification or based on historical data, consultants' reports, etc. Direct care hours may be added to indirect care hours to determine total hours of care needed. This can be converted to full time equivalents (FTE's) and split into shifts. Chapter 9, Financial Management, includes a section on budgeting that carefully depicts these calculations. Staffing may only be established by numbers of patients without consideration for patient acuity or variations in workload not related to census. A more reasonable approach is one in which staffing needs are evaluated from shift to shift based on patient classification data. This approach would consider not only the number of patients but also the severity of their illness to determine the number and mix of personnel needed to care for the patients. Especially in today's economic environment, the staffing program must be flexible enough to adjust staffing to those needs.

Staffing options that may improve flexibility are numerous. Float pools have been used for many years. Although they lost popularity for a time, the fluctuating patient census has resulted in their reappearance with multiple variations. Float pools may be specific for specialty areas or may be general. Float personnel may be paid incentives to work as "floats" and may be required to meet specific criteria. Flexible staffing options may also include "on call" personnel who work only as needed. Staffing options may also extend to variations in scheduling aimed at meeting certain departmental needs such as heavy workload times, workdays that are longer than 8 hours but are limited (e.g., 7 AM–5:30 PM), etc.

Scheduling

Scheduling may assume so many forms that it is not possible to cite all types or variations. However, scheduling will be discussed generally and several variations will be described. Scheduling of nursing staff is often difficult because of the factors that have been identified: fluctuations in patient census, personnel or staffing policies that influence scheduling, costs for staff, absenteeism, or other problems that result in non-predictable needs.

The major purpose of any scheduling system should be to ensure that the desired level of patient care can be delivered while maintaining productivity and cost-efficiency. Consistency and fairness to all personnel are other considerations in scheduling that cannot be overlooked. In any type of scheduling system, these needs must be met in such a way that personnel

S	M	T	W	TH	F	SS	M	T	W	TH	F	SS	M	T	W	TH	F	SS	M	T	W	TH	F	S
	X					XX			X				X					XX				X		
X			X				X					XX			X				X					X
		X				XX				X			X					XX				X		
X				X				X				XX				X				X				X
		X				XX				X				X				XX			X			
X			X				X					XX			X				X					X

FIGURE 17–4. Cyclical schedule.

satisfaction is maintained, if the long range goals related to stability in the department are to be met.

In developing a schedule for a unit or department, the first priority is ensuring adequate coverage 24 hours a day, 7 days a week, including holidays. This is based on the needs as determined through patient classification or preset ratios of staff as well as minimum numbers established to meet safety standards. Mix of staff is also a consideration in coverage. Included in coverage should also be continuity of care considerations. Long work stretches are not desirable generally by nursing staff members, but very short stretches reduce continuity. Some midpoint is best to ensure the most satisfactory arrangement.

Schedules must be flexible in their ability to adjust to vacation requests, holidays, or leaves of absence. This type of adjustment, as well as provision for appropriate weekends off, off days, and rotations, contributes to employee satisfaction and cannot be minimized. Staff members become very defensive about earned time off, especially when attempts are made to take control of such time totally away from the staff. Staggering vacation and holiday time can provide coverage while ensuring equitable treatment of nurses.

Coverage adjustment for weekends and holidays as well as variations on odd shifts must affect scheduling decisions. Although some variation between hospitals is evident, there is generally a reduced need for staff on weekends and holidays related to lack of availability of procedures. It is important to note that this has and will continue to change over time as hospitals consistently work to improve numbers of inpatient admissions by offering services every day that previously may not have been available on weekends. Examples include surgery, diagnostic procedures, and home health visits, all now often available routinely on weekends.

Scheduling is always difficult when all variables are considered. Experimenting with various options can assist a nurse manager in identifying the one most satisfactory to her unit's needs. Cyclical scheduling of some type tends to provide the most stable and easiest schedule for the nurse manager. In cyclical scheduling, off days are predetermined in some pattern that recurs in a cycle. An example of a cyclical schedule is found in Figure 17–4. Flexibility with this type of schedule is still necessary for holiday or vacation coverage.

Other important guidelines for scheduling may be helpful in maintaining the most satisfaction among staff. Advance posting of schedules to permit planning for off time is important to staff members. Changes in schedules should follow predetermined rules. For example, a nurse manager may permit schedule changes only before posting. Changes in the schedule after posting may be allowed only if the individual "swaps." These rules should be formalized and communicated to staff.

Scheduling may be centralized or decentralized or a combination. In centralized staffing, one individual has responsibility for scheduling for all nursing units. This provides the most consistency for scheduling. However, it is very problematic in that clinical considerations do not affect the scheduling, and there is a depersonalization that influences employee satisfaction. Decentralized scheduling provides for more input from staff, thus improving satisfaction, but often requires much of the unit manager's time. It does consider clinical problems and personal needs, and may therefore lack consistency. Additionally, it is often difficult to ensure coverage with a fluctuating census if there is no pool of float nurses who work only for that unit. A combination of decentralized and centralized scheduling probably resolves more of the problems identified. In this type of scheduling, the core staff for a unit is scheduled by the nurse manager, and the float personnel, utilized to fill in the holes when census rises or call-ins occur, are scheduled by the nursing office. This improves flexibility for the nursing department and requires cooperation and coordination between the nurse manager and house supervisor. There does, unfortunately, tend to be occasional problems with this method, too, since the goals of the unit manager (to cover her unit) and the house supervisor (to ensure the best coverage possible on all units with available resources) differ.

Other scheduling options include flexible alternatives that may be helpful in providing coverage, retention or recruitment of personnel, or meeting needs during census peaks. Options may include 10-hour shifts, 12-hour shifts, partial shifts, special weekend or weekday work weeks. Depending on the needs for a department, these options may or may not be helpful and may or may not be cost effective. However, these shifts may not be cost effective and may be detrimental in other ways.

Ten-hour shifts, for example, may work well in departments that have excessively high workload during certain hours or that operate for limited hours. An operating room, for example, may be utilized from 7 AM to 5:30 PM. Twelve-hour shifts result in fewer staff members needed to cover in a particular day, but overall may not require fewer personnel. For example, if four nurses are needed each shift in ICU, only eight nurses would be needed if 12-hour shifts were used. However, those eight nurses would only work seven shifts per two-week period, including 4 overtime hours each (total of 32 hours); to cover 14 days, 16 FTE's would be needed. To cover 14 days with 8-hour shifts, 16.8 FTE's of personnel would be needed, entailing no overtime. There is, therefore, no significant reduction in personnel or costs overall. There is also the problem of fatigue in nurses working 12-hour stretches consistently, which should be considered. Partial shifts may also be helpful during heavy load times but are otherwise not generally cost effective. For example, an extra nurse working 8 AM–12 noon, Monday through Friday, might be of great assistance in an active Labor and Delivery Department, which performs many non-stress tests, ultrasounds, or other procedures on outpatients during those hours.

Weekend versus weekday options, popular in the nursing shortage days, are very costly. These options entailed payment for more hours than actually worked. For example, an individual might work 24 hours and be paid for 40. The cost of such plans is tremendous. Seven on–seven off plans, in which individuals work seven days and are off seven days with payment for benefits and/or extra unworked hours, were excellent recruiting tools and provided stability for many 11–7 shifts. However, these, too, are not very cost effective.

Documentation

Documentation has been alluded to repeatedly throughout this chapter but must also be addressed separately because of its importance. Documentation of patient care has importance in the sense of being a legal document. As a legal document, that medical record may be subpoenaed and used as evidence in malpractice suits. Adequate documentation of facts related to the care of a patient may serve to defend a nurse or hospital against a claim of malpractice, and therefore cannot be minimized in importance.

More importantly, documentation serves as a device for communication between individuals or groups. Physicians document the medical orders and progress notes. Nurses must document that medical orders were carried out, that observations were made, and that nursing care was performed. Accuracy is essential, since future care may be based on the documentation. For example, even a weight becomes important when one considers that a physician may order a diuretic for a patient based on whether the patient has or has not lost fluid weight since yesterday. Legibility is important, since the record may be reviewed without benefit of the writer to interpret. Misreading or misinterpretation of a record may cause harm to the patient.

Although documentation is important, there is no universal requirement prescribing exactly how it should be done. This permits flexibility in the use of flow sheets or graphs, which may reduce the burden of documentation. Even computerized charting is acceptable. New computerized nursing information systems that allow care plan development, documentation, and profile information to be accomplished in coordination with requests for tests or procedures are very useful for documentation purposes. The primary goal is an accurate record of the care the patient has received. The method by which that goal is reached is left to the particular institution.

Several objectives for documentation should receive consideration. Documentation should assist in identifying patient problems and devising a care plan from that information. Documentation should also provide accountability for action by the nursing staff (O'Grady, 1977). Every professional nurse has responsibility for documenting actions, assessments, and responses. The detail of documentation is often left to the discretion of the nurse.

The nursing administrator may desire to devise a more consistent approach to documentation. Policy about documentation should clearly define expectations. Each procedure may realistically include a section on what should be documented in relation to the procedure. Leaving the details of documentation to the discretion of the nurse may result in inadequate documentation of events or observations.

Although a great deal of flexibility may be possible while maintaining the consistency desired, guidelines for documentation may specify minimally what should be charted and in what manner. All assessment data from history and physical examination are important, since this information will be needed throughout the patient's illness. The plan of care for the patient, including identified nursing diagnoses or problems, must be included. Any intervention performed or observed by the nurse is necessarily a part of the documentation. The patient's response to the interventions is another important aspect of documentation. Evaluation of responses, interventions, and plans may be included as well.

One of the most difficult aspects of the nursing administrator's job is achieving compliance with requirements for documentation. Quality assurance monitors may assist in determining compliance. Development of innovative approaches to motivate staff to document appropriately may require time on the part of the nursing administrator, but it will be worth the effort if goals for documentation can be met. The use of computerized nursing records is one such innovative approach that has and is improving documentation by nurses and improving productivity. Computer applications for documentation, then, may need to receive consideration by the nursing administrator.

Computerization

Computer literacy has become a major need among the nursing staff at nearly every hospital, and that need is likely to become even more important over the next few years. Computers, which have been commonplace in health care institutions' business offices, have become the current technology in nearly all hospital departments. From admission to discharge, hospital information systems play a role in those institutions that have planned ahead and have realized the need and benefit of computerization. The diversity of activities in health care institutions, the need for cost control and monitoring mandated by the health care environment, and the necessity for review and evaluation of care resulting from the changes in reimbursement systems have resulted in the need to obtain multiple data from numerous sources and to interrelate those data repeatedly. Without computerization, such a task would probably not be possible.

Computerization has evolved to its current state which is not only sophisticated but also planned for future updating as technology changes. Not only do hospital information systems provide financial reporting and patient data for billing; also, order entry, charging, and documentation have become integrated. For nursing, order entry was the initial step and provided sophistication in obtaining appropriate diagnostic studies. Reporting of diagnostic study results was associated and became an integral part of such systems in many institutions. More recently, the patient profile/care plan documents have been added. The patient profile data capture patient care events, physician orders, test results, and historical information as well as provide a means for development of patient care plans (Figure 17–5). Although the financial system and patient profile system were initially designed independently, it has become increasingly important for there to be an interrelationship between them (Halverson and Huesing, 1984).

The future direction for computerization is a total system that will integrate patient management and financial reporting systems. Control systems for materials management, diagnostic study reporting, and physician's office systems as well as quality monitoring systems and staffing and scheduling systems will continue to be integrated. The complexity of health care today and tomorrow will necessitate these changes. The implications are tremendous. Computerization may be used to track charges, maintain billing information, order diagnostic studies or supplies and charge them, report results, profile patient information, keep up with active orders, maintain a record of all orders, plan patient care, document patient care, communicate between departments, update files, schedule staff, determine staffing needs, classify patients, determine costs versus benefits, identify beneficial DRG's, cost nursing services, and so on. The nursing administrator, then, has an important responsibility to plan for these changes and to prepare her staff to meet the challenges of medical computerization. Never before has computerization offered so much for nursing. In an age of cost consciousness, every avenue must be explored to assist nursing departments in improving efficiency or maintaining quality care.

EDUCATION

Education's focus is to facilitate learning and hopefully to influence behavior when appropriate through that process. In the management of patient care, education can be divided into two specific areas—patient education and staff education. The majority of those at whom education is directed are adults and, as such, must be approached very differently than children if the education is to meet its objective. Education is an interactive process between the teacher and learner. The role of the teacher is to assess

PATIENT CARE PROFILE

BAY MEDICAL CENTER   1/9/87   8: 57 AM   PAGE: 1   SHIFT: 1

ACTIVITIES OF DAILY LIVING	0001 2121036 EDU
VITAL SIGNS Q 4H *See graphic*	#DUCK, DONALD Q SEX: M
NEURO. CHECKS Q 4H *See graphic*	ADM: 11/21/86 SRV: IM SMOKN
WEIGHT QD STANDING *8 A*	DOB: 9/30/46 40 COND: F LEVEL: 3
I & 0 RTN (DR. ORDER)	HT: 5/00 FI WT: 125/000 PO
FEEDING W/ASSIST *8-12*	009 MISC DOCTOR
BATH W/ASSIST *9 A*	ALG: FEATHERS, CATS
ORAL HYGIENE W/ASSIST *93¾*	DX: DIABETES W/WOUND INFECTION
BEDREST TURN Q 2H	L LEG

ACTIVITIES OF DAILY LIVING
VITAL SIGNS   Q 4H *See graphic*
NEURO. CHECKS   Q 4H *See graphic*
WEIGHT   QD STANDING *8 A*
I & 0   RTN (DR. ORDER)
FEEDING   W/ASSIST *8-12*   ⎫
BATH   W/ASSIST *9 A*   ⎬ *JB*
ORAL HYGIENE   W/ASSIST *93¾*   ⎪
BEDREST   TURN Q 2H
ELIMINATION   FOLEY CATH
ELIMINATION   BEDPAN
TRANSPORT   STRETCHER

ALL   SOFT *8 A 95% JB*
                      12 65% JB
PR: DIABETIC PATIENT
  : NO SMOKING
IS: WOUND AND SKIN — *JB*

ACTIVE ORDERS
   COMP BLD COUNT   1/09 *done by lab JB*
   SMA 6 PROFILE   1/09 *done by lab JB*
1: FASTING UNTIL BLD. DRAWN. H20 ALLOWED
   CHEST PA/LAT   1/10 A

TREATMENTS
1: RESP: (BBS)(CLEAR)UNLAB)ABN _X_
   CARDIAC: (REG)IRREG
Λ TELEMETRY: _X_
   PULSES: *R. brachial* (D, 1+, (2+), 4+)
   LOC: *Alert*   GI: *B/s hypoact.* GU: *urine clear*
2: *JB* ACCUCHECK: TEST BLD GLUCOSE
   Q4H SLIDING SCALE
   COVERAGE YES
3: *JB* D21/2 NS @ 50CC/HR
   IV SITE: (WNL)/ABN _X_
   HUNG *9A*, _X_
   CHECK QH *JB, JB, JB, JB,*
                    JB, JB, JB, JB
   RESTART ___ TUBING ___
   FILTER ___ DSG ___
4: *JB* FOLEY CATH TO BEDSIDE DRAINAGE.
5: *JB* GIVE CATHETER CARE:
   QD AND PRN. CATH INSERTED 1/7/.
   CATH CHG ___.
6: *JB* EGGCRATE MATTRESS TO BED
7: *JB* BETADINE DRESSING TO L LEG Q4H
              9A-1p·

NURSING GOALS
DG: RESTORATION OF NORMAL GLU-
     COSE LEVELS BY DIET THERAPY OR
     MEDICATIONS AND EDUCATION
     REGARDING DISEASE PROCESS,
     THERAPY, AND COMPLICATIONS.
DG: WILL HAVE HEALING OF INVOLVED
     AREA
PB: ELEVATED GLUCOSE LEVELS WITH
     RELATED SYMPTOMS.
GL: GLUCOSE LEVELS WILL BE RE-
     STORED TO WITHIN NORMAL LIMITS/
     COMPLICATIONS WILL BE AVOIDED.
PB: LOCAL AREAS OF INFECTION WITH
     HEAT, REDNESS, SWELLING, AND/
     OR DRAINAGE.
GL: HEALING OF AREAS W/O COMPLICA-
     TIONS. INSTRUCTION IN, AND UN-
     DERSTANDING OF, WAYS TO AVOID
     RECURRENCE.

NURSING INTERVENTIONS

1: *JB* ASSESS SKIN FOR IRRITATION
     AND BREAKDOWN.
2: *JB* ASSIST IN INCORPORATING
     DISEASE MANAGEMENT REGI-
     MEN INTO ADLS.
3: *JB* CONSULT WITH DIETICIAN.
4: *JB* DETERMINE DIET PREFER-
     ENCES.
5: *JB* EMPHASIZE IMPORTANCE: COM-
     PLIANCE W/ THE PRESCRIBED
     DRUG SCHEDULE.
6: _X_ ENCOURAGE DAILY EXERCISE.
7: *JB* INSTRUCT IN RECOGNITION OF
     ACUTE SIGNS AND SYMPTOMS.
8: _X_ NOTE ABRUPT OR UNUSUAL
     CHANGES IN BEHAVIOR.
9: *JB* OBSERVE FOR FATIGUE.
10: *JB* ASSESS AND EVALUATE FOR
      REDNESS, SWELLING, SKIN
      WARMTH, PURULENT

TIME	NURSING NOTES
2 p	*No change in initial assessment* —

INT	SIGNATURE	INT	SIGNATURE	INT	SIGNATURE
JB	*J. Bruneln*				

FIGURE 17–5. Computer documentation/care plan.

and promote learning, whereas the learner's role is directed at participation in the activities leading toward a behavior change (Redman, 1980).

The first step in education of either type is identification of the need. Assessment of needs may be accomplished in several ways. Direct questions are a common mechanism for this determination. Observation of behavior or condition is another way that need for learning may be assessed. Results of research or quality assurance studies may identify a need as well. Once the need is identified, the next step, readiness, must be determined.

Readiness for learning can be subdivided into motivation or willingness to learn and experiential readiness or actual ability to learn based on skills, attitudes, and experiences. Each of these facets of readiness may influence the others. Motivation to learn is influenced by ability to learn but may also be affected by physical condition, fears, anxieties, environment, or any one of numerous psychological factors. Experiential readiness is primarily related to development of specific skills or attitudes from experience. A child, for example, cannot learn to run if he cannot stand. Physical skills and experiences, then, may preclude certain learning. Assessment of readiness does require judgment on the part of the teacher, and questioning of the potential learner is needed before the judgment is made.

A person's beliefs and biases will influence his or her ability and the motivation to learn. These are part of the individual's receptivity to teaching. Several principles may be used to guide the educator in motivating the learner (Redman, 1980). The environment helps focus attention on what needs to be learned. Visual aids, for example, may capture the attention of the learner. Learning may be motivated by rewards, but self-motivation results in a more lasting type of learning. Readiness to learn is an important factor in effectiveness of learning. Learning is enhanced when material to be learned is well organized. Mild anxiety, which is normal with learning, improves learning, but severe anxiety prevents learning. Understanding those factors that influence learning readiness is very important in patient care management, since the desired outcome of learning is a change in behavior that may be essential to health or healing.

Once readiness has been assessed, objectives for learning may be determined. Objectives will guide the process and prevent confusion as to the desired outcome. Objectives should be behavioral and may be developed cooperatively between the teacher and the learner. Often, this type of development will enhance learning, since the learner feels more tied to the desired outcome. Objectives may be cognitive, or relate to knowledge, comprehension, application, analysis, synthesis, or evaluation. Objectives may also be developed in the affective domain, that is, resulting in an awareness, response, or value determination. Psychomotor objectives require performance of some action as the outcome of learning.

Adult learners must be ready to learn, must understand the desired outcome, and must recognize the value of that outcome. Also of importance is the need of many adult learners to utilize learned material immediately.

Adults have a wealth of knowledge as the basis for future learning. Unfortunately, many preconceived notions may also interfere with learning.

Learning can occur in a variety of settings. Like all communication, there may be barriers to learning, which need to be evaluated and removed if necessary. Finding the best setting for learning is a good idea, but it is often not practical or realistic. Planning and organizing material, then, must take into account the environment in which learning will occur. Any aids to learning may be evaluated in light of how effective they will be, given the environment.

Patient Education

The importance of patient education has increased in recent years as patients have demanded more information about their conditions and as patient behavior after discharge has been evaluated. Readmission or relapse related to non-compliance with treatment or lack of knowledge about care has had a significant impact, particularly as reimbursement issues come to the forefront of health care. Patient education programs, then, have been developed to reduce readmission, prevent relapse, and generally improve the outcome of health care interventions. Additionally, programs have been directed at wellness or prevention of illness.

Teaching programs for patients may be developed in specific categories in which patients commonly have problems with compliance or readmission. These categories include chronic illnesses such as diabetes, chronic lung disease, or heart disease. Other programs are directed at patients having specific treatments or procedures, such as surgery, heart catheterizations, or physical therapy. The programs are usually developed to provide consistent, reliable information about the topic. Often the classes are taught in group settings. However, education for patients who do not fall into a category that has a defined program cannot be neglected. It is essential that individual teaching/learning continue for every patient to the degree necessary to ensure, as is possible, understanding by the patient. These educational programs and individual patient teaching are an important part of discharge planning.

Several factors may influence the development of patient education programs. These may include the number and characteristics of the patient population, knowledge of which would be needed if appropriate planning for programs were to be accomplished. The cost involved in developing and presenting a patient education program is another factor. Costs for audiovisuals, booklets, closed circuit television, and staff time may be given consideration. Responsibility for the program's success or failure may be difficult to place, yet this would be an important factor in initiating a program. To ensure consistency in the education process, training would be needed for the teachers. Planning for this would be another important factor in the development of patient education programs. Finally, documentation of patient education is essential. Use of special education forms or simple inclusion of this in nurses' notes may accomplish this objective.

Patient education programs may be financed in numerous ways. Third party payers will generally pay for health education that is directly related to the admission diagnosis and that is essential to the care of the patient after discharge. Education for prevention of illness or for other conditions is usually not reimbursed (Rowland and Rowland, 1985). Of course, under prospective payment there is no additional funding available for education. Room rate charges often are used to cover such items as patient education. Because it is difficult to specifically identify a source of revenue for the education provided, nursing administrators may have difficulty in justifying expenditures to hospital administrators.

Patient education programs serve several very important functions that justify the costs for this development. Even under prospective payment, their value can be identified. Educational programs may reduce length of stay by training and educating patients pre-operatively for their post-operative course. For example, pre-operative training about coughing to occur post-operatively will prepare the patient for the procedure he might otherwise be too anxious about later. It has been repeatedly shown for many years that readmissions and complications may be minimized by education, since patient compliance will improve (Pratt, Seligmann, Reader, 1957; Simonds, 1967; Felton, 1976). All those points emphasize the value of patient education in overall reduction of health care costs.

Staff Education

Staff education is the other type of education important within the nursing department. Nursing is a continually changing profession and as such requires continued learning. Basic preparation for nurses varies from associate to master's level preparation for entry into nursing practice. Further complicating the problem of basic education is the lack of consistency from program to program at one entry level. As the base of nursing knowledge has grown, and nursing programs have attempted to keep up, some skill development and theory have been deleted from some nursing programs in order to have time for other knowledge and skills to be learned within the same time frame. The education-practice gap that has occurred is a very real problem for nursing administrators. That problem is preparing the graduate nurse for the practice of bedside nursing. Whether this problem realistically is one for the education or for the practice side of the gap may be a point of disagreement. There remains, however, a continuing problem of graduate nurses performing upon graduation at levels that are perceived to be lower than in the past. While this may be related to changes in patient acuity and to the growing body of nursing knowledge, the perception still exists.

Orientation programs, generally available in health care institutions, vary widely according to need and to funding. Budget constraints resulting

		Returns	
	Verbalizes	**Demonstration**	**Performs**
Skill	**Understanding**	**Competently**	**Independently**

TABLE 17–4
Orientation Checklist Sample

Unit: ICU   Employee: _____

Skill	Verbalizes Understanding	Returns Demonstration Competently	Performs Independently
1. Admit Patient to ICU			
2. Set up for Hemodynamic Monitoring			
3. Set up Ventilator			
4. Cardiac Output Monitor			
5. Calibration, Zero for Equipment			
6. ICP Monitoring			
7. Calculating SVR, CI			
8. Fluid Management, Including Calculation			
9. Management of Ventilator Patient			
10. Management of Open Heart Patient			
11. Streptokinase Infusion			
12. Chest Tube Setup/ Management, etc.			

from changes in reimbursement and drops in patient census have had a significant impact on orientation programs and on all staff education at a time when these programs are most needed. Orientation's purpose should be to acquaint the nurse who is new to the institution to the policies, procedures, and environment that will govern her practice. Orientation often must also provide for additional training or education for these nurses in order for them to practice at the level expected by the institution that has hired them.

Orientation programs have three major phases—orientation to the hospital, to the nursing department, and to the assigned nursing unit. Programs for the hospital and nursing department can be general and include policies and procedures. However, unit orientation programs should be very specific and should include an orientation checklist to document learning needs and/ or accomplishments. Table 17–4 is an example of an orientation checklist.

Inservice education is another aspect of staff education that is important in ensuring that staff members understand new policies and new equipment. Inservice may be voluntary, but often it is mandatory to ensure competence in practice. CPR, electrical safety, and fire and disaster review are often also included in this category. Some inservice programs are brief (15–20 minutes) but still serve the purpose of familiarizing staff members with new procedures or medications.

Continuing education programs are another dimension of staff education. These programs present new information important for the professional growth and development of the nursing staff. Continuing education may be available for staff members and for management and may be offered through seminars, institutes, workshops, or a series of classes. These may be available within or outside the institution. In the pursuit of excellence, there cannot be a replacement for this type of program.

Certification in specialties is one way in which there may be validation that standards of education, practice, and/or knowledge have been met. These standards may be developed by the specialty organization or by the ANA (American Nurses Association). Many specialty organizations offer certification programs that have variable levels of reliability as indicators of competent practice or of knowledge standards being met. Many certification programs do not and cannot validate competence in practice, since no examination or test for competent practice is included in the certification examination. However, certification does provide a mechanism by which the importance of education may be emphasized.

DISCHARGE PLANNING

The impact of prospective payment has been felt by many individuals in the health care institution. The discharge planner has felt this impact to a very large degree. With dollar incentives to reduce length of stay and prevent readmission, the discharge planner has motivation to plan a patient's discharge to meet these objectives. Who the discharge planner is within a particular institution may vary, but the goals of discharge planning are generally similar.

Discharge planning is directed at assisting the patient to return to society in a role as productive or normal as possible. This should be accomplished through involvement of the patient and/or family in the process and through individualized planning for the specific patient. An important aspect of this process is the coordination between the hospitalization and the recovery phase, which may involve multiple resources available to the patient.

The process of discharge planning is one that begins even before admission for many patients. Pre-admission testing, for example, may bring the patient into the system early in the process. Although formal discharge planning may require a physician referral within a particular institution, some plan for discharge must occur at some point in some manner, whether intentional or not. The first step after referral or identification of the patient's need for discharge planning is the interview. If the staff nurse is responsible for the process, she may obtain needed information during admission assessment. Information that may be pertinent to discharge planning includes family support, living arrangements, level of independence before hospitalization versus anticipated level of independence after hospitalization, and anticipated care requirements after discharge.

Conference or discussion with health team members about the patient's care requirements is an important step, since community resources may need to be identified. Once anticipated needs are identified, a plan for discharge is developed to be reviewed by all members of the team. Needs may be as simple as education or as complex as follow-up home visits, extended care facilities, or transfer to a specialty hospital for care. In each case, involvement of the patient and family cannot be overemphasized.

Implementation of the plan must begin before discharge to ensure that by the time of discharge the patient is ready. Continual evaluation of the components of the plan is necessary as well, to provide for change in the plan when indicated. Continuity of care is a major consideration in the implementation to ensure that each patient has the opportunity for maximum potential for recovery.

Discharge planning is somewhat dependent on several variables. Certainly, how ill the patient is may impact on his recovery. The anticipated outcome and the development of complications may also alter the success of discharge planning. The length of time involved in hospitalization and post-discharge care may have an effect. The type and availability of services or resources needed may influence discharge planning.

Given these variables, it is easy to understand the difficulty faced in planning for discharge. The nursing administrator may promote discharge planning through support of the process with policies and procedures as well as with dollars.

TOMORROW'S STRATEGIES

Management of patient care seems so basic that it may be difficult for a nursing administrator to think about strategies for tomorrow. However, as cost efficiency and productivity continue to gain importance, strategies for better patient care management must be emphasized. Nursing administrators must continue to monitor patient acuity as it relates to productivity to ensure that quality is maintained at a satisfactory level. That level will not be optimum in many cases, but rather the best possible care for the dollar spent. This may be difficult to determine. However, the use of quality monitoring to ensure that expected or desired quality is maintained as fewer dollars are spent will be helpful. The role of discharge planning and patient education will continue to be important as reimbursement issues or costs related to multiple factors have an impact. Continual evaluation of the mode of care delivery will be necessary as the nursing administrator considers alternatives or modifications to popular methods in order to improve productivity and reduce costs. Use of computerization to achieve support of the labor force will continue to receive consideration and support. Computer literacy will be among those criteria for future nursing positions as these changes occur.

Emphasis on education for staff and for patients will not decrease in the future, but will take on even more importance as discharge planning takes a dominant role in the nursing process. Growth and development of staff members through continuing education programs will also be improved as nursing staffs stabilize and adjust to the change in nursing practice.

The role of research in patient care management must be re-emphasized. Nursing research is significant for the future because of its potential effect on large numbers of people. Nursing research has and will continue to provide measurable benefits, including cost reduction in health care. Nursing research motivates nursing staff members to be innovative and challenges them to move nursing in a forward direction. The benefits of nursing research to the nursing administrator make it definitely a strategy for the future (Lindeman, 1984). Strategies for the nursing administrator in patient care management must begin and end with a close examination of the patient—his desires and expectations, his needs compared with the often limited resources available to serve him. All issues in patient care management will revolve around these key elements. The successful nursing administrator will be knowledgeable about the role nursing will play in relation to the conflicts identified.

References

Aduddell, P., and Weeks, L. (1984). A cost-effective approach to quality assurance. *Nursing Economics, 1,* 282.
Baer, C. (1984). Nursing diagnosis: A futuristic process for nursing practice. *Topics in Clinical Nursing,* January.
Betrus, A., Kane, E., Malloy, C., and Boro, L. (1985). Organizing for primary care in obstetrics. *Nursing Management,* 16(11), 31–38.
Billings, D. (1983). Patient classification in critical care. *Dimensions of Critical Care Nursing,* 2(1), 36–43.
Bulman, T. (1985). Ambulatory care: A practical way to quality assurance. *Nursing Management,* 16(12), 19–24.
Decker, C. (1985). Quality assurance: Accent on monitoring. *Nursing Management,* 16(11), 20–26.
Felton, G. (1976). Preoperative nursing interventions with the patient for surgery: Outcomes of three alternative approaches. *Int. J. Nursing Stud., 13,* 83–96.
Foley, W., and Schneider, D. (1980). A comparison of the level of care predictions of six long-term care patient assessment systems. *AJPH, 70*(11), 1152–1161.
Gebbie, K.M., and Lavin, M.A. (eds.). (1975). *Classification of nursing diagnoses.* Proceedings of the First National Conference held in St. Louis, Oct. 1–5, 1973. St. Louis: C.V. Mosby Co.
Gebbie, K.M. (ed.) (1976). *Classification of nursing diagnoses.* Summary of the Second National Conference. St. Louis: Clearing house, National Group for Classification of Nursing Diagnoses.
Giovannetti, P. (1979). Understanding patient classification systems. *JONA, 9*(2), 4–9.
Gordon, M. (1982). *Nursing diagnosis: Process and application.* New York: McGraw-Hill Books, Inc.
Halverson, C., and Huesing, S. (1984). Hospital information systems: The next three generations. *Healthcare Computing and Communications, 1* (11), 33–36.

Higgins, S., and Mercereau, K. (1985). Credentialling: Meeting the regulatory standards. *Nursing Management*, 16 (1), 25–29.

Hinson, I., Silva, N., and Clapp, P. (1984). An automated kardex and care plan. *Nursing Management*, 15(7), 35–43.

Huckabay, L., and Skonieczny, R. (1981). Patient classification systems: The problems faced. *Nursing and Health Care*, February, pp. 89–102.

Jackson, B., and Resnick, J. (1982). Comparing classification systems. *Nursing Management*, 13(11), 13–19.

JCAH (1986). *Joint Commission on Accreditation of Hospitals Accreditation Manual for Hospitals.* Chicago.

Johnson, K. (1984). A practical approach to patient classification. *Nursing Management*, 15(6), 39–46.

Kim, M., and Moritz, D. (1982). *Classification of nursing diagnosis: Proceedings of the third and fourth national conference.* New York: McGraw-Hill Books, Inc.

Kirk, R., and Dunaye, T. (1986). Managing hospital nursing services for productivity. *Nursing Management*, 17(3), 29–32.

Knowles, M.S. (1980). *The modern practice of adult education.* Chicago: Association Press.

Lagona, T., and Stritzel, M. (1984). Nursing care requirements as measured by DRG. *JONA*, 14(5), 15–18.

Lindeman, C.A. (1984). Theory and research as basic to nursing practice. *Issues in Professional Nursing Practice.* Kansas City: American Nurses Association.

O'Grady, T.P. (1977). Problem oriented charting: The educational and implementation challenge. *Supervisor Nurse*, 8(1).

Pratt, L., Seligmann, A., and Reader, G. (1957). Physicians' views on the level of medical information among patients. *Am. J. Public Health*, 47, 1277–1283.

Redman, B.K. (1980). *The process of patient teaching in nursing.* 4th ed. St. Louis: C.V. Mosby Co.

Rowland, H., and Rowland, B. (1985). *Nursing administration handbook*, 2nd ed. Rockville, MD: Aspen Systems Corporation.

Simonds, S.K. (1967). "The educational care" of patient with congestive heart failure. *Health Education Journal.* 25, 131–141.

Stanton, M. (1985). Teaching patients: Some basic lessons for nurse educators. *Nursing Management*, 16(10), 59–63.

St. Germain, D., and Meijers, A. (1984). Nursing workload measurement: An expanded future role. *Dimensions*, March, 18–20.

Vanputte, A., Sovie, M., Tarcinale, M., and Stunden, A. (1985). Accounting for patient acuity: The nursing time dimension. *Nursing Management*, 16(10), 27–36.

Zander, K. (1985). Second generation primary nursing: A new agenda. *JONA*, 15(3), 18–24.

TODAY AND TOMORROW

VI

This section proposes to be our crystal ball. We wish that it were, in order to see clearly into an uncertain future so that we might better prepare ourselves and our patients. Preparation represents the first 17 chapters. Conceptual, theoretical, and practical knowledge encourages analytical thinking and productive problem solving for dealing with social changes and their impact on society's health and nursing. Waves of major social changes have occurred within this society with increasing frequency since the beginning of the 1900's. These waves are now occurring with varying intensity on the average of every 8–10 years. These waves of social changes are brought about by such major events as wars, economic depressions, major inventions, or leaps in technology. It can be anticipated that such changes may begin to occur on an even shorter time frame. More rapid social change is possible, but given the political realities of governmental, corporate, and professional relations within our society, more frequent social change is unlikely. Therefore, our society will probably experience another major wave of social change, beginning around 1989. The nature of this coming wave of social change is speculative. Social change can result from wars, famine, endemic disease, political or economic collapse, and technological revolutions.

Chapter 18, Today's Issues and Trends, identifies six areas of problems, issues, and trends that we are currently experiencing. The six areas creating issues and trends are directly or indirectly related to one another, and the divisions are arbitrary. Individual rights and responsibilities, economic issues, and technological progress are three of these areas. Related to these areas are ethical issues, organizational issues, and professional issues.

Chapter 19, Tomorrow's Strategies, suggests three major strategies to address the six areas identified in Chapter 18. Within the three major strategies are several substrategies that need to be addressed, both at the national level as well as individualized down to the institutional level. The three main strategies consist of a professional strategy, an organizational policy, and a policy strategy.

It is hoped that as a result of these two chapters, nursing leaders will have a broad picture of the scope of issues and trends affecting their practice. Furthermore, the strategies will encourage further brainstorming and the identification of new alternatives and solutions to deal with tomorrow.

TODAY'S TRENDS
AND ISSUES

INTRODUCTION

The purpose of this chapter is to present six areas that are shaping and will continue to significantly shape the future of our society, the health care system, and the nursing profession. These key areas are either directly or indirectly related to one another, resulting in continual ongoing metamorphosis. The impact of these major issues and trends on nursing as well as on nursing leadership and nursing administration will be predicted. Strategies to deal with the effect of these issues and trends will be presented in the next chapter.

INDIVIDUAL RIGHTS AND RESPONSIBILITIES

Our society is experiencing an ever-increasing emphasis on individuals' rights, commensurate with associated responsibility (Bezold and Carlson, 1986). As an indication of a maturing society, this trend differs significantly from the individualism characteristic of the late 1960's and 1970's, which emphasized individual freedom. Labeled by some as consumerism, this trend does include an increased involvement of an individual in decisions

18

regarding the use of resources. However, the term consumerism is too limiting, in that it implies only external involvement of the individual in the selection of goods and services. The term consumerism also does not include the heightened awareness of the individual's control over his or her internal environment. Likewise, the term consumerism is not indicative of the concomitant responsibilities associated with this trend.

The trend of increasing individualism can be observed in several ways. Naisbitt (1982) points out that increasing technology leads to a sense of inhumanism, which is being compensated for by the need for increased personalizations. Simultaneously, as society becomes more global, individuals are made aware of their insignificance as well as their inability to control their environment. Events occurring 3000 miles away are now very familiar, and it becomes increasingly difficult to shut them out as terrorism, disasters, and hunger are interwoven themes throughout one's daily experiences.

Individual responsibilities are part of this trend and have also exhibited themselves in several ways. Society is beginning to realize that "there is no free lunch" and that everyone within society has a contribution to make in order to maintain society. This is expressed by the increasing emphasis on wellness. Continuation of life styles detrimental to a person's own self as well as costly to society is no longer condoned, but is increasingly met with outright disapproval and non-support. For those persons who through no fault of their own are in need, there are individuals who feel more responsible for assisting them to help themselves. Individual freedom is still important; however, the responsibility to build society is emphasized in several ways. Movements to help those in need, such as hunger victims, disaster victims, or victims of crime, are illustrations of this sense of responsibility. The judicial system's increasing use of restitution programs and community service as well as stiffer sentences for drunk driving and habitual offenders is another example of this sense of responsibility. Fairer tax laws, living within one's means, and efforts to preserve the environment and resources are also illustrations of this trend.

This trend of individual rights and responsibilities is also manifested by the explosion of self-help techniques in everything from hair care, dental care, and health care to self-hypnosis. Included also in this trend is a closer examination of who the individuals are and what their needs and contributions can be within society, hence the microscopic eye being turned on the baby boomers or Yuppies as well as on the significant impact of the elderly population on society. It is calculated that by the year 2000 over 13% of the U.S. population will be elderly and that by 2040 the elderly will compose 20% of the population. As individuals live longer, they are subject to more debilitating and chronic diseases. This results in the increased use of health services. Besides the increased and longer utilization of health services, there is also a corresponding increased need for other life and health needs, such as meals, personal hygiene, and social support (Fries, 1986). As society becomes more global and more mobile and as the elderly population becomes larger, the contributions the elderly can make will become more recognized and valued. Individuals will have the opportunity to pursue their second or third career. Younger generations will seek stabilization and a historical perspective for the fast paced twenty-first century from the older population, who have lived through a similar time warp.

The impact of this trend is already very apparent within the health care system. Individuals are much more involved in their own wellness, helping themselves in health care, the choices open to them, and the cost of the health products and services they consume. Litigation is frequently decided based on the individual's informed consent or lack of it. Shorter hospitalizations result in more self-care or the need for significant other support. Recognition of the important goals of hospice programs through reimbursement approval is also the result of this trend (Andrews, 1986).

What kind of impact will this trend have on nursing and nursing leadership? This should also be anticipated eagerly. Nurses are the epitome of "high touch" and of "caring" and thus are already the best qualified to maximize the benefits associated with this trend. Experience with holistic nursing provides nurses with the expertise to understand and integrate this trend into the health care delivery systems in which they operate (Shelton, 1985).

ECONOMIC ISSUES AND TRENDS

Another key trend is the application of economic models to the health care system. There are many experts, both within and outside of nursing, who would argue that this trend is the main one and the most significant because it determines all other trends and issues. Prior to the mid 1980's, there was not a great deal of emphasis on the cost of health care. The emphasis was on producing the greatest degree of health for every person. This model of health care emphasized the supply of health regardless of the demand or the resources required to produce it. It is now recognized that the system that evolved is not the most efficient, either from an economic standpoint or from a production or outcome standpoint. Although our society as a whole enjoys a standard of sophisticated health care second to none in the world, gaps and inequities are readily apparent. Of the nations with socialized medicine, only Canada is thought to have medical care equal to the United States. Other countries, such as Britain, Sweden, France, and Italy, spend considerably less on health care, but few Americans would choose to be hospitalized in these countries (Easterbrook, 1987). The cost of our health care is no longer a sleeping giant. Lauver (1985) tracked the effects of society's economic policy on the economy and welfare over the past century. Almost since its inception, the health care system has been exempt from the economic model applied to most other goods and services. The nature of health care was considered too personal, as well as an inherent right, to be subject to the forces of a free competitive market. The intervention of government, local, state, and federal, to ensure the achievement of this inalienable right further removed health goods and services from the forces of a competitive market. Now, the late 1980's is experiencing the economic realities of limited resources, necessitating that the health care system become more efficient. Carte blanche is no longer feasible nor desirable by individuals or governments bearing the cost. As a result, there are opposing arguments as to the best possible solution.

One argument endorses further government intervention and regulation in order to ensure equal access to minimum health care for all individuals. The obvious difficulties associated with defining what constitutes equal access, minimum, and health care are by themselves awesome problems. In addition, it is a well known economic reality that increased government regulations of other industries have only led to higher prices, less innovation, and greater inefficiencies (Feldstein, 1983).

The other argument emphasizes the advantages of the competitive market model. This model is characterized by a consumer who is free to choose those products and services that he values the most. An assumption of this model is that the consumer will make the best use of his resources, or in other words, maximize the utility of his resources. A competitive market model also states that demand will regulate the supply, which will be produced at the lowest cost possible. Another component of this model states that anyone can enter the supply market to produce goods and services. In other words, the supply market is not a monopoly or restricted. Obviously, the current health care system is a heavily government regulated, licensed, and restricted market. To change from the existing situations to a free market system would result in chaos and many undesirable effects. It is too simplistic to argue for one extreme or the other. Realistically, health is an entity of value to all individuals, but it is also very intimate and personal. The existence and welfare of society are also inextricably related to the health and welfare of its individuals. This implies a need for some form of safety net for individuals without resources to obtain health care; this is not a characteristic of a competitive market. In other words, the inequities and inefficiencies characteristic of the existing health care systems cannot be eradicated by either a completely regulated system or a freely competitive system. Government regulation is inevitable and desirable to achieve certain objectives. Historically, this regulation has been concerned with the supply side of health care. Emphasis is shifting and will continue to shift more to the demand side.

Alain C. Enthoven's (1978) consumer-choice health plan proposal consisted of a compromise between government regulation and competitive market forces. Canada currently utilizes many facets of this type of plan in its health delivery system. It goes without saying that no plan is without problems and pitfalls. However, Enthoven's proposal attempted to maximize the economic benefits associated with a competitive market while protecting the social requirements through some government regulation. Despite the passage of time since the publication of his proposal, the consumer-choice health plan retains relevance for tomorrow because some changes advocated by this proposal are now becoming evident in the health care system.

The consumer choice health plan (CCHP) attempts to organize the supply and demand systems of health through the use of various incentives to use resources wisely. The purpose of such a plan would be to "assure that all people have a choice among competing alternatives … good information on which to base their choice, and that competition emphasizes quality of benefits and total cost" (Enthoven, 1978). Through the use of vouchers that everyone would receive, individuals would decide how best to purchase the health care goods and services they valued the most. The vouchers would only purchase the equivalent of a basic health plan. Additional coverage would be the responsibility of the individual. This plan would also remove the tax exempt status of the health insurance premium contributions by employers, thus increasing the consumers' sensitivity to health care costs. Congress failed to make this change in 1986, although the issue was closely examined. Future efforts to tax health insurance premiums will probably be successful.

Providers of health care goods and services would be encouraged but governed by a set of rules. These rules would include periods of open enrollment to ensure equal access and minimize cream skimming. A qualified health plan would have to charge the same fee to all persons in the same risk group and have a minimum plan available. Another important safety regulation would include a limit on out-of-pocket costs. These out-of-pocket expenses include deductibles, co-payments, and any differences between coverage and actual costs. By this regulation, coverage for catastrophic medical expenses would be covered. For a more detailed explanation of how and why this particular approach could be effective, as well as evidence to support it, the reader is referred to the original article (Enthoven, 1978).

The economic issues of health care include a closer scrutiny by both government and business into the health care system. As the largest purchasers of health care goods and services, the federal government and private business have experienced an astronomical increase in the cost without realizing a comparable increase in services or benefits. As major payers, the federal government and businesses are exerting forces on health care providers to become more economically efficient. This pressure appears to be effecting changes without simultaneous concern for quality or comprehensiveness. The results of these forces are a significantly more competitive health care system. This competitive system is characterized by cutthroat competition maneuvers, joint ventures, and mergers. Survival of many health care providers and agencies is now in question. Hospitals are going out of business, reducing their personnel requirements to match decreasing patient census, or diversifying their services. Because the cost of health care has finally become unacceptable, alternative delivery methods and products are now being explored. The increasing use of home health care services and outpatient care is resulting in an increasing need for qualified nurses in these areas. However, prospective payment, the increasing age of the patient population, and restrictive admission policies have resulted in sicker patients in the hospital for a shorter period of time. Hospital administrators attempting to retrench their institutions have cut first into the most labor intensive department, namely nursing. Currently, in many situations, the non-professional staff is being reduced. The assumption underlying this activity is that the professional nurse is the most productive staff member because of a broader range of skills and abilities. If this assumption is not validated economically, other alternatives will be sought by health care administrators. As economic issues become even more significant, the impact of this trend on labor intensive nursing departments will become increasingly evident. Health care administrators will become more concerned with the issue of substitutability. There will be more efforts to substitute cheaper labor. Consumers will also promote substitutability in health care providers and will be more willing to use nurses rather than physicians. This will be offset to some degree by the surplus in some areas of physicians who will strongly resist this trend. Unfortunately, these trends will result in renewed interest in institutional licensure and credentialing (Andrews, 1986). This trend comes at a time when nursing is simultaneously attempting to further restrict its profession by upgrading its educational requirements to a BSN. Upgrading and restricting nursing will only be accomplished through continual, rigorous documentation of the cost efficiency of this change (Andrews, 1986).

The economic issues affecting health care may also result in the evolution of a three tier health care system in which the upper class has access to the highest level of health care, the middle class can access a minimum level of health care, and the poor and indigent have none, minimal, inconsistent, and unequal health care. The Gray Panthers are sufficiently concerned about the evolution of such a health care system that they have developed a national strategy to fight against it. Nurses are viewed as patient advocates and as such are not considered as proponents of such an inequitable health care system (Kuhn, 1985). Since historically nursing has not been considered very powerful or recognized for its economic potential, it will be necessary for nursing leadership to align itself with other groups such as the Gray Panthers to create a power base. Likewise, continued efforts to substantiate nursing's contribution to health and the attachment of a dollar value to that contribution will be achieved. Although there may be some nursing leaders who are reluctant to cost out nursing service for fear of what may be discovered, their voices of doom will be overshadowed by the vast majority of nurses, who want to prove their value to society. Nursing research, such as studies that correlate patient acuity and resource utilization, can make a significant contribution to the economic issues affecting the health care of our society and is urgently needed (Shelton, 1985; Bezold & Carlson, 1986).

TECHNOLOGICAL ISSUES AND TRENDS

Another trend, which three generations have already had to deal with in their lives, is the rapidity in which technology is changing the world. It is estimated that knowledge has increased at least three fold within the last 100 years, and it is expected to quadruple in the next 100 years. The twenty-first century is being forced upon society, and the twenty-second is not far behind. Naisbitt (1982) has labeled this the information age. Individuals possessing information possess power. Nurses accumulate vast amounts of information but are not very adept at utilizing it as a source of power. Because of the rapid changes in knowledge, information accrual, processing, interpretation, and communication will become increasingly important. Within a hospital, the center of information is the nursing unit and the patient's chart. Nurses are in the pivotal position to control this information, both for the patient and for the health care system. It is imperative for nurses to continue to control this information and turn it to their advantage. Nursing leaders should not transfer this source of power to another department but rather should move to consolidate patients' data files even more within nursing.

This attitude toward information control must be aggressive and positive. Any effort to computerize the information concerning the patient, including the data manipulated by nursing, should be encouraged. Placement of terminals at patient's bedsides or remote locations down hallways should be accepted with open arms by all nursing personnel as a means to increase their effectiveness and efficiency. Merging of nursing, medical, administrative, and fiscal data bases provides the best picture of the patient. Because it is the nurse who is at the bedside with the patient and computer, it is the nurse who is best able to put the total picture together, for both the individual and for the institution.

An intregral part of this technological trend is the impact of computerization on the health care system. All nurses must become computer literate for several reasons. In order to remain patient advocates, nurses must control and interpret the computerization of patient information. Computer literacy can improve nursing efficiency when applied correctly. Nurses who are not computer literate can be easily misled intentionally or unintentionally by other power seeking individuals or departments. Computer literacy will also be necessary to conduct the amount of research that will occur in nursing. More sophistication in methodologies and experimental studies can only be accurately conducted with the use of computers (Milio, 1986).

The technological process that is being experienced by individuals in society will only serve to increase their sense of isolation and inhumanism. There again, one can understand the importance of the caring and compassionate "high touch" nurse. Nursing leadership can market both the economic efficiencies of professional nurses and the holistic personal care they provide.

ETHICAL ISSUES AND TRENDS

Ethical issues are already becoming increasingly apparent to both consumers and providers of health care. These ethical issues are being brought about as a result of the economic and technological issues and trends. There are many similarities between economic theory and ethical decision making, mainly because they both deal with the allocation of limited resources (Andreoli and Musser, 1985).

Ethical issues concerning allocation of limited resources are generated by several situations. Limited bed capacity in intensive care units is one example. Limited availability of organs for transplantation is another ethical dilemma. The expense of artificial organs for the benefit of a few individuals as opposed to increasing the nutritional status of indigent children is just another example.

Increasing technology creates further ethical dilemmas because of the ability to create and sustain life. Quantity of life versus quality of life will become a more prominent issue in society as more and more individuals are personally touched by this dilemma. With further technological innovations, initiation of life as well as determination of death will become increasingly sophisticated but not necessarily easier. Research and experimentation will become more important and rigorous. But, at the same time, protection of human rights will become more blurred.

The majority of these ethical decisions will not be made in the courts. As before, moral law evolves before judiciary law. This means that most ethical decisions will be made individually as the situation occurs. The situations described usually include nurses. How staff nurses participate in these situations is largely determined by their nursing leaders. Conflict of values will be experienced by all participants. Support, counsel, and rational decision making will provide the mainstay of determining a successful outcome for those involved.

ORGANIZATIONAL ISSUES AND TRENDS

Economic issues and technological trends as well as the increasing awareness of the individual's rights and responsibilities are having a significant impact on organizations, both outside and within health care (Detmer, 1986). Words such as "retrenchment" and "product line management" are the buzz words of today. Application of theories X, Y, and Z is being synthesized in order to create the productive, rewarding working environment of tomorrow. Diversification of services competes with "sticking to the knitting" of what one organization excels at producing. Alternative sources of revenue necessitate mergers or joint ventures. All of this activity has resulted in a disintegration of traditional organizational lines. Decentralization was popular in the late 1970's and early 1980's. However, productivity and efficiency concerns have resulted in a feeling of loss of control by many chief executive officers. Mergers and product line management have resulted in the need for reshuffling of management functions and responsibilities. Matrix models are considered the organizational structure of the present and of the future. Matrix organizations are viewed as being able to respond more rapidly to change. Collaboration between product lines and experts is encouraged and facilitated in this type of structure. Matrix models also retain the advantages of a flatter, leaner organization that enables those best qualified to be in charge of the product.

Product or service line management is an organizational opportunity for nursing leaders. Because of the services they provide and their location within the organization, nurses function as coordinators of patient care; nurses possess the most and relevant information relating to patients; they interface the most with the majority of related departments and services; and they are in a position to evaluate and initiate changes in a timely manner. All of these attributes qualify nursing leaders to assume product/ service line management positions. As product line managers, nursing leaders must be experts on the product as an entire concept, understanding the principles associated with marketing the product; be responsible for the profitability and coordination of the product; and be accountable for the planning and forecasting of the product (Anderson, 1985). Product/service line trends in health care organizations are really not unfamiliar territory for nurse leaders, although product/service line management is a new organizational approach that requires change, flexibility, and adaptability.

Emphasis is also being placed on networking, which can be considered an informal organization. Networks are especially efficient when it comes to processing information. Nurses historically are very adept at networking and should utilize this expertise in a variety of ways. Nursing leaders usually have established networks with health care providers outside of the acute setting. Joint ventures to increase efficiency and productivity are appropriate objectives of such networks. Concomitantly, mentoring of nurses by one another goes hand in hand with networks. It is also appropriate for nurses to seek mentors outside of nursing.

Nurses are also one of the most subspecialized group of health professionals. This subspecialization provides nurses with the expertise to be involved in every type of health care product line management.

PROFESSIONAL ISSUES AND TRENDS

The professional issues and trends occurring at this time are fertile ground for involvement of nursing leaders and nursing administrators. To ignore them is to help condemn nursing to extinction. Nursing administration does not occur solely behind the high walls of an acute care institution. The institution has had to move beyond its walls, and so must the nursing service administrators.

The largest issue facing nursing at this time concerns preparation of the professional nurse (Bezold and Carlson, 1986). As mentioned earlier, renewed efforts will be made to initiate institutional licensure, certification, and substituting of health care providers (Andrews, 1986). These efforts are very dangerous for nursing. They will originate in the hospitals. Therefore, the nursing service administrator must be well prepared to identify the necessary preparation of the professional nurse and to prove her value.

As the professional association (ANA) moves to upgrade the educational requirements for a professional nurse to BSN and thereby restrict entry into nursing, several arguments will be voiced. One existing concern is that restricting entry will worsen the nursing shortage. Severe shortages will in turn result in an artificial increase in the salaries, which increases health costs. Another argument involves the outcome of the educational process. Should the basic BSN graduate be a generalist and the master's prepared graduate nurse a specialist, or should the baccalaureate student specialize in her last 12–18 months of school? The generalist versus specialist argument will only create further disunity within the profession. Now that the BSN appears to have become relatively well accepted as the inevitable, a new argument has risen to take its place. Nursing cannot afford to spend another 12 years debating the generalist-specialist issue. The nursing product needed will be determined by the evolving health care system. This product of nursing education will need to meet the needs of older, sicker patients in a variety of settings. The most efficient and effective way to produce this nursing product needs to be decided now (Andrews, 1986; Bezold and Carlson, 1986; Kuhn, 1985).

Any discussion of the educational preparation of nurses must also involve the cost of that education. Research into the true cost of nursing educational programs should be a high priority among nursing deans. These data are critical to the strategic planning of nursing education in the future. Historically, nurses have enjoyed significant governmental support through the various nurse practice acts. As a result, many nurses, both at the graduate and undergraduate level, have received scholarships. Additionally, schools of nursing have also received substantial funding. As a result the true costs of educating a professional nurse have not been experienced by those involved. The emphasis has been on quantity of nurses. This is no longer true. Economic issues will result in decreased funding for schools of nursing and nursing scholarships. Nursing is in the best position it has ever been in to wean itself from the public dole. If nursing continues to be profiled as seeking funding for itself, it will be met with public skepticism. Efforts to obtain funding for nurses should be highly specific and limited. Nurses should be viewed as voluntarily reducing their drain of governmental resources. When the true cost of a nursing education is finally determined, there will be fewer individuals who can afford it. Standards for entry into nursing schools must remain high, and the profession must continue to be regarded as a highly desirable and worthwhile career. The availability of advanced specialized nurses will be important to increase the professional status of nurses.

Increasing the professional status of nurses is an important issue for nurses at this time because of their primary role of patient advocate. Nurses must be recognized as important professionals if they are to be effective in protecting the rights and procuring the needs of their patients (LeRoy, 1986; NLN, 1985, Barthowski and Swandby, 1985).

Within the professional issues of preparation and the nurse's primary role as patient advocate, the issue of nursing's image will become increasingly important. Nursing can no longer be considered a powerless, low paying occupation that performs under the direction of the physician. This image is not effective, either for the recruitment of new nurses or for patients' confidence in the nurses' capacity to be their advocate. The professional association (ANA) is moving forward in a number of ways to enhance the image of nursing. Recognition of media that promote a good image of nursing is one of their efforts. Likewise, consultation in the development of nursing characters in media productions is encouraged and available. Nurses are assuming more leadership roles that are increasingly visible to the public eye. Examples of these visible leadership positions include Sister Rosemary Donley, Executive Vice President of the Catholic University of America, and Sheila Burke, Deputy Chief of Staff, Office of the Senate Majority Leader, Senator Robert Dole. These nurses are the role models and image of nursing leadership for the 1990's.

SUMMARY

Six major issues and trends are significantly affecting both the nursing profession and its leadership and will continue to do so. Within each of these issues and trends are many subissues as well. The role of women is not identified as an issue for the future, for several reasons. The majority of that battle has been exposed, identified, and fought during the last 10 years. It is an ongoing struggle. Comparative worth will always be an issue. Tremendous gains have been accomplished. To continue to make it an issue will not achieve the results that are desired. Rather, a recognition of the issues involved can be sufficient to gain due process. In other words, society recognizes the inequalities and problems that exist in regard to women. It is no longer necessary or effective to beat the drum. Women will have to continue to prove themselves every day in order to maintain the progress that has been made and to make any more. That is the reality of the situation. Instead, focus on the major issues described in this chapter is of primary importance. It is through an understanding of these trends and issues and their impact on society and more specifically on nursing that the nursing administrator may develop her strategies for a successful tomorrow.

References

Anderson, R.A. (1985). Products and product-line management in nursing. *Nursing Administration Quarterly, 10*(1), 65–72.

Andreoli, K.G., and Musser, L.A. (1985). Trends that may affect nursing's future. *Nursing & Health Care, 6*(1), 47–51.

Andrews, L.B. (1986). Health care providers: The future marketplace and regulations. *Journal of Professional Nursing, 2*(1), 51–61.

Barthowski, J.J., and Swandby, J.M. (1985). Charting nursing's course through *Megatrends. Nursing & Health Care, 6*(7), 375–377.

Bezold, C., and Carlson, R. (1986). Nursing in the 21st Century: Conclusion. *Journal of Professional Nursing, 2*(1), 69–71.

Detmer, S.S. (1986). The future of health care delivery systems and settings. *Journal of Professional Nursing, 2*(1), 20–26.

Easterbrook, G. (1987). The revolution in medicine. *Newsweek, 109*(4), 40–74.

Enthoven, A.C. (1978). Consumer-choice health plan (Part I and Part II). New England Journal of Medicine, *298*, 650–658.

Feldstein, P.J. (1983). *Health care economics*, 2nd ed. New York: John Wiley and Sons.

Fries, J.F. (1986). The future of disease and treatment. *Journal of Professional Nursing, 2*(1), 10–18.

Kuhn, M.E. (1985). Nurse and patients—together we can heal the sick health care system. *Nursing & Health Care, 6*(7), 363–364.

Lauver, E.B. (1985). Where will the money go? Economic forecasting and nursing's future. *Nursing and Health Care, 6*(3), 132–135.

LeRoy, L. (1986). Continuity in change: Power and gender in nursing. *Journal of Professional Nursing, 2*(1), 28–38.

Milio, N. (1986). Telematics in the future of health care delivery: Implications for nursing. *Journal of Professional Nursing, 2*(1), 39–49.

National League for Nursing (NLN) (1985). Mission and goals, 1985–1987 Biennium. *Nursing & Health Care, 6*(8), 408–409.

Naisbitt, J. (1982). *Megatrends*. New York: Warner Books.

Shelton, J. (1985). Can nursing options cut health care's bottom line? *Nursing and Health Care, 6*(5),251–253.

TOMORROW'S STRATEGIES

In order for nursing leadership to deal effectively with the issues and trends identified in the previous chapter, several strategies need to be developed and implemented. These strategies, if effected, will enable nursing to meet the challenges it is encountering and provide a solid basis for moving into the next century.

A PROFESSIONAL STRATEGY

A professional strategy encompasses several areas, including basic preparation of professional nurses; preparation of specialists, including nursing administrators; and activities within the profession itself (Bezold and Carlson, 1986a; Lancaster, 1986). ANA's long established endorsement of the baccalaureate degree as the basic level of preparation must be instituted within this decade. Intensive effort must be directed at this move in order to make it timely and successful. Failure to act on this issue could forever doom nursing to an occupational status. Stiff competition is being encountered from associate degree advocates. Organizations such as the American Association of Junior and Community Colleges have well directed offensive strategies to combat this move. This internal dissension has wreaked havoc long enough within nursing. Nursing must move on; it cannot tread water any longer.

Funding efforts for nursing should emphasize graduate nursing education. Emphasizing the points made by the Institute of Medicine (1983) report on the importance of graduate nursing education will make efficient use of

19

that alliance. Historically, nursing has successfully aligned itself with powerful groups in order to achieve its objective. This is another example of such an opportunity. It must be recognized, however, that alignment may be viewed suspiciously owing to the threatening changes in health care. A win/win situation should be outlined and promoted. Studies indicate a significant shortage of graduate nurses prepared in geriatrics and administration. Instead of spreading resources thinner, existing programs and faculty with declining enrollment should be abolished or converted to specialties designed to meet the changing needs of society.

There also remains controversy over the preparation of the nursing service administrators. Allied schools such as hospital, health service, or public administration are preparing graduates who will actively compete for the same jobs as nursing administrators. These other programs are also actively recruiting nurses as students. Filerman (1985) argues that only one approach will ensure effective preparation of nurse managers, and that is in the school of business. McClure (1985), on the other hand, argues for an integrated approach that prepares the nurse administrator for her dual role of administrator and of nurse. McClure states, "It is precisely the nurse administrator's clinical background ... that makes her contribution to administrative decisions unique." Current research is examining the type of curriculum needed by nursing administrators to manage a clinical discipline. Students of nursing administration should receive the needed educational preparation from the best sources possible. This means nursing from nursing and business from business. It is not effective or efficient to insist that nurses receive their education from other nurses who have neither the knowledge nor the expertise to teach them. The stakes are too high and the competition is too fierce for this to work. Nursing administrators should be prepared from a collaborative model that provides nurses with the best of both worlds (Jones and Poulin, 1983; AACN/AONE, 1986; Price, 1984; McClure, 1985).

Both graduate and undergraduate nursing programs will have to take into consideration the population and needs of their students in order to attract the cream of the crop (Bezold and Carlson, 1986b). Although the majority of nurses will continue to be female, the number of male students will continue to increase. Nursing has already changed to a more career-oriented profession. However, as there are fewer nurses and as they become better educated, they will achieve greater autonomy. Nursing as a second career is becoming more popular, and undergraduate recruitment strategies should reflect this potential market. These older, wiser, and more mature individuals will require different teaching strategies than the 18–21 year olds (Bednash, 1985). Nursing recruitment should emphasize the initiative and personal aspects of nursing as a career. Nursing increases an individual's ability to know more about herself and help herself stay healthy. In a world of automation, standardization, and computerization, nursing can emphasize its unique contribution to an individual's fulfillment (LeRoy, 1986).

Since nursing education will become increasingly expensive, it will be necessary to design a strategy to revamp the educational process. This is an ideal opportunity for collaboration between nursing service and nursing education through the use of adjunct faculty positions and the teacher-practitioner models. Leaders from both spheres can develop a cost efficient model of both undergraduate and graduate nursing education that is streamlined, can accommodate a wide variety of students and prepares nurses to deal with the future (Moody and Henry, 1986).

Within this professional strategy, it will be necessary for nursing to examine its practice models. Previously, nursing has operated primarily under a *goal-driven model* of total patient care. In this model, goals are set, resources are marshalled, and action is implemented, which is then followed by evaluation. It is now necessary to provide total patient care using a *resource-driven model*. In this model, goals are set only after consideration of the resources available and only if the goals represent the best use of those resources (Stevens, 1985). This approach will be more realistic in tomorrow's limited health care system. It will also be extremely frustrating to nurses who are conditioned to unlimited resource utilization in the achievement of idealistic goals. Nevertheless, the adoption of this strategy is necessary for nursing to exist in the economic environment of tomorrow's health care.

In order to effectively design academic programs and clinical practice models, a professional strategy should include an increasing emphasis on and support of research. Tremendous strides have been made in nursing research. From unprofessional and unscientific starts, research has improved to the point at which it now fills professional nursing research journals and is published in many other scholarly and professional journals. The support of Sigma Theta Tau and the Division of Nursing in the Department of Health and Human Services has been instrumental in the flourishing of research activities. Acquisition of grant money from a variety of sources has also encouraged nursing research. The establishment of a National Institute of Nursing in 1986 should also further facilitate nursing research. Nursing research is essential if nursing theory is to develop and define the unique body of knowledge that is nursing.

In order for nursing research to proliferate and be implemented, the professional strategy must emphasize collaboration between service and education. Nursing service and nursing education cannot continue to be divided in philosophy or practice. Collaboration enables the educator to remain competent and use her knowledge to improve clinical practice. The clinician brings to education her expertise of dealing in the actual setting and the application of research findings. Research can more easily be accomplished because of the blending of the educator's research experience and methodological expertise with the clinician's problem identification and readily available setting. Research emphasis should include the impact of nursing on the elderly, cost effectiveness of nursing services, effectiveness of nursing in health promotion and education programs, and the impact of technology on patients and on nursing (Andreoli and Musser, 1985). As stated in earlier chapters, the largely untouched area of nursing administration theory and research is greatly needed. Research into nursing organizations, politics, etc., can also contribute to theory development in other disciplines.

Nursing, as a profession and as individual professionals, should develop specific strategies to enhance its image to society. Society's perception of nursing and its value to society are the result of individual experiences as well as media messages. Sister Donaley, in her address during Sigma Theta Tau's 1987 teleconference on knowledge building, emphasized the importance of nurses being perceived as "knowledge workers." In an information, highly technological age, nurses will not be valued for their "high touch" alone. As caring, compassionate workers in society, working for the welfare of society, nurses will be valued for their intelligent use of information and technology in a warm, caring, and compassionate manner. This is the image to be promoted at all levels of nursing. The "knowing" nurse at the bedside manages an individual's care to enhance the person's participation and control of his own life. The "knowing" head nurse utilizes data analysis in conjunction with quality care indices to staff the unit to maximize efficiency and job satisfaction. The director of nursing service facilitates product line management by sharing information and problem solving across department lines. The nurse executive educates the health care administrator, as well as the public, in the specific contributions that nursing makes to positively affect health care in primary and secondary health care settings, in addition to the tertiary setting.

ORGANIZATIONAL STRATEGIES

The second major type of strategy to be developed concerns organizations and other systems. The last chapter identified the changes in the traditional organizational structures and emphasized the benefits associated with matrix models. Another organizational process encouraged was networking. Additionally, the importance of collaboration and alliance cannot be underestimated. This type of organization includes the triad of administrator-nurse-physician, possibly along product lines. When all leaders are on equal footing, there is a shared interest in achieving a common goal. Nurses will have no trouble shouldering their share of responsibility in this type of situation.

Another possible organizational strategy that is being proposed as an effective, professional way to manage nursing in the next century is that of shared governance (Porter-O'Grady and Fennigan, 1984). Possibly even more difficult to initiate than the triad, shared governance for nursing offers a model of professional nursing practice from the nursing administrator down to the individual staff nurse.

Whatever organizational strategy is chosen will depend on the individual institutions, and thorough study should precede any attempted change. Immature organizations will have difficulty with these more complex and radical models. These organizations or departments might do better to simplify their existing structure.

POLICY STRATEGIES

Policy strategies are those actions by individuals that identify relevant policies to be effected and then develop activities to effect them. Health policies or nursing policies are the object of these strategies. Diers (1985) pointed out that although the world one lives in may not always seem rational, it is usually not random. Policy strategies are designed to give nurses more control over their world through the examination of a policy that is essentially nothing more than a decision. Decisions or policies are based on data that are not always accurate. These policies occur at the unit level, the institutional level, all the way to the national level. The magnitude of the policy will determine the strategy designed to effect it. Politics are an inevitable companion of policies and cannot be ignored in the development of any policy strategy.

Nurses are not usually comfortable with policies because they do not feel privy to the vocabulary often associated with policy. This objection is only a smoke screen and should be discarded. Understanding policy formulation at any level should be incorporated into all levels of nursing education in order to dispel the mystique associated with it. Then nursing will be better prepared to involve itself in effecting policy decisions at all levels. Andreoli and Musser (1985) emphasized the importance of nursing leadership's visible and active participation in health policy at all levels. Nurses control the majority of information that has to do with the health care products used and the services that occur in acute care settings. It is the responsibility of nursing leadership to organize this information into a power base to effect institutional as well as national health care policies (Bezold and Carlson, 1986b).

A progressive and bold vision of nursing's future state in the next century has been set before us by Myrthle Aydelotte of the American Academy of Nursing (Selby, 1987). The basics of nursing—its intimacy and helping nature—will not change. Nurses of the twenty-first century will operate with autonomy of practice, fully accountable for their choices and decisions. Autonomy will also be demonstrated through self-governance as individuals and as groups. The role of the nurse will be clear and well defined to the public and other health care providers. As a highly valued group within society, nurses will be adequately remunerated and have concomitant power and prestige. Functioning within this visionary state of nursing will be four major roles for nursing: the provider of direct services to clients, the researcher and developer of new knowledge and techniques, the case manager, and the executive. This visionary state will not happen automatically or evolve given present circumstances. Nurses will have to earn this state and create it through planned change, hard work, and risk taking. The majority of roles suggested in this future state will all be directly related to or impacted on by nursing leadership. The strategies that have been suggested are ways for nursing administration to achieve nursing's preferred future.

References

American Association of Colleges of Nursing (AACN), and American Organization of Nurse Executives (AONE) (1986). Joint position statement on graduate education in nursing administration. *AACN Newsletter*, 12(1), 3.

Andreoli, K.G., and Musser, L.A. (1985). Trends that may affect nursings' future. *Nursing & Health Care*, 6(1), 47–51.

Bednash, R.C. (1985). Insights from the past portray nurses of the future. *Nursing & Health Care*, 6(9), 496.

Bezold, C., and Carlson, R. (1986a). Nursing in the 21st century: An introduction. *Journal of Professional Nursing*, 2(1), 2–9.

Bezold, C., and Carlson, R. (1986b). Nursing in the 21st century: Conclusion. *Journal of Professional Nursing*, 2(1), 69–71.

Diers, D. (1985). Health policy and nursing curricula—a natural fit. *Nursing & Health Care*, 6(8), 421–424, 433.

Diers, D. (1986). To profess—To be a professional. *The Journal of Nursing Administration*, 16(3), 25–30.

Filerman, G.L. (1985). Nurse managers: Preparing for the future. *Nursing & Health Care*, 6(2).

Jones, D.A., and Poulin, M.A. (1983). Having it both ways. *Nursing Outlook* 31(2), 119–122.

Lancaster, J. (1986). 1986 and beyond: Nursing's future. *The Journal of Nursing Administration*, 16(3), 31–37.

LeRoy, L. (1986). Continuity in change: Power and gender in nursing. *Journal of Professional Nursing*, 2(1), 28–38.

McClure, M.L. (1985). Educational preparation for nursing administration. *Nursing & Health Care*, 6(5), 231.

Moody, L.E., and Henry, B.M. (1986). Futurist approaches in nursing education. *Nursing Economics*, 4(3), 134-137.

Porter-O'Grady, T. (1985). Health versus illness: Nurses can chart the course for the future. *Nursing & Health Care*, 6(6), 319–321.

Porter-O'Grady, T. and Fennigan, S. (1984). *Shared governance for nursing*. Rockville, MD: Aspen Systems.

Price, S.A., (1984). Master's programs preparing nursing administrators: What are the essential components? *The Journal of Nursing Administration*, 14, 11–17.

Selby, T. (1987). Academy looks at nursing's preferred future. *The American Nurse*, 19(1), 12.

Stevens, B.J. (1985). Tackling a changing society head on. *Nursing & Health Care*, 6(1), 27–30.

INDEX

Note: Page numbers in *italics* refer to illustrations; page numbers followed by (t)refer to tables.

Ability, and power, 79
Absenteeism, 364
Abuse of drugs, by personnel, 363–365
Acceptance of change, 277
Access to health care, 287–288
Accountability, 379–382
Accounts, uncollectible, on financial statement, 196
Accounts receivable, 198, 225
Accreditation (JCAH), 379–381
Acid test ratio, 202
Ackoff, R., on planning, 167, 168
ACP (average collection period), 201
Acquisition of power, strategies for, 82–84
Acting, in value clarification, 12
Action, and power, 79
  bias for, in successful businesses, 163
  in mentor-mentee relationship, 108
Action plan, for implementation of objectives, 183
  in quality assurance, 390–391
Activity, administrative, in risk management, 332–333
  units of, department-specific, 208(t)
Acuity, patient, 288, 381
Acuity system, 381
  in salary expense budget, 212
Adaptability, in strategic management, 170
Adjourning stage, in group development, 113
Adjustment of rates, 224
Adjustments and allowances, on financial statement, 196–197, 197(t)
Administration. See *Nursing administration*.
Administrative activities, in risk management, 332–333
Administrative Behavior, 119

Adopters of change, 278–279
Advantage, relative, and change, 272
Advertising, 257
Affect, in mentor-mentee relationship, 108
Agent(s) of change, 278, 279
Aggression, passive, 310–312
Alcohol and drug abuse, by personnel, 363–365
Alderfer, C., needs theory of, 91
Allocation, of costs, 203–204, 205(t)
  of financial requirements, 223, 224
  of resources, ethical choices and, 24, 28, 423
Allowances, on financial statement, 196–197, 197(t)
Alternatives, analysis and selection of, and change, 274
American Medical Association (AMA) principles of medical ethics, 23
American Nurses Association (ANA), on BSN entry level, 149
  on definition and scope of nursing, 50
American Nurses Association (ANA) Code for Nurses, ethical standards in, 23
Analysis, budget variance, 218–219
  capital expenditure, 226–227
  cost/benefit, of capital expenditures, 226
  data, in forecasting, 222
  environmental, concept of organizational culture in, 174–176. See also *Organizational culture.*
  in strategic management, 170, 173–178
  feasibility, 188–190, 189(t)
  financial statement, 194–202
    adjustments and allowances in, 196–197, 197(t)